EMANCIPATORY KNOWING

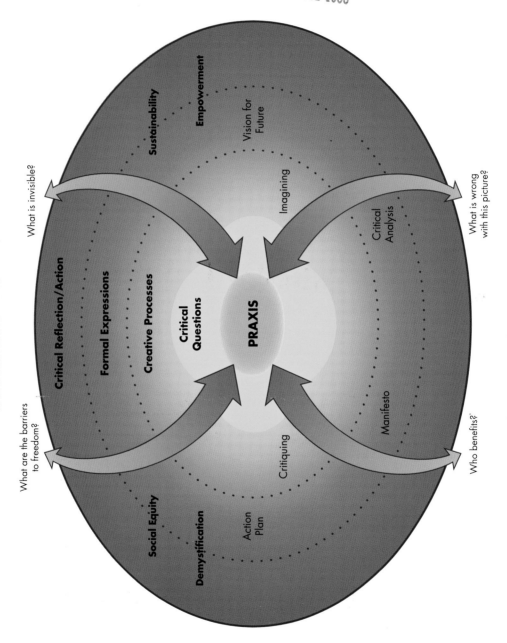

INTEGRATED THEORY AND KNOWLEDGE DEVELOPMENT IN NURSING

Seventh Edition

ELSEVIER

evolve

∴ *To access your Student Resources, visit:*

http://evolve.elsevier.com/Chinn/knowledge

Evolve® Student Resources for **Chinn/Kramer:** *Integrated Theory and Knowledge Development in Nursing,* **7th Edition** offer the following features:

Student Resources (NOTE: Instructors also have access to student material.)

- **Appendix A: Interpretive Summary: Broad Theoretic Frameworks Defining the Scope, Philosophy, and General Characteristics of Nursing**
  Further study that encapsulates needed information on broad conceptual models and frameworks in nursing.

- **Appendix B: Interpretive Summary of Selected Middle-Range Theories**
  Additional information on a variety of approaches used to develop middle-range theories and how middle-range theory addresses specific clinical phenomena.

- **Weblinks**
  Up-to-date links to sites relevant to nursing theory for expanded study.

INTEGRATED THEORY AND KNOWLEDGE DEVELOPMENT IN NURSING

Seventh Edition

Peggy L. Chinn, RN, PhD, FAAN
Professor Emerita
School of Nursing
University of Connecticut
Storrs, Connecticut

Maeona K. Kramer, APRN, PhD
Professor of Nursing
University of Utah
Salt Lake City, Utah

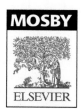

MOSBY

ELSEVIER

MOSBY
ELSEVIER

11830 Westline Industrial Drive
St. Louis, Missouri 63146

INTEGRATED THEORY AND KNOWLEDGE   ISBN: 978-0-323-05270-2
DEVELOPMENT IN NURSING

978-0-323-05270-2

Acquisitions Editor: Yvonne Alexopoulos
Developmental Editor: Heather Bays
Publishing Services Manager: Jeffrey Patterson
Senior Project Manager: Mary G. Stueck
Design Direction: Kim Denando

Printed in the United States of America

Last digit is the print number: 9   8   7   6   5   4   3   2

PREFACE

In this, the seventh edition of our book, we have introduced a new pattern of knowing that we have termed *emancipatory knowing*. In addition to this major revision, there is new material on evidence-based practice and many other additions consistent with emerging trends in nursing. This revision includes a significant number of additional examples that clarify our thinking, and we made changes suggested by the comments of three thoughtful and capable anonymous reviewers.

From the beginning our view of the theory development enterprise was considered a bit radical. We believed that multiple approaches and unconventional ways of thinking were needed to develop ideas about what we know and how we know it. In our first edition entitled *Theory and Nursing*—published in 1983—we grounded our work in a Basic System of All Sciences that originated in psychology (Piotrowski, 1971). This model that "started it all" described four processes—largely scientific in nature—that reflected the focus of knowledge development in the social sciences at the time. Despite its focus on the more scientific processes associated with theory and research, the model appealed to us because it deliberately addressed the nontechnical and abstract processes of science that are part of the theory building process, such as concept analysis. The model spoke to our inclinations about the importance of ideas and abstract thinking, as well as about the uncertainty of truth in the development of theory for nursing as a practice discipline.

The Piotrowski model remained the foundation for our second edition, but by the publication of the third edition, Barbara Carper's (1978) groundbreaking work identifying four fundamental patterns of knowing extracted from the nursing literature of the time had appeared in the professional journal *Advances in Nursing Science*. Carper's naming of nonempirical ways of knowing was powerful for us because it provided a way to begin to think about the diverse and necessary approaches needed for creating knowledge in nursing. At some level we knew that empirical science, while important, was an inadequate knowledge foundation for a practice discipline such as nursing. At that time we were not prepared to address the methodologic aspects of the fundamental patterns (other than empirics) beyond the important insights that Carper provided. We knew however, that this was a direction we wanted to pursue, so we each began to address the patterns in our teaching practices. We also launched investigations and engaged in formal academic study that would further develop an understanding of the aesthetic, personal, and ethical patterns of knowing.

In the fourth edition, we were ready to introduce our early thinking concerning methods for pattern development and use for each of the fundamental patterns of knowing. Still our ideas remained in the very early stage of projecting possibilities. By the time of publication of the fifth edition, we each had completed projects that brought us closer to a more complete description of the development of aesthetic, personal, and ethical knowing.

The fifth edition contained full chapters devoted to the aesthetic, personal, and ethical patterns of knowing in nursing, and included descriptions of methods that we envisioned and have used to develop knowing and knowledge within these patterns. We recognized that the book remained heavily focused on empirics and empiric theory, which was the dominant mode of investigation in use in nursing at the time. Although we conceptualized empirics as broadly as we think is feasible, we realized it was still "empirics," and we also understood that important knowledge structures were coming to the fore that did not fit within it or within the other patterns of knowing.

As the time for revision into a sixth edition approached, we contemplated the addition of another knowing pattern that would include various critical and poststructuralist approaches to inquiry. By this time we had been exposed to the nature of emancipatory knowing through completion of academic coursework, participation in the Critical Social and Feminist Theory Conferences, our personal writing, activist work, and research projects. Although both of us were convinced of the need for nursing to develop emancipatory knowledge and for nurses to develop as emancipatory knowers, we were concerned that our experiential background was not yet sufficient to substantially develop the pattern.

When the time for this revision into a seventh edition arrived we still questioned our ability to conceptualize emancipatory knowing, but decided to "take the plunge" and introduce this new pattern of knowing. Our commitment to the importance of emancipatory knowing and knowledge for both the profession of nursing, those we care for, and for the world community in general energized this work. This is a time when nursing is developing curricula for a professional doctorate, while seemingly moving away from a focus on theory in its practice, curricula, and research. The current focus on evidence-based nursing practice clearly is much more than the application of empirical research in practice. For these reasons, we believe it is more critical than ever to return to serious thought about what constitutes knowledge and knowing, about who we are and should be as knowledge developers, and about what we wish to accomplish as a profession.

As we go to press with this edition we also acknowledge that the emancipatory knowing pattern as we have conceptualized is only a beginning effort. The full range of possible patterns of knowing and approaches to knowledge development remain to be developed, and those currently named require refinement. As we finish this revision, our commitment to the view that multiple patterns of knowing, including those we hope are named in the future, are imperative for the development of disciplinary nursing knowledge. Once scholars and scientists assume a perspective that fully embraces all patterns of knowing, the emphasis shifts away from formally defined empiric theory as knowledge, to an emphasis on knowledge that is broader than that produced by the usual forms of research. The naming of this book reflects this commitment to broad forms of knowledge, but also reflects the need to refocus and strengthen the value for discipline appropriate theory in nursing.

Consistent with our desire to focus on knowledge development broadly while retaining value for theory as a significant knowledge form, this edition changes the chapter structure we introduced in the fifth edition. Chapter 1 continues to overview nursing's fundamental patterns of knowing and introduces emancipatory knowing as a pattern that encompasses Carper's fundamental patterns. In this chapter we present our model of the essential interrelationships between knowing and knowledge in nursing for each pattern and as a whole. We have made some minimal changes in the language of our model that are more consistent with our current thinking and are more inclusive of the variety of empirical knowledge development approaches. In Chapter 1 we overview the ontology (the "being/knowing" aspect of nursing) and epistemology (the "knowledge development" aspect) for each pattern, using our model for knowledge development as a guide. The nature of praxis as a process integral to emancipatory knowing and knowledge is included.

Chapter 2 still provides an overview of the historical development of nursing, with a particular focus on knowledge development. We integrated new information on current knowledge development trends, including translational research, evidence-based practice, and practice-based evidence. After much thought we retained the information on broad conceptual models as proposed during the 1950s to 1980s. We expanded the section on values and resources, incorporating examples that illustrate how values and resources affect knowledge development. In general, we reorganized and streamlined this chapter consistent with reviewers comments to improve its readability and flow.

We have reordered the remaining chapters in this edition. Rather than beginning with the pattern of empirics, Chapters 3, 4, 5, and 6 are now devoted to the nonempiric patterns of knowing. Chapters 7, 8, 9, and 10 retain the classic content on empiric theory development from previous editions.

Chapter 3 describes the emancipatory knowing pattern, detailing how it interrelates with the four fundamental patterns developed by Carper. Praxis as the process of emancipatory knowing is also described. Chapter 4, devoted to ethical knowledge development, includes new content on ethical decision trees. Chapter 5 discusses personal knowing and Chapter 6 covers aesthetic knowing; these chapters remain generally intact except for minor updating and editorial changes.

Chapter 7 describes the processes of conceptualizing and structuring theory using the processes of creating conceptual meaning and structuring and contextualizing theory. Chapter 8 addresses the description and critical reflection of theory. Chapter 9 focuses on validating and confirming empiric knowledge through research that generates and tests theoretic relationships. Chapter 10 focuses on validating and confirming empiric knowledge through practice by deliberative use of empiric theory.

This edition includes an updated glossary, reflecting the ongoing challenge of keeping word definitions current and adding words newly introduced in this edition. We moved the former Appendices to the Evolve website: http://evolve.elsevier.com/Chinn/knowledge. Appendix A remains an overview of historically important, broad conceptual models and frameworks in nursing, some of which are still undergoing active development. Appendix B provides examples of selected middle-range theories in nursing. We have retained and revised our discussion of the nature, development, and importance of middle-range theory in the text, referring readers to some of the excellent sources in the literature that contain the most recent examples of middle-range theories in nursing. Importantly, one major change throughout this edition is the integration of examples that, hopefully, will provide helpful illustrations of our intent. The need for examples was an important and consistent point raised by reviewers and we have taken their suggestions to heart.

Finally, in this edition we have added questions at the end of each chapter to stimulate readers to think about the content of the chapter and come to a deeper appreciation of the text as it relates to their own experience. The questions in each chapter also highlight the interrelatedness of all patterns of knowing, prompting the reader to consider all dimensions of knowing while focusing on the specific content of a chapter. In particular it is our intention that the questions will sharpen the reader's understanding of the emancipatory knowing process of praxis—critical reflection and action that transforms experience.

NOTATIONS ON LANGUAGE

Since the third edition we have continued to make shifts in the language used in this text. In general, these shifts are now reflected in most scholarly and scientific literature in nursing and other disciplines. However, because of the radical thinking that much of our language represents, it remains a struggle to fully incorporate linguistic changes that are consistent with our intentions. Many of these shifts carry significant but subtle meanings, and so we include here the notations on language that are included in prior editions.

Our initial aim was to shift the writing style to a clearer, more accessible, and more readable format. From reader comments, we believe we have had some success in this area. We have always maintained that language needs to be a vehicle for healing within the profession and should connect those who develop knowledge with those who use knowledge. Until we no longer need a language that identifies nurses as either academics or practitioners, nurses who work in academia and nurses who work in practice need to communicate better with one another. Consistent with this commitment, we began the editing process with the intent to eliminate words and phrases that depend on or assume a style typically reserved for the academician. We began by simplifying sentence structure, eliminating pretentious words when a common word would do, shifting to the active voice as much as possible, and limiting the use of pronouns to instances in which an agent is clearly identifiable.

As we worked, we became aware of more flaws in the underlying structure of the language and tried to address them as consistently as possible. We became conscious of value assumptions and connotations inherent in the language. Many terms commonly associated with the practice of scientific methods carry antagonistic, adversarial, objectifying, and militaristic connotations that are contrary to the intents of a human science. Some terms we found to occur with impressive frequency were *competing images, judgments, capture, aim, target, operation, boundaries, argument,* and *debate*. Even when the strict meaning of a word was adequate for the text, we sought to shift the language to words that carry a similar literal meaning but a more human and caring value connotation. For example, instead of the militaristic phrase "defend your position," we use "share your ideas."

There were other subtle meanings that we built into the language and structure of earlier editions, some of which were contradictory to our intent. We did not intend to prescribe "set" or "best" metatheoretic approaches or to convey a strict adherence to linearity. Yet much of what we presented resulted in an approach that was authoritarian, prescriptive, and linear. In later editions we shifted from a prescriptive, criteria-based approach to theory description and evaluation, to a mode of questioning and considering alternatives. We have continued to refine and enhance this approach. We deleted references to the "first," "second," or "third" "step" in a process and instead wrote of issues or alternatives that could be addressed in the context of process.

Another shift we made in the language is informed by our intent to reframe traditional relationships between people. We have sought to directly engage and empower the reader. We speak directly to the reader as "you," with the intent to encourage your own abilities and ideas rather than impose the authoritative voice of the text. We raise questions intended for you, the reader, to address in your own way and in your own context rather than looking to the authoritarian text for an answer.

The problem of language once again surfaced in the fourth edition, where we introduced our ideas about personal and aesthetic knowing and knowledge. Language around emancipatory knowing posed similar challenges. We understand that much of the content introduced in these chapters will feel strange to many—and we endeavored to use language that is understandable as well as provide illustrative examples. We continue to try to make the content of this book accessible and understandable, but we realize language that effectively expresses some of these abstract and elusive ideas is not readily available. We hope our struggles to make these ideas accessible ultimately reflects language that is clear and concise, yet rich with meaning.

The language shifts we have made and continue to make have led to profound differences in how we think about the processes for developing knowledge. We invite you to join us in the process of deepening an understanding and awareness of the ways in which language creates and shapes our collective values, knowledge, and indeed our reality.

ABOUT THE AUTHORS

The introduction of emancipatory knowing in this edition carries with it a responsibility to disclose our personal standpoints that shaped the development of this work. Such disclosure is standard for scholars who produce critical theoretical work of various types. Personal disclosure of the authors' perspectives is important so readers understand the motivations and interests that undergird the work. Certainly the content of our entire book is politically motivated, but our production of an emancipatory knowing pattern and what we have said about it implies an agenda for change; that is, it implies an emancipatory interest. Thus it is important for you to know something about how we came to the place from which the chapter was written.

To an observer, we would appear to be very different women; we are distinctly different personalities, we each have our own unique approaches to our work, and distinct ways of interacting with friends and family. We have different life experiences and grew up in different cultures (Hawaii, Michigan). However, when we examine those essential things that form a perspective on a work like this one, we are remarkably similar. Like many of you, we have experienced discrimination and oppression as well as privilege. We both enjoyed the privilege of being white and felt the oppressions shared by all women. As lesbians, once married with children, we also acutely experienced the discrimination that attends the denial of basic rights based on sexual identities. Discrimination based on religious beliefs has also been part of our experiences.

Accidents of birth located us both in loving but materially poor families. Inherent personality traits that questioned authority coupled with innate intelligences and abilities motivated us to question and rebel from the beginning. An openness to new ideas and a willingness to change also shaped our professional paths. Learning and academic advancement came to each of us easily and were made possible through government subsidies and work opportunities available at the time. Thus we both found ourselves in academic settings early in our professional careers. Our professional lives have been spent primarily within academic settings. Academia, with its focus on an exploration of ideas, tempered as well as illuminated how our lives had been formed by both privilege and lack of privilege.

Though rebels from the outset, it was through study, academic and otherwise, reflected against our lives experienced as nurses and women that galvanized the formal pursuit and embracing of critical thought and activities. We found that the radical literature we were reading and studying made perfect sense in relation to our experiences of the world. As feminists for example, we saw the pronouncements of feminist theory play out in our everyday academic lives and in the lives of nurses in all professional roles. The explanations embodied in critical social theory came alive as we tried to secure societal resources for nurses, women in our communities, elders, and socially disadvantaged children. In short, our connections with a variety of underserved groups and the formal knowledge we were exposed to increasingly validated our lived experience. We came to believe the processes and products associated with emancipatory knowing are critically important and powerful tools to shape and change nursing, ourselves, and the world community. Despite its power and potential to create real change, emancipatory knowing and knowledge is still largely misunderstood, disvalued, and ignored in nursing. For all of these reasons we are inspired to share our vision of emancipatory knowing as well as knowledge and knowing in general with you.

IN THANKS

When we first conceived the essential elements of this book, we had both recently completed our doctoral programs and were beginning our academic careers. During a 2-year period of our early academic lives we were both employed at the University of Utah, where we collaborated professionally and discovered our mutual interests in theory and knowledge development. Despite living in different geographical locations we have since maintained an ongoing professional association. We now have completed our active teaching careers and continue our personal growth as we begin to experience our "resignation" from formally appointed academic life. We owe so much of our ability to change and mature in our thinking to those who enrolled in our classes and labored with us to push the edges of knowledge and venture into that which is possible but not yet fully real. It is to each of you who have worked with us in classrooms that we owe our greatest debt of gratitude. Without your continual prodding for clearer explanations, your challenges to our ideas, and your insistence in pushing us beyond our preconceived notions, much of what has emerged in this book would not have been possible. Indeed, in the classroom you became our teachers and we give to you our deepest appreciation.

Our many academic colleagues—within the institutions where we taught and studied as well as those around the world—have contributed to our thinking by being an informed, critical, and thoughtful audience. Our close friends and chosen families have continued to provide the love and support so essential to this type of work—our deepest thanks and gratitude to you.

To the three formal reviewers who thoughtfully read and commented on this work, we are grateful. Each of you provided insights that were helpful in this revision. For the most part we made each of the changes you suggested and feel confident that your careful critique, both positive and negative, has produced a stronger volume. We truly appreciate your effort.

We extend deep appreciation to those who provided substantive comments on early drafts of Chapter 3 and our conceptualizations of emancipatory knowing: Drs. Beverly Hall, Jeanne DeJoseph, Mickey Eliason, and Carla Randall. Your thoughtful reading of our drafts, questions, and challenges were invaluable as we refined the chapter to express as clearly as possible our intended meanings.

We are also grateful to Dr. Patricia Gray who provided insightful critique on several chapters and made helpful suggestions concerning the integration of content related to evidence-based nursing practice.

As much as we feel deeply the ways in which this work depends on our interactions with each of our colleagues, we acknowledge that the content of this book remains our own doing and our own responsibility. We have taken the responsibility to represent and acknowledge the work of others as openly and honestly as possible. We hope there are no errors in the text, yet we expect there will be. We are learners and make no claim to having final answers. We ask that you understand and honor our wish not to be seen as an authoritative voice, but rather a voice among many to be challenged and moved beyond. We began our professional collaboration in 1972 and continue to provide for one another the challenges and the grounding that are inherent in conceptualizing and co-writing a work of this type. It is our mutual respect and appreciation for one another, as well as our inherent differences, that sustain this type of relationship over time. We are grateful to each other for these mutual gifts. We offer this work, always in progress, to you in the hope that it will continue to provide a perspective that is worthy of critique and that deepens your understanding and inspires your own thoughts and actions.

Peggy L. Chinn

Maeona K. Kramer

Reference List

Carper, B. A. (1978). Fundamental patterns of knowing in nursing. *ANS. Advances In Nursing Science, 1*(1), 13–23.

Piotrowski, Z. A. (1971). Basic system of all sciences. In H. J. Vetter & B. D. Smith (Eds.), *Personality theory: a source book* (pp. 2–18). New York: Appleton-Century-Crofts.

CONTENTS

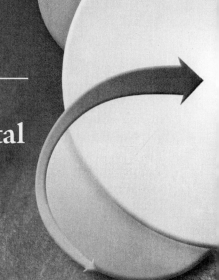

CHAPTER 1

Nursing's Fundamental Patterns of Knowing

It is the general conception of any field of inquiry that ultimately determines the kind of knowledge that field aims to develop as well as the manner in which that knowledge is to be organized, tested and applied. . . . Such an understanding . . . involves critical attention to the question of what it means to know and what kinds of knowledge are held to be of most value in the discipline of nursing.

Barbara A. Carper (1978, p. 13)

KNOWLEDGE FOR A PRACTICE DISCIPLINE

This text is devoted to exploration and discussion of ways in which knowledge is developed in nursing. It includes traditional ideas of empiric theory development but moves beyond traditional views of theory to a contemporary, more inclusive view of knowledge and knowing for a practice discipline.

In addition to empiric science as a means for developing knowledge, this book addresses the development of knowledge linked to personal knowing, ethics, aesthetics, and the pattern of emancipatory knowing. We are introducing and explaining emancipatory knowing for the first time in this edition. However, it is not altogether new; it has a long tradition expressed in nurses' efforts to understand and enact a high quality of care. It is reflected in nursing's understanding that the social context in which care is given determines the nature of care provided and affects the health and well-being of individuals and groups.

Nursing involves processes, dynamics, and interactions that can only be fully understood when science, ethics, aesthetics, and personal and emancipatory knowing come together. Best practices in nursing are those that arise from praxis—critical reflection and action to change what has been in the past and to create a future that enables health for all. Praxis is the process of emancipatory knowing. Praxis involves the shaping and creation of the future and requires a vision of the future you want to create. The vision is not limited to any one pattern of knowing but rather requires development of knowledge in all knowing patterns to form a whole of integrated knowing.

Praxis requires the bringing together of knowledge in all patterns, but the methods for developing knowledge and the expression of knowing are unique to each of the patterns. The methods required for one pattern cannot be used to develop knowledge within another pattern. The scientific methods of empirics, for example, cannot be used to develop personal, ethical, aesthetic, or emancipatory knowledge.

Although we discuss the unique features of developing knowledge and enacting knowing for each pattern, we return again and again to the complementarity of the processes for each pattern and their contribution to the whole of knowing. We also focus on asking critical questions that move away from the unquestioned use of rules, methods, and principles to perspectives that value imagining what is possible for the future.

KNOWING AND KNOWLEDGE

The term *knowing* refers to ways of perceiving and understanding the self and the world. Knowing is an ontologic, dynamic, changing process. The term *knowledge* refers to knowing that is expressed in a form that can be shared or communicated with others. In a discipline, knowledge represents what is collectively taken to be a reasonable and accurate understanding of the world as it is understood by the members of the discipline. The "knowledge of the discipline" is that which has been collectively judged by standards and criteria shared by members of the disciplinary community. The ways in which knowledge is developed is an epistemologic concern that reveals how nurses come to know and how nurses acquire shared knowledge in the discipline.

As nurses practice, they know more than they can communicate and use insights and understandings that they often take for granted. Much of what is known is expressed through actions, movements, or sounds. These every-day actions reflect the whole of knowing. What is expressed in a nurse's actions embodies a simultaneous wholeness that textbooks and theories can never portray. What happens in practice can only be shared in the moment and typically is not available to a broader audience.

We believe that much of what nurses know has the potential to be more fully expressed and communicated than it has been in the past and that this can happen when all forms of knowing are integrated and valued. Written language and other symbols that are used to convey empiric knowledge will only partially reflect the whole, but when you move beyond the traditional limits of empirics, it is possible to convey a more complete picture of what is known within the discipline as a whole.

Sharing knowledge is important because it creates a disciplinary commu-nity, beyond the isolation of individual experience. Once this happens, social purposes form, and knowledge development and shared purposes form a cyclic interrelationship that moves us toward prospective, value-grounded change or praxis.

OVERVIEW OF NURSING'S PATTERNS OF KNOWING

Since Nightingale first established formal secular education for nurses, nursing has depended on formal knowledge as a basis for practice. The nature of knowledge changes with time, yet overall the fundamental values that guide nursing practice have remained remarkably stable (Clements & Averill, 2006; Fawcett, 2006).

Carper (1978) examined early nursing literature and named four funda-mental and enduring patterns of knowing that nurses have valued and used in practice. One of the patterns is the familiar and respected pattern of empirics, the science of nursing. In addition, she identified ethics, the com-ponent of moral knowledge in nursing; personal knowing in nursing; and aesthetics, the art of nursing.

Our conceptualization of emancipatory knowing is based on nursing lit-erature that addresses the social and political context of nursing and health care, and on critiques of the four fundamental patterns of knowing that take issue with the omission of these contextual concerns. The dominant conceptualization of, and theorizing about, nursing has involved the care of individuals who are sick or at risk for health problems. Knowledge devel-opment addressing social context and political activism as central to nursing practice has been limited, but these concerns have long been acknowledged in the work of activist nurses. These nurses have recognized serious social barriers to health and well-being. They set about to change the conditions that limit health and well-being, and they wrote accounts of their experiences, insights, and actions (Hagedorn, 1995; Hall, 1963, 1964, 1966; Kinlein, 1977; Milio, 2000). Several nurse scholars have provided insightful critique and viable adaptations of earlier conceptualizations of the knowing patterns that touch on emancipatory knowing (Fiandt, Forman, Megel, Padieser, & Burge, 2003; Munhall, 1993; Silva, Sorrell, & Sorrell, 1995; Wainwright, 2000; White, 1995; Wolfer, 1993). Our conceptualization of emancipatory knowing in this text draws on prior accounts of nurse activists and critiques of writings related to nursing's patterns of knowing, as well as on our own scholarly and activist experience.

The fundamental patterns of knowing as identified by Carper remain valuable in that they conceptualize a broad scope of knowing that extends beyond the limited boundaries of empirics. We retain our discussion of each of these fundamental patterns in this text. Our descriptions of the development of empiric knowledge remains consistent with the prevailing approaches to empiric knowledge development.

The emancipatory, personal, ethical, and aesthetic patterns have not been as well developed within the discipline, reflecting a neglect of these patterns of knowing and an overvaluing of empirics as the knowledge of the discipline (Fawcett, 2006; Fawcett, Watson, Neuman, Walker, & Fitzpatrick, 2001). However, methods for developing knowledge related to ethical, personal, aesthetic, and empiric knowledge are beginning to be systematically described and reflected in literature that identifies the value of a broader scope of knowing and knowledge in practice (Clements & Averill, 2004; Fiandt et al., 2003; Gramling, 2006; Lane, 2006; Weis, Schank, & Matheus, 2006). Because of this shift, we have reordered the presentation of each pattern of knowing to first discuss emancipatory knowing, followed by ethics and personal and aesthetic knowing, and ending the text with our conceptualization of the more traditional approaches to empiric knowledge development.

We have extended the understanding of Carper's descriptions based on our ideas and research and the insights of other nursing scholars. In the following sections we provide an overview of our conceptualization of each of the patterns of knowing in nursing. Each pattern has the following two forms of expression: formal expressions in language and writing, and expressions in actions—or in practice—without words. In addition, these sections introduce the methods we propose for developing each of the patterns.

Emancipatory Knowing: The Praxis of Nursing

Emancipatory knowing is the human capacity to critically examine the social, cultural, and political status quo, and to figure out how and why it came to be that way. From this pattern of knowing, people come to identify inequities embedded in social and political institutions, and to clarify the cultural values and beliefs that need to change to create fair and equitable conditions for all. Emancipatory knowing requires an understanding of the nature of knowledge and the ways in which knowledge itself, or what is taken to be knowledge, contributes to larger social problems. This understanding takes into account the power dynamics that create knowledge, and the social and political contexts that shape and influence knowledge and knowing. This kind of knowing seeks freedom from institutional and institutionalized social and political contexts that sustain that which is unjust—that perpetuate advantage for some and disadvantage for others.

Emancipatory knowledge grows out of critical analysis of the status quo and visions of the changes that are needed to create change toward equitable and just conditions that support all humans in reaching their full potential. Formal written expressions of emancipatory knowledge describe the conditions that limit human potential, the circumstances that create and sustain those conditions, what is required to change the status quo, and what needs to be created in place of the status quo. Emancipatory knowledge is also expressed in actions that are commonly recognized as activist projects directed at changing existing social structures and establishing practices and structures that are more equitable and favorable to human health and well-being.

The process of emancipatory knowing is praxis; the product is the emancipatory changes that are shaped by praxis. Praxis, at the collective and individual levels, requires both critical reflection and action. Praxis occurs at the individual level when people recognize conditions that unjustly limit their abilities and experiences, reflect on the situation with a growing realization that things could be different, and take action to change the circumstances of their lives. As actions emerge, individuals remain continually attuned to the ideals they seek and critically reflect on conditions emerging from the actions that they take to transform their experience.

Praxis as collective endeavor requires reflection and action in concert with others who are engaged in the personal and collective struggle involved in creating social and political change. When groups of people collectively share their individual insights and experiences, everyone's realizations grow and develop and possibilities for change multiply. When members of a discipline such as nursing engage in praxis at a collective level, their cooperative reflections and actions can create substantial change. Praxis at the collective level creates emancipatory knowledge that can be authenticated and understood by members of the discipline. As a community of critical reflectors and actors, nurses collectively begin to act on their insights and take action to transform nursing and health care. In this way the critical reflections and actions that constitute praxis continue to change in the direction of creating emancipatory knowledge, making visible how equitable and just social structures can be enacted. The cycle of praxis (action and reflection to undo unjust social practices) and the emancipatory changes it produces is an ongoing process. As praxis produces change, that change undergoes further action and reflection in relation to the envisioned outcome.

Ethics: The Moral Component of Knowledge in Nursing

Ethics in nursing is focused on matters of obligation: what ought to be done. The moral component of knowing in nursing goes beyond knowledge of the norms or ethical codes of nursing. It involves making moment-to-moment judgments about what ought to be done, what is good and right, and what is responsible. Ethical knowing guides and directs how nurses conduct their practice, what they select as important, where their loyalties are placed, and what priorities demand advocacy.

Ethical knowing also involves confronting and resolving conflicting values, norms, interests, or principles. There may be no satisfactory answer to an ethical dilemma or moral distress-only alternatives, some of which are more or less satisfactory. Ethical knowing in nursing requires an experiential knowledge of social values and mores from which ethical reasoning arises and knowledge of the formal principles and codes within the discipline (Carper, 1978). Like all other patterns of knowing, ethical knowing is expressed in nursing actions—what we call moral/ethical comportment. Others can observe nursing actions based on ethical knowing, and the underlying ethical knowledge can be discerned and examined.

Ethical principles and codes are set forth in the philosophic ideals on which ethical decisions rest. Ethical knowledge does not describe or prescribe what a decision or action should be. Rather, it provides insight about which choices are possible, and it provides direction toward choices that are sound, good, responsible, or just.

Ethical knowledge forms are like empiric theory and formal descriptions in that they reflect some dimensions of experience and express relationships between phenomena. However, empiric theory relies on observations that can be confirmed by others. Ethical codes and principles cannot be tested in this sense because the relationships expressed in codes and principles rest on underlying philosophic reasoning that leads to conclusions concerning what is right, good, responsible, or just. The reasoning can include description of experience to substantiate an argument, but the conclusions are value statements that cannot be perceived or confirmed empirically.

Personal Knowing in Nursing

Personal knowing in nursing concerns the inner experience of becoming a whole, aware, genuine self. Personal knowing encompasses knowing one's own self and the self of others. As Carper (1978, p. 18) stated, "One does not know about the self, one strives simply to know the self." It is through knowing one's own self that one is able to know the other. Full awareness of the self, the moment, and the context of interaction makes possible meaningful, shared human experience. Without this component of knowing, the idea of therapeutic use of self in nursing would not be possible (Carper, 1978).

Personal knowing is most fully communicated as an authentic, aware, genuine self. Other people perceive the existence of a unique person by physical characteristics but also come to know the person as a unique personality. As personal knowing emerges more fully throughout life, the unique or genuine self can be more fully expressed and becomes accessible as a means by which deliberate action and interaction take form.

It is possible to describe certain things about the self in personal stories and autobiographies, which are the formal written expressions of personal knowing. These descriptions provide sources for deep reflection and a shared understanding of how personal knowledge can be developed and used in a deliberative way. Descriptions about the self are limited in that they never fully reflect personal knowing, and they are retrospective in that they can describe only the self that was. However, publicly expressed descriptions can be a tool for developing self-awareness and self-intimacy and for communicating to others valuable possibilities for developing personal knowing (Hagan, 1990; Nelson, 1994).

In a sense, all knowing is personal; each individual can know only through personal senses and sensibilities. For example, empiric theories can be learned, but their meaning for the individual comes from personal reflection and experience with the phenomena of the theory. Ethical codes and moral beliefs are likewise personal in nature. We recognize this broad meaning of personal knowing, but our focus is the aspect of personal knowing that delves into the processes of knowing the self and of developing self-knowing through healing encounters with others.

Aesthetics: The Art of Nursing

Aesthetic knowing in nursing involves deep appreciation of the meaning of a situation and calls forth inner creative resources that transform experience into what is not yet real, bringing to being something that would not otherwise be possible. Aesthetic knowing makes it possible to move beyond the surface—beyond the limits and circumstances of a particular moment—to sense the meaning of the moment and connect with depths of common human experience that are unique for each person (sickness, suffering, recovery, birth, death). Aesthetic knowing in practice is expressed through the actions, bearing, conduct, attitudes, narrative, and interactions of the nurse in relation to others. It also is formally expressed in art forms such as poetry, drawings, stories, and music that reflect and communicate symbolic meanings embedded in nursing practice.

Aesthetic knowing is what makes possible knowing what to do and how to be in the moment, instantly, without conscious deliberation. It arises from a direct perception of what is significant and meaningful in the moment. The nurse's perception of meaning is reflected in the action taken. The meaning is often shared without conscious exchange of words and may not be consciously or cognitively formed. Sometimes what a situation means to the nurse comes from the nurse's own experience and knowledge, making it possible for the nurse to bring into the situation possibilities that are new for a particular situation. The nurse brings the new possibilities into the situation through actions—movements and verbal expressions—shaping the experience into what would not otherwise exist. The nurse's actions take on an element of artistry, creating unique, meaningful, often deeply moving interactions with others that touch common chords of human experience. We refer to this aspect of nursing practice as the transformative art/act.

Aesthetic knowing is expressed in the moment of experience-action (Benner, 1984; Benner & Wrubel, 1989) in the transformative art/act. Aesthetic knowledge is formally expressed in aesthetic criticism and in works of art that symbolize experience. Aesthetic criticism is the written expression of aesthetic knowledge that conveys the artistic aspects of the art/act, the technical skill required to perform the art/act, knowledge that informs the development of the art/act, the historical and cultural significance of specific aspects of nursing as an art, and the potential for the future development of the art form.

Empirics: The Science of Nursing

Empirics is based on the assumption that what is known is accessible through the physical senses, particularly seeing, touching, and hearing. Empirics can be traced to Nightingale's precepts concerning the importance of accurate observation and record keeping. The science of nursing emerged during the late 1950s (Carper, 1978). Empirics as a pattern of knowing draws on traditional ideas of science. For empirics, a collective or individual reality exists and truths about it can be understood through inferences based on observations and understandings that are verifiable or confirmable by other observers.

Empiric knowing is expressed in practice as scientific competence—competent action grounded in scientific knowledge, including theory. Scientific competence involves conscious problem solving and logical reasoning, but much of the underlying empiric knowing that informs competent reasoning remains in the background of awareness. What remains in the background usually can be brought to awareness when attention turns to the reasoning process itself.

Empiric knowledge is formally expressed in the form of empiric theories, statements of fact, or formalized descriptions and interpretations of empiric events or objects. The development of empiric knowledge traditionally has been accomplished by the methods of science. Often this has involved testing hypotheses derived from a theory that offers a tentative explanation of empiric phenomena. Many types of formal descriptions and theories that express empiric knowledge in nursing are linked to the traditional ideas about what is legitimate for developing the science of nursing. In addition, newer methods have been developed to include activities that are not strictly within the realm of traditional empiric methodologies such as phenomenologic or ethnographic descriptions or inductive means of generating theory and formal descriptions.

PROCESSES FOR DEVELOPING NURSING KNOWLEDGE

Nursing's patterns of knowing are interrelated and arise from the whole of experience. Nurses learn a portion of the knowledge of the discipline in their basic education and continue to build on their acquired knowledge as they practice (Benner, 1984). It is the experience of nursing that gives nursing knowledge its richness, depth, and meaning. Formally expressed nursing knowledge is developed using methods of inquiry that are grounded in practice, and in formal scholarly methods specifically designed for each pattern. Figures 1-1 and 1-2 illustrate interrelationships among each of the patterns.

As shown in Figure 1-1, emancipatory knowing surrounds and connects with each of the four fundamental patterns of knowing. The four fundamental patterns are represented in the figure by the central sphere (yellow on the color version [see color insert inside front cover]) surrounding the core of practice/praxis (purple on the color version [see color insert inside front cover]). The central location of the fundamental patterns and the arrows that extend from the center through the outer spheres represent two aspects of emancipatory knowing in relation to the other patterns of knowing. One is an inward view that examines nursing knowledge and

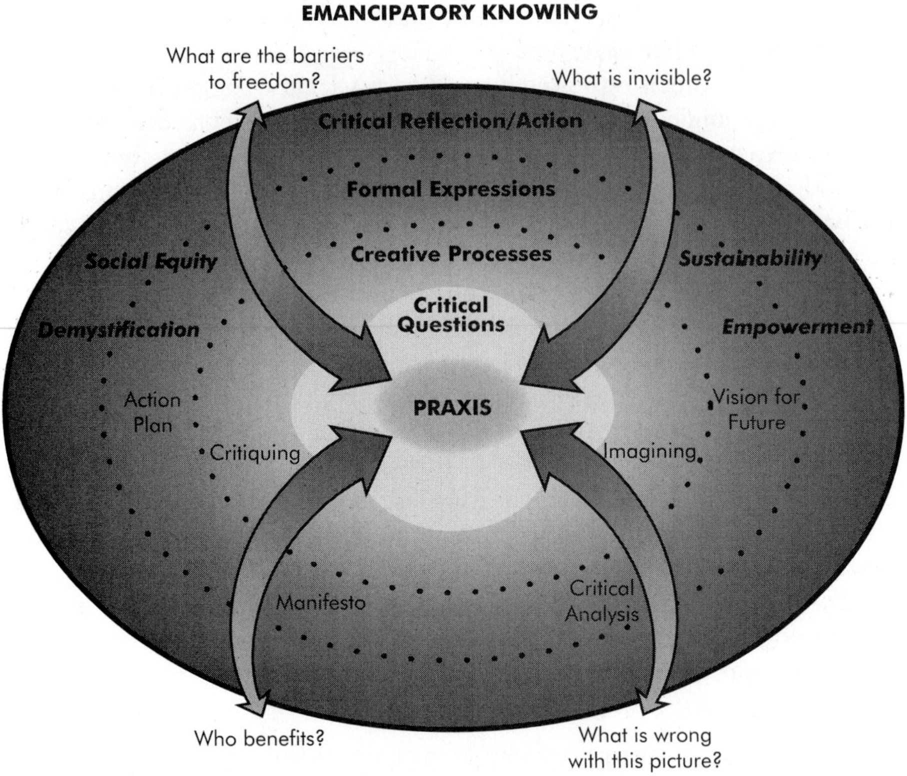

EMANCIPATORY KNOWING

What are the barriers
to freedom?

What is invisible?

Critical Reflection/Action

Formal Expressions

Social Equity

Creative Processes

Sustainability

Demystification

Critical
Questions

Empowerment

Action
Plan

PRAXIS

Vision for
Future

Critiquing

Imagining

Manifesto

Critical
Analysis

Who benefits?

What is wrong
with this picture?

FIGURE 1-1   Processes for developing emancipatory knowledge.

the practice of nursing. The other is an outward view that examines social
and political practices that form the background for development of
nursing knowledge and practice. The inward view critically examines all of
the methods used in developing and using nursing knowledge, and the
nature of knowledge that is taken as authenticated. The outward view considers the social and political contexts in which nursing knowledge is developed and in which nursing is practiced, whose interests nursing serves, and
ways in which nursing shapes and is shaped by its context and history.

The critical questions of emancipatory knowing are shown external to
the outer ring of critical reflection/action. These questions are asked in
relation to the greater social context of nursing and health care, as well as
in relation to disciplinary knowledge and knowing expressed in nursing
practice arising from each of the four fundamental patterns, as depicted
by the four double arrows. The critical questions illustrate the kinds of realizations that awaken and sustain emancipatory awareness and suggest what
needs to change. The critical questions arise from a nurse's personal

experience, either in practice or some other aspect of life that affects practice. Examples of the questions themselves are placed outside the boundaries of the model to represent the fact that critical questions also come from awareness of larger social and political context. The arrows that extend from the center to the outer realm of the model and beyond represent the ongoing, constant, and synchronous nature of praxis that arises when you or other nurses ask and act in relation to the critical questions.

The three outer spheres that encircle the fundamental patterns of knowing represent the creative processes used to develop emancipatory knowledge, the written forms of expression of emancipatory knowledge that assist and enable praxis, and the reflection/action that creates emancipatory change. The creative processes used to develop emancipatory knowledge are critiquing the status quo and imagining what might be different to create a better world—one that is more equitable for all. The critique can be approached using one or more of several possible lenses—such as the lens of race, ethnicity, socio-economic status, sexual identity, age, culture, religious belief, or political orientation—to uncover the subtle ways in which injustice is sustained, and to deepen awareness of what needs to change. From the critique emerges a vision of what could be, and ideas about the actions that are needed for change. Formal expressions of the critique, such as critical analyses that are published in scholarly journals or action plans that are communicated electronically or in writing, provide a shareable account of the creative processes of critiquing the status quo and imagining for the future. Formal expressions communicated as emancipatory knowledge also provide insights concerning the processes of praxis for emancipatory change—knowledge that can be applied in other situations that call for similar kinds of changes.

Praxis, the critical reflection/action dimension of emancipatory knowing, is at the very center of the model, and is also represented as critical reflection/action in the outermost sphere. The inner sphere of praxis is the local, individual expression of critical reflective nursing practice, a place where new awareness of problems often begins to take shape, where consciousness shifts to a realization that your experience and your situation are problematic. The outer sphere of praxis is critical reflection and action that are situated in and directed to the larger social, political, and economic contexts of nursing practice.

The outcome of emancipatory knowing is the social change that arises from praxis. The discipline authenticates emancipatory knowing by demonstrating that social change, and the formal disciplinary expressions that explain those changes, accomplishes imagined and intended shifts that end injustices and inequities. The authentication processes examine the sustainability of the change and the presence of social equity, demystification of processes that sustain inequities, and empowerment for all; these processes are shown in bold black within the two outer spheres of Figure 1-1.

Figure 1-2 provides the detail of the central circle in Figure 1-1 and is a representation of the unique processes and expressions of each of nursing's fundamental patterns of knowing originally proposed by Carper (1978). In Figure 1-2, each of the fundamental patterns is represented as a quadrant. At the periphery of each quadrant are critical questions that development of knowledge and knowing within each pattern requires. In the center of each quadrant, a large arrow represents the forms of expression of knowledge within each pattern. These arrows point to the inner sphere, showing the practice or action expression of knowing that is associated with the pattern.

The inner sphere of Figure 1-2 is shown as a whole, without quadrant boundaries, representing our view that in nursing practice knowing is experienced as an integrated whole and can never be experienced as discrete patterns. It is within the central circle that individual praxis (critical reflection

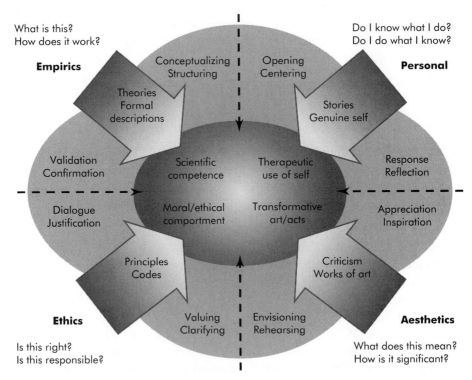

FIGURE 1-2 Processes for developing ethical, personal, aesthetic, and empiric knowledge.

and action in practice) occurs. Along the vertical axis, represented by vertical broken arrows, are the processes for developing the formal written and communicable knowledge expression for each pattern. Along the horizontal axis, represented by horizontal broken arrows, are the collective processes used within the discipline for validating or authenticating what is known.

Critical questions for each of the four fundamental patterns appear in the outer area of Figure 1-2. The inner sphere shows the action expressions of knowing. These two areas—the outer critical questions and the inner action components—comprise the experience of knowing, or the ontologic dimensions of knowing/being in the moment of practice. The processes shown along the vertical and horizontal arrows represent the epistemologic dimensions of processes for developing and authenticating knowledge.

We have chosen to embed the model of the four fundamental patterns within the pattern of emancipatory knowing as shown in Figure 1-1. We believe that the critical questions asked and enacted in the moment of practice, as well as the disciplinary approaches to knowledge development, need to be examined and understood in relation to how they enable or disable praxis and emancipatory change.

Another way of conceptualizing the processes for all five patterns of knowing is shown in Table 1-1. The following dimensions are shown in the table:

- Critical questions
- Creative processes for developing knowledge
- Formal written expressions of knowledge
- Authentication processes
- Integrated expressions of knowing in practice

Each dimension is unique to each pattern of knowing. You cannot create empiric theory, for example, by using the creative processes of ethics, personal, aesthetic, or emancipatory knowing. In practice, knowing is experienced as a whole, but you can observe and describe the unique dimensions related to each pattern that arise from the whole.

Critical questions address the kind of understanding that emerges within the individual patterns. Emancipatory knowing addresses the critical questions "Who benefits?" "What is wrong with this picture?" What are the barriers to freedom?" and "What is invisible?" Personal knowing addresses the critical questions "Do I know what I do?" and "Do I do what I know?" Ethics addresses the critical questions "Is this right?" and "Is this responsible?" Aesthetics addresses the critical questions "What does this mean?" and "How is this significant?" Empirics addresses the critical questions "What is this?" and "How does it work?"

TABLE 1-1 Dimensions Associated with Each of the Patterns of Knowing

Dimension	Emancipatory	Ethics	Personal	Aesthetics	Empirics
Critical questions	What are the barriers to freedom? What is hidden? What is invisible? Who is not heard? Who benefits? What is wrong with this picture?	Is this right? Is this responsible?	Do I know what I do? Do I do what I know?	What does this mean? How is this significant?	What is this? How does it work?
Creative processes	Critiquing Imagining	Valuing Clarifying	Opening Centering	Envisioning Rehearsing	Conceptualizing Structuring
Formal expressions	Action plans Manifestoes Critical analyses Visions for the future	Principles, codes	Stories Genuine self	Aesthetic criticism Works of art	Formal descriptions Theories
Authentication processes	Social equity Sustainability Empowerment Demystification	Dialogue Justification	Response Reflection	Appreciation Inspiration	Confirmation Validation
Integrated expressions in practice	Praxis	Moral/ethical comportment	Therapeutic use of self	Transformative art/acts	Scientific competence

These critical questions and others like them are implicit in practice. They can be, and often are, asked consciously or deliberatively to bring to light a better understanding of what is happening or to initiate some form of inquiry to find an answer that seems elusive. The process of posing a question and seeking answers or solutions improves practice and advances the knowledge on which practice is founded.

The creative inquiry processes lead toward formal expression of knowledge. The creative processes for emancipatory knowing are critiquing the status quo and imagining alternative social structures. Personal knowledge is developed by opening and centering the self. Opening and centering are the processes involved in coming to know the unique, genuine self. Development of ethical knowledge uses processes of clarifying and valuing issues of rights and responsibilities in practice. Aesthetic knowledge is developed by envisioning possibilities and rehearsing art/acts that can be called on to transform experience. Empiric knowledge development uses the reasoning processes of conceptualizing and structuring empiric phenomena.

From these processes, formal written forms of expression are created that can be presented to members of the discipline. Emancipatory formal expressions include critiques of existing social and political circumstances that redefine that which is problematic in society and suggest a vision for the future. Action plans focus on how to change those conditions. Manifestoes include impassioned statements of the values and perspectives that lead to the critical need for social change, and visions for the future.

Ethical inquiry leads to ethical principles and codes and to other expressions, such as precepts that guide ethical conduct in practice. The critical questions for personal knowing and knowledge development lead to the creation of autobiographic stories and the lived expression of the nurse's being in nursing care situations. The experience of authentically being who one is conveys the genuine self. Aesthetic inquiry leads to works of art that symbolize nursing experience and to aesthetic criticism that reveals deep meaning embedded in nursing art/acts. Empiric inquiry leads to the development of theories; formal descriptions models; and constructions such as statements of fact, models, thematic descriptions of experience and conceptual frameworks.

The formal expressions of each pattern, once they are available to the members of the discipline, make possible certain kinds of formal inquiry processes that depend on the community or on the collective efforts of several members of the discipline. These are the processes for authenticating knowledge. Emancipatory knowledge is authenticated through a collective process of critical reflection to ascertain how fully the ideals of social equity have been achieved, and if these ideals have been sustained. These authentication processes suggest that collectively the discipline has a continuing responsibility to return again and again to the critical questions that initiate social change, examine the outcomes of actions in light of the change that was envisioned, and once again re-form actions to continue the human struggle toward full human potential.

For the patterns of ethical, personal, aesthetic, and empirical knowing, the processes for authenticating knowledge are shown in Figure 1-2. Ethical principles and codes lead to collective dialogue and justification of the soundness of the principles in addressing nursing's ethical and moral dilemmas. For personal knowing, autobiographical stories and the expression of the genuine self lead to reflection and response from others in the discipline with the intent of discerning the value and adequacy of personal insights. Aesthetic criticism and works of art lead to formation of collective appreciation of aesthetic meanings in practice and become a source of inspiration for development of the art of nursing. In the empiric pattern, statements representing empiric events and perceptions are subjected to inquiry that can be confirmed or validated in similar but different situations.

All knowing is expressed in action, in ways of being and doing that convey powerful symbolic representations of what is known. For emancipatory knowing, this is the process of praxis, represented in Figure 1-1 as the outermost sphere of critical reflection/action in relation to nursing's social context, and in the innermost sphere in relation to the practice of nursing. Praxis is synchronous critical reflection/action that is directed toward transforming social conditions toward full human health and well-being for all. The innermost sphere in Figure 1-2 represents the action forms of expression of knowledge for each of the four fundamental patterns—that which is enacted in the practice of nursing. Individual nursing praxis involves continually noticing what is happening in practice, asking critical questions about that practice, creating changes to shift practice in a desired direction, and noticing what happens as a result. Nursing praxis also involves the continual process of questioning the social and political contexts that limit full human potential, and acting to change social and political policy. Praxis inspires the formal inquiry processes that ensure ongoing knowledge development and energize emancipatory change.

Our view of praxis is informed by a postmodern perspective, meaning that one can never fully embrace knowledge within any of the patterns as the final "truth." The confirmation, justification, inspiration, and reflection processes that authenticate disciplinary knowledge within each of the patterns are ongoing processes that provide greater clarity and understanding as new conditions and circumstances unfold. Given this perspective, knowledge is taken to be a construction that varies across time, place, and person. Knowledge is constructed not only by us, but also for us, through social practices and systems of language and discourse. It is the processes inherent in praxis that ensure knowledge is never understood as "truth." Rather, nurses employ their best understandings in their current practice, but also continually challenge what is currently understood to shed light on new possibilities for helping people move toward health and healing. Nurses also join others who notice larger social and political circumstances that limit what is possible for all, and take deliberate action to create circumstances in which health and well-being can flourish.

All of the processes involved in developing nursing knowledge are inter-active and nonlinear, and there is no one starting point. Nurses in practice and nurses who primarily engage in the formal inquiry processes all contrib-ute to the activities that are involved in creating nursing knowledge. Each nurse engages in activities that make possible critical reflection/action, scientific competence, moral/ethical comportment, therapeutic use of self, and transformative art/acts.

To illustrate how these processes interact, suppose you have an empiric problem concerning what nursing approaches to relieving pain are effective in practice and why. You might begin to address this problem by locating evi-dence related to nursing approaches to relieving pain, and subsequently planning a research program to systematically study two different approaches to pain relief for which there is not yet sufficient evidence. You would identify the theoretic explanations associated with each approach and develop a research plan that tests selected hypothetic relationships. Whereas the empiric questions are the starting point and remain the focus of your method, your approaches and methods are influenced by awareness of social, political, and cultural attitudes and practices involved with the experience of pain and its alleviation, practices that might create ample or limited funding for your proj-ect. Aesthetic meanings of pain and suffering relief for various cultural groups in your study will affect how you choose and use measurement tools. Personal meanings concerning the experience of pain will shape how you report find-ings, whereas ethical values around what is best or right to do when the potential for addiction arises will influence how and when pain relief is given and received.

Personal knowing commonly is the avenue through which awareness emerges of possibilities that are not yet fully understood. For example, sup-pose you come to realize and appreciate the unique perspective of an immi-grant family who is receiving pre-surgical care in the clinic. The family has been labeled "difficult" and "uncooperative" by other nurses. As you encounter them, you sense that something has not seemed to fit for the family and just has not felt right. As you open yourself to trying to understand their behavior, a growing appreciation of the family's perspective gradually brings a new insight that the entire family would like to stay with their member during her hospitalization for an upcoming surgery. The nurse shares this awareness with the family, and the relationship shifts to bring the family's perspective to the center. Although having several family members occupy a single room during recovery is not feasible, a plan is put in place whereby one or two family members can be with their member in her room, and others can occupy a nearby waiting room. Personal knowing is the starting point to bring a situation to awareness, but as you explore your awareness, your knowledge of the social and cultural context of an immigrant family in a hospital clinic sharpens your sensitivity to social inequities and injustices that create barriers to understanding the family's perspective. You also use empiric theories about fear and anxiety as a tool in understanding the significance of the situation, within a frame of ethical principles that require both caring and justice for other hospitalized patients in the vicinity of their family member. How and when to confirm your hunches about what concerns the family requires aesthetic sensibilities to discern the meaning of the experience.

Suppose you want to address an ethical question concerning what is right in a situation where a physician asks you to withhold information related to the stage of her disease from a woman hospitalized for treatment of a malignant tumor. You might begin with the focused, creative activities of making explicit the personal and group values (valuing) that should guide your actions, clarifying the positions you find in ethical codes and principles that inform the issue and setting forth how the application of these principles would function with the people with whom you work. These processes would lead you to a dialogue and justification of your ideas, primarily based in ethical reasoning. When you begin to share your ideas with colleagues, the questioning and discussion that result will bring to awareness the personal insights of others engaged in the dialogue. Your dialogue brings to light empiric evidence about what various stages for malignancies mean in relation to treatment effectiveness. You will explore the range of aesthetic significances that are possible in this and similar situations, for example meanings around treatment options in relation to recovery. Your dialogue will also illuminate the nature of social processes and institutionalized values, such as a value for screening mammograms that carry a risk of radiation injury, in which the ethical problem is situated.

Aesthetics as a starting point, like personal knowing, often begins with the nurse's own awareness, but the expression often takes an art form that shows what the nurse envisions about the situation. The art can be in the form of the nurse's action in a situation. Suppose you feel a connection to the experience of chronic pain in a elderly woman with dementia. In a moment of caring for the person, you act from a deeply developed knowing of the meaning of chronic pain in a way that connects with the person's own experience. Understanding and acting aesthetically in relation to the meaning of pain requires the integration of empiric knowledge about the subjective nature of the pain experience in older persons and ethical principles related to the relief of pain as a caring act. Personal knowing from having suffered unnecessary pain yourself also contributes to the expression of aesthetics by shaping how expressions of pain are interpreted and how you act in relation to those interpretations. Emancipatory knowing contributes when you understand that the person in pain, being elderly and demented, has little social value and probably is not receiving pain medication routinely as needed. This understanding is important for aesthetic practice because your reflection and action in relation to this understanding (having a nursing conference that illuminates the situation of undertreated pain in the demented elderly) enables changes that create possibilities that were not previously present (appropriately managed pain for this and other socially devalued persons).

Emancipatory knowing is a common starting point for nurses because of the value that nurses typically place on understanding the cultural and social contexts that influence people's experience of health and illness. Suppose that you become increasingly uncomfortable with legal restrictions influencing the dispensing of medications for pain, and aware that these restrictions are so focused on preventing drug abuse that unnecessary restrictions are being placed on legitimate uses of drugs to alleviate pain. Together with other concerned health care providers and patients, you embark on a project to change the political and legal structures so that access to pain relief is not unnecessarily limited. You draw on empiric evidence concerning both drug misuse and pain relief, people's personal experiences and expressions of pain, aesthetic portrayals of experiences of pain and drug misuse, and ethical principles that guide decisions and actions related to drug use and misuse. You gradually form a plan of action and begin the project of changing the political/legal structures, continually integrating new awareness and insights and remaining open to shifting the action plan as you reach toward your vision of the future.

PATTERNS GONE WILD

When knowledge within any one pattern is not critically examined and integrated within the whole of knowing, distortion, instead of understanding, is produced. Failure to develop knowledge integrated within all of the patterns of knowing leads to uncritical acceptance, narrow interpretation, and partial utilization of knowledge. We call this "the patterns gone wild." When this occurs, the patterns are used in relative isolation from one another, and the potential for synthesis of the whole is lost.

Emancipatory knowing removed from the context of the whole of knowing produces an extreme political standpoint that is unjustly imposed on others. Even when a particular political system has the potential to benefit people and create a more equitable social order, if it is imposed on others in the extreme it has potential to create another form of oppression and injustice. Failure to constantly critically question one's own political standpoint is counter to emancipatory knowing and leads to this pattern of knowing gone wild. Remaining critically reflective and open to empirical, ethical, personal and aesthetic insights is central to emancipatory knowing.

Empirics removed from the context of the whole of knowing produces control and manipulation. Ironically, these have been explicit traditional goals of the empiric sciences. When the validity of empiric knowledge is not questioned, one danger is its potential use in contexts in which it does not belong. When you recognize how all the patterns contribute to the validity of empirics, you begin to see the unquestioned goals of control and manipulation as a distortion or misuse of empiric knowledge.

Ethics removed from the context of the whole of knowing produces rigid doctrine and insensitivity to the rights of others. This happens when you simply set forth personal ideas concerning what is right or good and advocate a position on reasoning derived from personal perspectives. You may present a justification for a perspective to others but not take seriously the processes of dialogue that the justification invites. In the absence of this integrating process, the person's position remains isolated, with little or no opportunity for empiric, personal, or aesthetic insights to give meaning and social relevance to the ideas.

Personal knowing removed from the context of the whole of knowing produces isolation and self-distortion. When this happens, your self remains isolated, and knowledge of self comes only from what is known internally. Self-distortions can take a wide range of forms, from aggrandizement and overestimation of self to destruction and underestimation of self.

Aesthetics removed from the context of the whole of knowing produces indulgence in self-serving expressions and lack of appreciation for the fullness of meaning in a context. Human actions emerge from and are represented by the tastes and desires of the individual alone, without taking into account the deep cultural meanings inherent in an authentic art/act. Your attempts to enact art/acts are not artful, but self-serving, shallow, arrogant, and empty actions. Self-serving preferences grow out of a failure to comprehend the deeper cultural, historical, and political significance of the art/act itself. Inauthentic meanings are assigned to another's experience, or a self-serving posture is assumed with respect to another person.

To illustrate "patterns gone wild" in a nursing situation, imagine Ruth, an elderly woman who is now living in an extended care facility. Ruth has lived a life rich in experience and activities and loves to verbally explore her past, making sense of what it means and how it relates to her present life. Having always been physically active, she takes a nightly stroll before going to bed. She walks the halls, unsteady but determined, smiling and peering into other rooms. Hearing other residents talking or moaning, she sometimes goes into their rooms and tells them stories or talks with them to ease their troubled nights. She does not willingly retire to her own room, and her nightly excursions often disturb others who are trying to sleep or who want to be left alone.

Consider what might happen if any one of the patterns of knowing were isolated from the context of the whole of knowing. Emancipatory knowing alone might lead you to defend Ruth's individual right to do as she wishes regardless of how this affects others, based on a liberal political philosophy of the primary rights of individuals. Ethics taken alone might impose your view of what is good for Ruth, leading to a prescription in her care plan that would confine her to her bed after the lights are out and creating a rigid, rule-oriented atmosphere that is insensitive to what others see as right or good for Ruth, or that Ruth sees for herself. Personal knowing in isolation could impose your perspective that Ruth is a nuisance who is interfering with the time needed to complete the charting for the night. Aesthetics alone would impose your own tastes, preferences, and meanings on the situation. You might attempt to confine Ruth to her room and play your favorite new-age music without considering whether Ruth can hear the music or whether she finds the music soothing or appealing. Empirics isolated from the other patterns of knowing might require giving Ruth a drug that would be effective in bringing sleep, thereby controlling the situation and manipulating her into compliance, regardless of other concerns.

When you, being the good nurse you are, act so that emancipatory knowing, ethics, aesthetics, personal knowing, and empirics come together as a whole, your purposes for developing knowledge and your actions based on that knowledge become more responsible and humane and create liberating choices. A whole understanding of Ruth and the meaning of her life means you have taken into account the social and political prescriptions for long-term care, Ruth's safety, the needs of other residents, Ruth's personal life history and that which gives her pleasure, ethical dimensions of moral development and caring for others, the aesthetic meanings of her actions in the cultural context of aging, and the personal perspectives of the nurses who care for her. Many choices remain open in addressing Ruth's situation, but all of these considerations together would lead you to nursing approaches that would differ from any of the approaches taken from one knowing perspective alone.

WHY DEVELOP NURSING'S PATTERNS OF KNOWING?

As is shown in Figures 1-1 and 1-2 and from our discussion of the knowing patterns, the fundamental reason for developing knowledge in nursing is for the purpose of creating expert and effective nursing practice. Nursing's unique perspective and the particular contributions nurses bring to care come from the whole of knowing, a wholeness that has survived despite a cultural and contextual dominance of empiric knowing (Clements & Averill, 2006; Fawcett et al., 2001; Fry, 1992). In a sense the discipline of nursing can be viewed as the empiric pattern of knowing gone wild in that the majority of formal knowledge development efforts have focused on empiric knowledge development methods. Moreover, knowledge has been equated with empiric forms to the exclusion of any other forms of expression, and the basis for best practices in nursing has come to be associated almost exclusively with empiric evidence.

The idea that knowledge development is separate from practice can be seen as deriving from the dominance of empirics. Empiric theory is inadequate to represent the complexity of the practice world. In fact, the methods of science traditionally require controlling or eliminating the uncontrolled and unpredictable contingencies in the practice realm, which makes the findings of empirics questionable when used in a practice context. The practice implications of empiric theory are often not direct or immediately obvious, and empiric theory often uses a different language from that used in practice.

A shift to a balance in knowledge development to reflect each of the patterns of knowing in nursing holds potential to bring the realm of knowledge development and the realm of practice together. Bringing together "knowing" and "doing" is praxis—the synchronous, thoughtful reflection and action to create a desired future of emancipatory change. Images of a desired future are not confined to any one pattern but rather are reflected in all knowing patterns.

Methods for developing emancipatory, aesthetic, personal, and ethical knowing compel immersion within the realm of practice. Giving attention to these aspects of knowledge development shifts how empirics itself is viewed. Empirics becomes part of a larger whole, and its value takes on different meanings in this context. In addition, as greater attention is given to methods other than empirics, many of the traditions and assumptions that underlie empiric methods are challenged, opening the way for creating empiric methods that better accommodate the contingencies of practice.

Formally expressed nursing knowledge provides professional and disciplinary identity, which in turn conveys to others what nursing contributes to the health care process. Professional identity that evolves from distinct disciplinary knowledge provides a basis from which nurses can create certain aspects of their practice. The knowledge that forms nursing practice provides a language for talking about the nature of nursing practice and for demonstrating its effectiveness. Once nursing practice is described, it is made visible. Moving to a conceptualization of knowledge that more fully embraces the whole of practice will serve to impart value to what has been intangible. Also, when nursing's effectiveness can be shown, it can be deliberately shaped or controlled by those who practice it.

On an individual level, nursing knowledge can provide self-identity and confidence because you will have a firmer base when your ideas are questioned. As you become familiar with the language and processes of knowledge development, you can begin to think about how assumptions, definitions, and relationships within each of the patterns of knowing can be challenged. The study and understanding of knowledge development will provide a basis on which to take risks, act deliberately, and improve practice.

Imagine yourself as a nurse who is using massage to ease chronic pain for a hospitalized person. A physician notices that you are using this method of care. Because this approach is unfamiliar to the physician, she asks you about it. You explain your reasoning, which is based on nursing knowledge. You can cite research evidence of the effectiveness of massage and how you have integrated that evidence into a clinical decision to use it. You convey to the physician information about the positive results that the person is experiencing. You explain the ethical importance of providing relief from suffering, the aesthetic components of the meaning in the situation, and what you have learned about the therapeutic use of self in giving a massage. You explain the societal shift toward accepting and expecting complementary therapies to be included in any approach to care and the social practices that labeled alternative practices "quackery" that kept this valuable therapy suppressed. You also cite facts concerning the nurse practice act in your region that includes massage as a legitimate nursing care practice. Your explanation leads to an informed discussion about various approaches to caring for people with pain and why your approach seems to be effective for this person. As other practitioners learn of your knowledge in this area, they seek your consultation in caring for people with pain. Your knowledge of empiric pain theory and what is effective in caring for people with pain, as well as your emancipatory, ethical, aesthetic, and personal knowledge, provides a valuable resource for developing and improving practice.

Nursing's formally expressed body of knowledge also provides the discipline with a coherence of purpose. Coherence of professional purpose is closely linked to professional identity. Coherence of purpose contributes to a collective identity when nurses agree on the general practice domain. The processes for developing nursing knowledge serve as a means for resolving significant disagreements among practitioners about what is to be accomplished. Varying points of view concerning the general purpose of nursing are reflected in the following questions:

- Should nurses address prevention of illness?
- Should nurses treat human responses to illness?
- Should educational programs be structured around nursing process? Nursing diagnosis? Patterns of knowing? Critical thinking? Evidence-based nursing practice?
- Should nurses view health and illness as opposites?
- Can ill or diseased people also be healthy?
- Is political activism part of nursing's responsibility to society?

As nurses develop individual and collective responses to these questions, our directions for developing knowledge will be clearer, and in turn our knowledge development efforts will contribute to clarifying responses to questions such as these. Nursing knowledge facilitates coherence by examining such questions as a basis for deliberate choices. When nurses examine and agree about professional purposes and develop knowledge related to those purposes, the public and other practitioners will recognize nursing's expertise in relation to those arenas. The fact that nurses are responsible for certain situations will be directly and indirectly communicated to society, and professional identity and coherence of purpose will continue to evolve. By shifting to a balance in the development of all nursing's knowledge patterns, a sense of purpose can develop that is grounded in the whole of knowing that shapes and directs nursing practice.

REFLECTION AND DISCUSSION

In this chapter we considered nursing's patterns of knowing and introduced ideas about how the whole of knowing emerges. We have described traits of each of the following patterns: emancipatory, ethical, personal, aesthetic, and empiric. We introduced ideas about how the inquiry processes for each pattern form the knowledge of the discipline. The central message of this chapter is that all patterns of knowing form an integrated whole, and the whole of knowing is essential as a basis for best practices in nursing.

To deepen your appreciation of the whole of knowing, consider the following questions related to the content of this chapter:

1. Recall a difficult situation in your own nursing experience. What contextual factors contributed to this situation? Were there institutional policies, social structures, or cultural expectations that influenced your experience? What were the ethical problems of the situation? What personal opinions or values did you bring to the situation? Were there any creative solutions or possibilities that you recognized as a nurse that might have changed the situation? Are you aware of empiric facts or theories that might explain the situation?

2. Which components of nursing practice are the most challenging for you: Scientific competence? Therapeutic use of self? Moral/ethical comportment? Transformative art/acts? Praxis? What kinds of experiences or knowledge do you need to more fully develop each of these components of practice?

3. Have you experienced a situation in which one of the patterns of knowing "went wild"? Describe this experience and discuss it with your colleagues. Identify how the whole of knowing would bring about a transformation in the situation.

4. Describe a nursing care interaction that is particularly memorable for you. Reflecting on this interaction, address each of the critical questions for each pattern of knowing:

From an *emancipatory perspective:*

1. What might be wrong with this picture?
2. Who benefited in this situation?
3. What were the limits to full human potential for everyone involved?
4. What was not visible or perceived at the time?

From an *ethical perspective:*

1. Were things right and just in this situation?
2. Were the actions of those involved responsible actions?

From a *personal perspective:*

1. Did I know what I did, and did I do what I knew?
2. Did I do something unintentionally, good or bad, that I now understand?

3. Did I act in a manner consistent with my inner knowing, or did I betray myself?
4. Would I act differently understanding what I now know about myself?

From an *aesthetic perspective:*

1. What were the meanings of the situation for those involved?
2. How was this situation significant for those in the situation?

From an *empiric perspective:*

1. What empiric knowledge was being used during the interaction?
2. Was empiric knowledge used appropriately?
3. Did the interaction suggest the nurse was scientifically competent?

Reference List

Benner, P. A. (1984). *From novice to expert: Excellence and power in clinical nursing practice.* Menlo Park, CA: Addison-Wesley.

Benner, P. A., & Wrubel, J. (1989). *The primacy of caring: Stress and coping in health and illness.* Menlo Park, CA: Addison-Wesley.

Carper, B. A. (1978). Fundamental patterns of knowing in nursing. *ANS. Advances in Nursing Science, 1*(1), 13–23.

Clements, P. T., & Averill, J. A. (2004). Patterns of knowing as a method for assessment and intervention for children exposed to family-member homicide. *Archives of Psychiatric Nursing, 18*(4), 143–150.

Clements, P. T., & Averill, J. A. (2006). Finding patterns of knowing in the work of Florence Nightingale. *Nursing Outlook, 54,* 268–274.

Fawcett, J. (2006). Commentary: Finding patterns of knowing in the work of Florence Nightingale. *Nursing Outlook, 54,* 275–277.

Fawcett, J., Watson, J., Neuman, B., Walker, P. H., & Fitzpatrick, J. J. (2001). On nursing theories and evidence. *Journal of Nursing Scholarship, 33*(2), 115–119.

Fiandt, K., Forman, J., Megel, M. E., Padieser, R. A., & Burge, S. (2003). Integral nursing: An emerging framework for engaging the evolution of the profession. *Nursing Outlook, 51,* 130–137.

Fry, S. T. (1992). The role of caring in a theory of nursing ethics. In H. B. Holmes & L. M. Purdy (Eds.), *Feminist perspectives in medical ethics.* Bloomington, IN: Indiana University Press.

Gramling, K. L. (2006). Sarah's story of nursing artistry. *Journal of Holistic Nursing, 24*(2), 140–142.

Hagan, K. L. (1990). *Internal affairs: A journalkeeping workbook for intimacy.* New York: Harper & Row.

Hagedorn, S. (1995). The politics of caring: The role of activism in primary care. *ANS. Advances In Nursing Science, 17*(4), 1–11.

Hall, L. E. (1963). A center for nursing. *Nursing Outlook, 11*(11), 805–806.

Hall, L. E. (1964). Nursing: What is it? *The Canadian Nurse, 60*(2), 150–154.

Hall, L. E. (1966). Another view of nursing care and quality. In K. M. Straub & K. S. Parker (Eds.), *Continuity in patient care: The role of nursing.* Washington, DC: Catholic University Press.

Kinlein, L. (1977). *Independent nursing practice with clients.* Philadelphia: Lippincott.

Lane, M. R. (2006). Arts in health care: A new paradigm for holistic nursing practice. *Journal of Holistic Nursing, 24*(1), 70–75.

Milio, N. (2000). *9226 Kercheval: The storefront that did not burn.* Ann Arbor: University of Michigan Press. (Original work published 1971.)

Munhall, P. L. (1993). "Unknowing": Toward another pattern of knowing in nursing. *Nursing Outlook, 41*(3), 125–128.

Nelson, G. L. (1994). *Writing and being: Taking back our lives through the power of language.* San Diego, CA: LuraMedia.

Silva, M. C., Sorrell, J. M., & Sorrell, C. D. (1995). From Carper's patterns of knowing to ways of being: An ontological philosophical shift in nursing. *ANS. Advances in Nursing Science, 18* (1), 1–13.

Wainwright, P. (2000). Toward an aesthetics of nursing. *Journal of Advanced Nursing, 32*(3), 750–756.

Weis, D., Schank, M. J., & Matheus, R. (2006). The process of empowerment: A parish nurse perspective. *Journal of Holistic Nursing, 24*(1), 17–24.

White, J. (1995). Patterns of knowing: Review, critique, and update. *ANS. Advances In Nursing Science, 17*(4), 73–86.

Wolfer, J. (1993). Aspects of reality and ways of knowing in nursing: In search of an integrating paradigm. *Image: The Journal of Nursing Scholarship, 25*(2), 141–146.

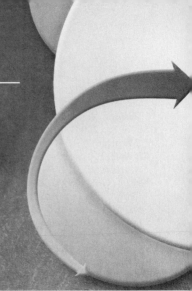

CHAPTER 2

The History of Knowledge Development in Nursing

Nursing history was taught, but never accorded much importance . . .
a casual interlude . . . and even more disheartening not valued.
Lacking historical record the profession is poorly informed . . .
a void in self awareness that affects the stature and growth of nursing
as a vital, essential service.

Myra Levine (1999, p. 214)

The history of knowledge development in nursing is a vast subject indeed. In this chapter we can only touch upon some of the key events that are part of nursing's rich knowledge development heritage. Our purpose is to trace major historical trends that undergird serious inquiry around each of nursing's patterns of knowing and to spark interest in further study of the subject.

Well before the advent of modern nursing in the United States, as marked by the beginning of the Nightingale era in the early 1900s, nursing existed in many forms that shared a common core. What the word *nursing* means and the functions of nurses have shifted to reflect the social order of the time and the demands placed on nurses. Despite shifts in functions, nurses have played a role in the care of the ill since the beginning of recorded history. Nursing has been fundamentally linked with a nurturing role toward the infirmed, ill, and less fortunate. Much of nursing's history is tied to the history of medicine, which has dominated the accounts of changes in care of the sick throughout time. Although much of nursing's unique history has been obscured or lost, there is substantial evidence that supports the value and strength of nursing in the delivery of care and the promotion of health.

Early conceptions of nursing knowledge were grounded in a wholistic view of health and healing. Nurses writing about nursing between the late 1800s and 1950s addressed all aspects of knowing, perhaps without recognizing it. These nurses wrote about the importance of observation and recording of facts, of bringing a sense of virtue to the care of the sick, and of the characteristics of a good nurse. Early writings also addressed the art of nursing and called for responsible social action that would better the lot of the sick. With increasing interest in promoting the study of science during the 1950s in the United States, nursing shifted toward a focus on empirics as the primary concern of the discipline. However, even during this period in nursing's history, threads of philosophic and practical commitment to wholistic practices and to other patterns of knowing persisted. As the 21st century approached, nurses gave serious attention to wholistic approaches in practice and to knowledge and development of methods for all patterns of knowing.

Today's knowledge development approaches will undoubtedly continue to "change with the times" as societal values and resources alter. Despite changes, strong evidence exists to support the claim that nurses have, throughout time, developed and used knowledge to improve practice. This chapter reviews some of the key events in nursing's knowledge development trajectory from antiquity to the present. It also addresses how societal values and resources operate to create nursing's history.

FROM ANTIQUITY TO NIGHTINGALE

There is ample evidence that long before the work of Nightingale, nurses assisted in the routine care of the sick and, in some societies, independently provided healing care (Achterberg, 1991; Donahue, 1995; Ehrenreich & English, 1983). The care provided by these early nurses was influenced by the healing traditions within society. Pagan healers such as shamans, as well as midwives and other folk healers, linked disease to influences within a spirit world. These early healers used rituals, ceremonies, and charms to dispel perceived evil and invoke good. Plants and herbal remedies also were used for healing. Nurses provided assistance to others in carrying out healing traditions but were also independent providers of care.

Early Christian traditions often attributed disease to divine wrath, and punishment was meted out for the sinful transgressions that brought about disease states. With the advent of early forms of scientific thought dating from the mid-1500s to the mid-1700s, pagan and early religious views of illness underwent challenge. The work of scientists and philosophers such as Copernicus, Galileo, Bacon, and Newton began to lay the groundwork for a view of disease as the result of natural rather than spiritual causes. As society's understanding of disease etiology changed, approaches such as invoking the spirits with charms, or punishment for religious transgressions, began to subside. It was nurses who were there to provide nurturing and assistive services consistent with the view that disease was linked to natural causes. The early religious orders offered a respectable avenue for sisters and monks to provide care to the ill and infirmed. In some societies, nursing care was also provided by people who were being punished for civil offenses, people who were homeless and needed shelter, people addicted to drugs and alcohol, and women who were prostitutes. Nurses also included women who bore primary responsibility for the care of their ill family members.

NIGHTINGALE'S LEGACY

Although nursing as a nurturing, supportive activity always has existed, it was Florence Nightingale who advocated and promoted the need for a uniformly high standard of nursing care that required both education and certain personal characteristics. Recognition of nursing as a professional endeavor distinct from medicine began with Nightingale. Her actions and writings on the subject of nursing and sanitary reforms earned her recognition as the founder of modern nursing (Dossey, 1999). For our purposes, modern nursing refers to nursing that followed the work of Nightingale. Nightingale spoke with firm conviction about the nature of nursing as a profession that could provide an avenue for women to make a meaningful contribution to society (Nightingale, 1969). In the mid-1800s, women cared for the sick as daughters, wives, mothers, or maids. These socially prescribed roles influenced Nightingale's conviction that nursing should be a profession for women, but this cultural tradition was secondary to her philosophy. Her primary concern was the more pervasive plight of Victorian women. Women in her era were poverty-stricken and forced to work at menial labor for long hours for little or no pay, or else they were, as was the case with Nightingale, idle ornaments in the households of wealthy husbands or fathers. In either case, there was no avenue for women to use their intellect, passion, and moral activity to benefit society (Nightingale, 1979).

Nightingale spent the first decade of her adult life tormented by a desire to use her productive capacities in a way that would benefit society.

She eventually defied the wishes of her family and broke free of the oppressive social prescriptions for her life. She obtained training as a nurse with the protestant sisters at Kaiserswerth Hospital and subsequently agreed to serve in the Crimean War (Dossey, 1999; Nightingale, 1979; Tooley, 1905; Woodham-Smith, 1983). After her service in the war, Nightingale wrote *Notes on Nursing* (1969), in which she set forth the basic premises on which nursing practice should be based and articulated the proper functions of nursing. Though written for the lay nurses of the time, *Notes* contains timeless wisdom still appropriate for today's professional nurses. In her view, nursing required astute observation of the sick and their environment, the recording of these observations, and the development of knowledge about the factors that promote the reparative process (Cohen, 1984; Nightingale, 1969). Nightingale's framework for nursing emphasized the utility of empiric knowledge. She is recognized for using the statistics she gathered in a way that would further the cause of health care in England and throughout the world (Dossey, 1999).

Firmly committed to the idea that nursing's responsibilities were distinct from those of medicine, Nightingale maintained that the knowledge developed and used by nursing must be distinct from medical knowledge. Medicine, wrote Nightingale, focused on surgical and pharmacologic "cures," a tradition that relied heavily on empiric science. Nursing, however, was broader. Nursing was to assist nature in healing the patient. This was to be accomplished by managing the internal and external environments in an assistive way—in a way that was consistent with nature's laws. Nightingale also had a great influence on nursing education and founded St. Thomas School in London after her return from the Crimea. She insisted that women who were trained nurses control and staff early nursing schools and manage and control nursing practice in homes and hospitals to create a context supportive of nursing's art. Nightingale's influence on nursing education was felt within schools of nursing in all of the British Commonwealth, the United States, and many other parts of the world. The first Nightingale schools were autonomous in their administration, and nurses held decision-making authority over nursing practice in institutions where students learned.

Instruction in Nightingale schools emphasized the powers of observation, the necessity of recording observations, and the potential for organizing nursing knowledge gained through observation and recording. Students also learned proper techniques of nursing. Nightingale's strong beliefs about the character and values that should be cultivated in nursing were reflected in the admission standards and educational programs of early schools (Dennis and Prescott, 1985; Dossey, 1999). Nightingale regarded nursing as a calling and vehemently opposed registration practices of the day as a way to ensure the quality of practitioners. She argued that testing and subsequent registration might ensure a minimal knowledge base but would not guarantee the quality of moral disposition within the individual nurse. Nightingale advocated that nursing was much more than knowledge of facts and techniques. These were important, but to her, nursing also required a certain ethical and moral disposition, a certain type of person, and an ability to act artfully. Nightingale also addressed emancipatory knowing and was concerned about the social-political context within which nursing occurred. For example, in *Notes on Hospitals,* as well as in other documents addressed to military administrators, she outlined the need to rectify unsanitary environmental conditions in hospitals in order to create a proper environment for healing (Nightingale, 1859).

FROM NIGHTINGALE TO SCIENCE

The period from the beginning of the 1900s to about 1950 was a time of great change in nursing that still continues to mold and shape knowledge development processes. Three major themes mark this period and reflect societal change patterns in the United States as they pertain to hospitals, the role of women in society, and the nature of nursing education.

Loss of the Nightingale Ideal

Despite Nightingale's insistence that nurses rather than hospital administration or physicians control nursing care, many circumstances came together in opposition to her model for schools of nursing in the United States. The medical care system developed as a capitalist, for-profit business. This system provided the context for rapid technologic development and a complex institutionalized system to support medical interventions. Early in the 1900s, as the Nightingale era was ending, medical care was taking shape as a science. Women were viewed as incapable of practicing medicine and unqualified to be scientists. With industrialization, large populations of people moved to urban areas, and the number of hospitals increased dramatically in these areas.

Physicians and hospital administrators saw women as a source of inexpensive or free nursing labor who could further their economic goals. Many women entered nursing, providing student labor for hospitals in exchange for receiving apprenticeship training to become nurses. Many were working-class women with limited opportunities for education and meaningful work. Once trained for nursing in hospital schools, many found themselves without employment as new student recruits filled available staff positions.

Nurses were exploited both as students and as experienced workers. They were treated as submissive, obedient, and humble women who were "trained" in correct procedures and techniques. Ideally, they fulfilled their responsibilities to physicians without question. Nurses' positive desire to help people in need, coupled with their relative lack of educational preparation and social or political power, led to an extended period in history when nursing was practiced primarily under the control and direction of medicine (Group and Roberts, 2001; Lovell, 1980).

The Entrenchment of Apprenticeship Learning

Despite strong leaders who followed the Nightingale tradition and viewed nursing knowledge as unique, nursing knowledge has not always been regarded as distinct from medicine. The control of nursing education and practice was transferred from the profession to hospital administrators and physicians during the early 1900s, when most of the Nightingale-modeled schools in the United States were brought under the control of hospitals (Ashley, 1976). Strong efforts to move nursing to institutions of higher learning were not enough. Consistent with the social history of women, nursing was viewed and treated increasingly as a role supporting and supplementing medicine and certainly not one that required a unique knowledge base (Hughes, 1980; Lovell, 1980; Roberts & Group, 1995). Although training was acceptable and even necessary, true education for women and nurses was discouraged, discouraging, and limited. Indeed, education was counterproductive for women who, as nurses, were expected to follow orders and serve the needs and interests of physicians in providing care (Melosh, 1982; Reverby, 1987).

Economic independence for women in the United States was not possible until the mid-1900s. Even a woman who earned an income was not able to have a bank account, own property, or conduct financial transactions in her own name. Normal schools were established for the training of teachers, and nursing schools were available for training nurses, but to obtain long-term security, women were required to conform to the role of wife or daughter. Throughout the early part of the 20th century, nursing practice was based on rules, principles, and traditions that were passed along through limited apprenticeship forms of education. Nursing practice also included an ever-increasing array of delegated medical tasks that were acquired as medical knowledge expanded—tasks performed by nurses as extensions of physicians. Higher education for nurses was not available. What evolved as nursing knowledge was wisdom that came from years of experience. Nursing was viewed primarily as a nurturing and technical art that required apprenticeship learning and innate personality traits congruent with the art (Ashley, 1976; Group & Roberts, 2001; Hughes, 1980). Tradition as a basis for nursing practice was perpetuated by the nature of apprenticeship education (Ashley, 1976). Nursing students were presumed to learn at random through long hours of experience, with limited exposure to lectures or books, and to accept without question the prescriptions of practical techniques. The novice nurse acquired knowledge of what was right and wrong in practice by observing more experienced practitioners and by memorizing facts about the performance of nursing tasks. Nurse recruits also learned what sort of "person" a nurse should be through the imposition of rigid rules that regulated most aspects of behavior, including sleeping, eating, socializing, and dress—both inside and outside the hospital walls. Rules were strictly enforced with severe penalties for those who strayed outside the rules' boundaries.

Persistence of Nursing Ideals

Despite social impediments to the development of nursing knowledge, nursing philosophy and ideology remained committed to the idea that nursing requires a knowledge base for practice distinct from medicine (Abdellah, 1969; Hall, 1964; Henderson, 1964, 1966; Rogers, 1970). This commitment grew from the consistent recognition that, although the goals of nursing and medicine were related, the central goals and functions of nursing required knowledge not provided by medicine or by any other single discipline outside of nursing.

Although social circumstances limited possibilities for nursing education, early nursing leaders sustained ideals that reflected Nightingale's model of education and practice. Because most nursing service was provided as free labor by students in hospitals, those who graduated secured jobs as independent practitioners who were engaged by families to assist in the care of the sick in homes and hospitals. Many nurse leaders were active in confronting a wide range of community-based social and health issues of the time, including temperance, freedom for enslaved people, the right to vote for the disenfranchised, and control of venereal disease. These experiences cultivated and required a broad view of nursing knowledge and a desire to change the future of nursing. These were women for whom technical training did not "take." Despite that training, they saw nursing as independent, vital, and based on a firm knowledge base.

As nurses developed community-based practices, their work and writings reflected the multiple patterns of knowing in which their efforts were grounded. There is substantial evidence that graduate nurses in the early part of the 20th century had ethical and moral commitments that contributed substantively to improving health conditions in hospitals, homes, and communities. Not only did they develop health knowledge as they practiced, but they were politically committed to finding ways to distribute this knowledge to people who needed it (Wheeler, 1985). Consistently throughout the early 20th century, nursing leaders in the United States worked together nationally and internationally in strong connecting networks and called for a social and political ethic that would restore the control of nursing practice to nurses and promote the health and welfare of citizens.

Margaret Sanger, Lillian Wald, Lavinia Dock, Susie Walking-Bear Yellowtail, Mabel Staupers, and Ada Thoms are among those nurses who were challenged by specific needs in society and set about to change problematic practices affecting health care. They observed the circumstances of people in their work environment, identified health-related needs, and worked with others to meet those needs. Integrating ethical commitment with scientific knowledge, they acted to improve health care practices.

Sanger, for example, developed knowledge about reproduction and birth control. She fought against great odds to distribute birth control information to women who were desperate to obtain it and established a foundation for family planning programs that remains viable today in the form of Planned Parenthood (Sanger, 1971). Wald became concerned about child care and family health in the context of extremely poor conditions of sanitation in the crowded immigrant tenements of New York City. She established the Henry Street Settlement in New York City, which is still operating today. Based on concepts of community health nursing and social welfare programs, Wald developed stations from which safe milk was distributed to families with young children and centers for educating mothers in the care of their families (Silverstein, 1985; Wald, 1971). Dock was an ardent suffragist and pacifist who worked for much of her professional life with Wald at the Henry Street Settlement. She campaigned actively for changes in labor laws that would benefit women and children. Twenty years of her life were devoted to gaining enfranchisement for women in the United States; she reasoned that if women could vote, the oppressive laws that affected them could be changed (Christy, 1969).

Notably, many influential nurses among minority groups in the United States also took equally significant actions to improve the health and well-being of their people, but they are far less known. Susie Walking-Bear Yellowtail was a midwife who traveled throughout North American Indian reservations to assess the health, social, and educational problems of Native Americans and recommend solutions (Yellowtail, www.ana.org/hof/yellowtail.htm). She was instrumental in ending abuses of women, such as involuntary sterilization, that were occurring within the Indian Health

Care System (Yellowtail, www.missoulian.com/specials/100montanans/list/062.html). Mabel Staupers worked for improved access to equitable health care services for African American citizens (Staupers, www.ana.org/hof/stauperm.htm). Her research investigating health care needs in Harlem led to the founding of the first facility in Harlem for treating tuberculosis in African Americans (Staupers, www.workingworld.com/magazine/viewarticle.asp?articleno=392&wn=1). Ada Thoms was among the first nursing leaders to recognize public health as a new field of nursing, and in 1917, she added a course on the subject to New York's Lincoln School for Nurses curriculum (Thoms, www.ana.org/hof/thomab.htm). She also founded the Blue Circle Nurses, a group of African American nurses who worked with local communities and provided instruction on sanitation, diet, and appropriate clothing. Ada Thoms also organized a campaign to encourage members of the National Association of Colored Graduate Nurses to vote following passage of the 19th amendment that gave women the right to vote (Thoms, http://tjsworldforreal.blogspot.com/2006_02_01_tjsworldforreal_archive.html).

Like contemporary scholars, these and other early nursing leaders kept alive the ideals of practice as chronicled by Nightingale and used multiple ways of knowing to ground improvements in health care and nursing practice. They were women of strong personal character who lived their ethical conviction that nurses can and should control nursing practice. Their ethical and moral ideals of nursing practice required making observations and organizing the knowledge that came from their observations. Art and emancipatory knowing was central to their practice as they orchestrated complex system changes—changes that required a sense of how to interpret and maneuver through the social and political environments in which they found themselves.

KNOWING PATTERNS IN THE EARLY LITERATURE

Also, during the period of time between about 1900 and about 1950, nurses and others were writing about nursing and patient care in the journals of the time. These early journal articles reflected all knowing patterns; however, the patterns were not named until the late 1970s, with the publication of Barbara Carper's doctoral research (Carper, 1978). An examination of nursing literature published before the 1950s is rich with detail about how nursing embodies, reflects, and requires multiple ways of knowing. The following sections provide some examples of how early writings addressed each pattern of knowing, including the pattern of emancipatory knowing.

Emancipatory Knowledge and Knowing

The early literature's attention to emancipatory knowing was reflected primarily by the recognition that inequities exist as well as descriptions of situations that create inequities and injustice. The early literature also included directives about what nurses must do to change unfair social conditions. Whereas some of these early writings were contributed by nurses, others were written by physicians and non-nurse educators and published in nursing journals and books or presented to nursing audiences.

The existence of social inequities was acknowledged by Effie Taylor in a speech given at the opening session of a national nursing organization meeting. Taylor (1934) noted that the "nations of the world are sick mentally and socially and need to be enabled to live better, think better and act better." (p. 474). How injustices are created is embedded in an eloquent quote of Lavinia Dock (1902–1903), who noted in an early *American Journal of Nursing* article that

> after one has worked for a time healing wounds which should not have been inflicted, tending ailments which should not have developed, sending patients to hospitals who need not have gone if their homes were habitable, and bringing charitable aid to persons who would not have needed it if health had not been ruined by unwholesome conditions, one longs for preventive work ... something that will make it less easy for so many illnesses to occur, that will bring better conditions of life. (1902–1903, p. 532)

Kinloch, a Scottish physician and Chief of the Department of Health in Scotland, echoes Dock when he notes that "were our efforts unified ... we need not be concerned with signs and symptoms, but with proper nurture, replacing the need for treatment" (1932, p. 714). Another cause of social injustices was "anxiety over material necessities," as mentioned in a 1913 physician's address to graduates of the El Reno Sanitarium. Such anxiety "precludes living the ideal, full, free and independent effective life" (Young, 1913, p. 266). Though this physician was addressing graduating nurses, the precept would likely have applied to others as well.

Marion Faber, a registered nurse, noted that it is "effects of the environment that cause deformation of the personality" (1927, p. 1048), whereas Joseph Mountin, a physician and then assistant surgeon general of the United States, stated that the "hospital hierarchy tries to provide social service according to the rules of private competitive enterprise" and this "requires a financial sleight of hand to keep the institution going" (1943, p. 34). These hierarchies, according to William Kilpatrick, a doctorally prepared educator, resulted in a "factory system that reduces individuals to a non-entity amid the bigness of the organization" (1921–1922, p. 791).

Concerns over increasing levels of education of the time led two doctorally prepared academic educators to suggest that "vested interest will preclude the development of professionalism (in nursing) as hospitals will not be able to adjust to the loss of student work hours" (Bixler & Bixler, 1945, p. 732). Isabel Stewart, a nurse and faculty member at Columbia University, wrote that "custom and training are the great authorities and are rigid and static" (1921–1922, p. 908). Stewart further noted that "authority becomes entrenched and does not allow for change in the individual" (p. 908). Allen Gregg, a physician and Director of Medical Sciences at the Rockefeller Foundation, attributed injustices to "envy and malice and hate and violence" (1940, p. 738). Paul Johnson, a doctorally prepared person whose credentials were not cited, stated in an address to the Massachusetts State League of Nursing education that

> the first and most powerful influence upon human minds is the unconscious operation of social custom . . . the question of what to teach is superfluous . . . what is taught is the product of long experience of moral custom. (1928, p. 1087)

Johnson (1928) also suggested how to address the conditions of social injustice. Nurses must

> seek by criticism and appreciation to broaden the bypath . . . to decrease moral provincialism which makes men blind to good beyond their own . . . this [moral provincialism] may be overcome by historical and cultural sympathy with others and understanding and appreciation of values that have appealed to other people. (1928, p. 1087)

Elizabeth Wright, presumably a nurse, in a transcript of a talk given to a state nurses' association, wrote that "the nurse must possess imagination and perception of individual differences, and have the power to place oneself at the central point of other people's experiences" (1953, p. 451).

Katherine McClure, a nurse professor, noted the need to "improve the environment and conditions of the persons she nurses without remaking them to suit ourselves" (1951, pp. 221–222), whereas nurse Janet Geister wrote that "the real wisdom of human life is compounded out of the experiences of ordinary men" (1937, p. 261). These nurses apparently recognized the importance of acting in relation to the needs of others while understanding that effective change must come from a grass roots position. Bixler and Bixler (1945) stated that nurses' social attitudes should reflect the conception that "every citizen is entitled to health care" (p. 753), whereas Taylor (1934) wrote that nurses must have a "broad sense of justice" (p. 475) and should "not know color or creed" and "be for the poor as well as the rich" (p. 473). Kilpatrick further addressed how to undo social injustices by stating we should "seek the development and expression of each in relation to all, and cause others to grow" (1921–1922, p. 795), whereas Stewart (1921–1922, p. 908) stated that "knowledge, culture, individual development, freedom, health and expertness are used in service of the social group," emphasizing that "education has a social purpose and nursing is no exception."

Noted anthropologist Margaret Mead, in an address to a convention of the American Nurses Association, stated that "nursing stands between those who are vulnerable and the community that may forget them, not care for them" (1956, p. 1002). Genevieve Noble, a graduate nursing student, understood that nurses must notice injustice when she stated that the "nurse cannot be indifferent to the welfare and happiness of the undernourished child in the street or the maid working in her corridor" (1940, p. 161). Esther Lucille Brown, a researcher for the Russell Sage Foundation who authored reports about nursing, recognized that "nursing must create alliances with problems outside the privileged home and hospital, and should be concerned with those who have chronic disease, are aged and physically handicapped" (Goostray & Brown, 1954, p. 720). Finally, Elizabeth Porter, who was president of the American Nurses Association, in 1953 summarized many of the social conditions that create social injustices and inequities—the focus of emancipatory knowing. Porter noted that "hunger, poverty, injustice and disease are the enemies of peace" and that when

> man arrogates to himself blessings that he denies others, these blessings begin to slip through his fingers . . . and . . . a chain around another's neck means there is a chain about your own . . . and that passivity or acquiescence to the chains of others means you enslave yourself. (1953, p. 948)

For Porter (1953), necessary actions included "supporting humanitarian programs on a worldwide scale" (p. 948), taking responsibility to change the "conditions in which men live and the conditioning of their mind" (p. 948), and "putting the good of the world and community before the selfish interest of individuals or specialized groups" (p. 949).

To summarize, the early nursing literature addresses the importance of emancipatory knowing by recognizing that social injustices existed as well the conditions that created them. This literature is replete with directives for nursing actions required to rectify societal injustice and conditions that privilege one group over another. Injustices were not hidden or mystified. Rather, perhaps concurrent with the expansion of nursing into community-based practices, the necessity to recognize social inequalities and take strong measures to rectify them was emphasized.

Ethical Knowledge and Knowing

Before the 1950s, ethics primarily was represented as virtues possessed by the nurse. Nurses were expected to be moral individuals, who, it follows, do the right thing. Virtue and responsibility were paramount for nurses. Duty and responsibility included protection, truth telling, and imparting specialized knowledge (Conrad, 1947; De Witt, 1901; Warnshius, 1926). An editorial in the *American Journal of Nursing* noted that "the doctor is responsible for the general conduct of the case, but the nurse is responsible for the honest performance of her own duties" (De Witt, 1901, p. 15). This editorial further noted that "born qualities added to training" were critical for ethical conduct (p. 15). Duty often was expressed in religious admonitions to love, live right, and have faith. Duty was seen as a sacred obligation, as illustrated by a lay author who wrote "a good nurse will die before admitting she is even tired [for] loyal service is one of the articles of the profession's religion" (Drake, 1934, pp. 137–138). Moral fitness for nursing was important, and moral examinations were recommended. Agnes Riddles (1928), a nurse, stated that "women [nurses] should hold their position only after a moral examination as well as a technical one" (p. 29). Riddles listed a variety of moral infractions attributable to nurses of the time, including lack of consideration for the patient, neglect of aseptic precautions, disrespect for human life, and lack of proper experience in assembling needed nursing materials.

Charlotte Aikins (1915), presumably a nurse educator, outlined an entire curriculum for teaching ethics in *Trained Nurse and Hospital Review*. The curriculum included knowledge of "the customs and laws of the hospital world which she (student) must be admonished to accept meekly" (p. 136) and "personal virtues of importance such as reticence, tact, and discretion in order that she may do no harm" (p. 136). "Health, carriage, voice, manner, habits and general deportment" (p. 136) also were important. During the junior year, ethics would cover "handling of supplies and appliances, avoiding accidents, use of good surgical technique, wise use of recreation and holidays, and the necessity of a good conscience" (p. 137). Another early nurse mentioned the need to keep preconceptions and prejudices to a minimum as a part of ethical conduct (Oettinger, 1939).

Paul Johnson (1928), in an address to a statewide gathering of nurses, asked: "What should ethics teach?" (p. 1084). He differentiated ethics and morality. Ethics, according to Johnson, is the "science of right conduct" (p. 1085). Ethics investigates "boldly" what this is by "questioning moral tradition, examining moral facts, and searching out moral values" (p. 1085). Ethics requires "careful investigation, open-minded judgment, the practice of reasonableness and intelligent doubting" (p. 1085). Ethical sensitivity, rather than the rules approach of "laying down exact rules for conduct" (p. 1084), was important to cultivate. Such an attitude questions the establishment of rules as the basis for biomedical ethics and validates a relational perspective for ethical conduct. Johnson's early article also challenges virtue ethics, the position that relies on the good person to do the right thing, by differentiating ethics and morality and calling ethics the "science" of right conduct.

Early authors imparted a variety of goals for ethical knowledge and knowing, including protection of patients' privacy and rights, advocacy, and minimization of patients' discomfort and inconvenience. Broader goals also were mentioned, such as increasing tolerance and respect by respecting the individual worth, autonomy, and dignity of individuals; assisting in the development of the individual; strengthening society and self; developing economic security; and promoting peace.

In summary, the early periodical literature reflects a view of ethical behavior and comportment as conforming to individual virtues. Such virtues were evidenced by religious living, self-sacrifice, and a nearly blind duty to others' rules and prescriptions. The seeds of relational ethics are found in the questions raised concerning the cost to the individual and the profession of blind adherence to rules and prescriptions. Although most of what is termed ethical comes from religious traditions and authoritative trust in others, writers also discussed questioning traditions and making responsible judgments, studying what one doubts, and analyzing and criticizing basic precepts.

Personal Knowledge and Knowing

The importance of the person of the nurse is evident in that the prevailing ethics of the time called for a virtuous person. However, qualities of person beyond virtue also are found in the early literature. Margaret Conrad (1947), writing about the nature of expert nursing care, recognized the necessity for a well-balanced, integrated personality to contribute to the care of others. Allen Gregg (1940), a physician, in an address to three national nurse meetings, asked nurses to "seek honestly and earnestly to find what really matters to us and what beliefs and convictions we hold" (p. 738). Gregg also redefined virtue as "the inner life as well as the outer in consistency of behavior with one's own thoughts and feelings" (p. 740) and further stated that "motives and conduct must harmonize" (p. 740). Motives must be sound or there is no virtue in the great sense, no independence, and no self-confidence (p. 741). The fundamental importance of personal knowledge is acknowledged in that "only when a person is something to herself can she become anything to anybody else" (p. 741). Gregg's article, written in the postwar period, recognized that science cannot provide personal knowledge because "the social wisdom of man does not derive from chemistry and physics and mechanical skill. Decency does not visit our common dwelling place without invitation" (p. 739). Genevieve Noble (1940), writing as a student in "The Spirit of Nursing," emphasized the need for an inherent inner self-discipline rather than an imposed discipline for adequate nursing care. Katherine Oettinger (1939) gave equal importance to personal knowing and empirics by stating that "the personality of the nurse is quite as important as the distinctive facts she learns" (p. 1224).

Important personal characteristics included acceptance of self that is grounded in self-knowledge and confidence. Personal integrity and honesty, as well as enthusiasm, versatility, courageousness, stability, and emotional diversity, were important features of personal knowledge. Such knowledge is created by engagement with life, finding out what really matters, and reflecting on it. Nursing practice requires a depth of personal knowing that acknowledges the validity of feelings, openness to freely discussing feelings, and examining reciprocal emotions in dialogue and relation. A nurse of high personal character evidences an inner and outer harmony and commands respect of self and others. As Oettinger (1939) put it, such a nurse is "free from conscript minds giving conscript thoughts" and is "free to change the status quo" (p. 1244). In summary, a whole host of personal attributes that go beyond virtuous behavior, including self-discipline, knowledge of self, and an openness to the processes of reflection in order to create actions with integrity, are basic to good nursing care.

Aesthetic Knowledge and Knowing

A sense that nursing has an artistic component is clearly evident in early periodical literature. L. F. Simpson (1914), another physician speaking to nurses, stated that "real nursing is an art; and a real nurse is an artist" (p. 133). Conrad (1947) stated that the art of nursing included such things as "knowing what the patient wants before she is asked" (p. 162). It arises from "combining instinct, knowledge and experience" (p. 162). According to Conrad, art depends on imagination and resourcefulness and requires "true perspective" (pp. 162–163). Furthermore, art requires practice, and some nurses "never acquire it" (p. 135). Experience was seen as important to develop aesthetic knowing. As Austin Drake (1934), a layperson, put it:

> Circumstances alter cases ... the nurse adapts her roles at will according to her patient's physical state and particular mode ... if he is able and desires ... she talks, otherwise she is silent, intent upon her duties ... the severity of the illness does not determine this. (1934, pp. 136–137)

Art in the more traditional sense was recognized as important to the art/ act of nursing. In 1923 Lois Mossman (1923), an assistant professor of education, acknowledged that "science cannot explain what happens when we respond to beauty of form or motion but the response is pleasurable and influences what we are doing" (p. 318). Mossman asks novice nurses to "experience beauty, to see it in the commonplace, to learn of books, poems, pictures, and music that interpret beauty and draw from them to fit the needs of those we serve" (p. 319). According to Mossman, "Life is rhythmical and lights must be set off by the shadows" (p. 319). Edward Garesche (1927), a Roman Catholic priest, eloquently expressed the elusiveness of assessing our art and the importance of distinguishing it from empirics. He stated: "The service of the learned professions does not bear measuring while it is being rendered" (p. 901).

In summary, the early literature represents aesthetics as a combination of knowledge, experience, intuition, and understanding. Aesthetic knowing was creative and intuitive and consisted of exquisite judgments without conscious awareness but sensed intuitively by unexplained insight and hunches. Aesthetic knowledge was gained through appreciation of the arts and by subjective sensitivity to individual differences. Aesthetic knowing also was gained by personal imitation of those who possess the art. Aesthetic knowing required speculation, imagination, and the superimposition of impressions on facts. The practitioner who had a sincere intentionality and the ability to carry out sophisticated assessment could act artfully. It was through the interpretation of interaction that each succeeding interaction became more meaningful.

Empiric Knowledge and Knowing

Before the era of "science" in the mid-1950s, there was clear recognition of scientific knowledge as a source of power. A physician who addressed the annual meeting of the Michigan Nurses Association acknowledged that scientific knowledge had increased and asked nurses to acknowledge its power and value for producing knowledge. The physician cautioned against quackery and portrayed science as a source of legitimate criteria for selection of information provided to patients (Warnshius, 1926). Despite the value of science, he also emphasized the importance of a central focus on the welfare of the patient.

Empirics commonly was represented as knowledge of underlying principles and techniques associated with nursing. According to Margaret Conrad (1947), a baccalaureate-prepared professor of nursing, this required an understanding of the laws of nature and the principles of physics, chemistry, physiology, and psychology. In other early articles the procedural and technical aspects of nursing were emphasized, including bed making; food tray handling and feeding; carrying out personal hygienic measures such as bed baths and oral hygiene; and managing delegated medical procedures such as drains, catheterizations, enemas, alcohol baths, vital signs, and medication administration (Brigh, 1944; Mountin, 1943). Muriel Burgess (1941), a nursing student, outlined the "facts of care," which included diagnosis; social factors such as heredity, environment, and education; and medical factors such as past history of family and history of present illness, symptom onset, physical examination, and laboratory and x-ray findings. She further noted that the plan should include the progress of the patient and use graphs whenever possible. Treatments prescribed and the continuing plan for care also were important. Genevieve and Roy Bixler (1945), two doctorally prepared educators, addressed the development of empirics and wrote "the elements of science should be defined and organized, gathered from every science contributing to nursing and arranged in the most convenient order for thought" (p. 730). Bixler and Bixler stated that scientific compartmentalizations were artificial, arbitrary, and to be avoided by nursing science. Nursing science existed apart from practice, but its use in the service of professional practice represented a "new synthesis." Science, they asserted, needs to be integrated as an art.

Formal observation also was established as a valued technique and a skill critical for the development of nursing empirics. A 1947 editorial in the *American Journal of Nursing* admonished nurses to develop keen observation skills because "the lack of descriptions or records of nursing care based on actual experience is appalling" (Conrad, p. 655). Written observations could form the basis for a complete patient study to provide an interpretive picture of present-day nursing ("Changes in Nursing Practice," 1947). In a speech at a student nurse convention, Blanche Pfefferkorn (1933), who was identified only as a registered nurse, stated that empiric knowledge came from questionnaires, detached observation, and field studies. According to Pfefferkorn, a scientific attitude was important. Scientific knowledge included "facts that were organized into a form or structure that were not dynamic and reports of field studies" (p. 260). Regardless of source, scientific knowledge served as a skeleton and answered questions about "what." Good science represented the "what" well. Pfefferkorn noted that the nurse needed to know how, not just what, and stated that field studies could "enliven fact gathering by providing knowledge of how" (p. 260). Agnes Meade (1936), a nurse who wrote an article titled "Training the Senses in Clinical Observation," cautioned about the following pitfall of scientific bias: "A distinguishing feature of scientific observation is that the observer knows what is being sought, and to a certain extent what is likely to be found" (p. 540).

In summary, in the early literature the nature and importance of science for nursing were clearly reflected. Early authors envisioned ways for empiric knowledge to be created and displayed. Although scientific-empiric knowledge could come from disciplines outside of nursing, there was recognition of the unique nature of nursing science. Principles, facts gleaned from observation, and procedural guides to action were important forms of empirics that were necessary for completing routine hygienic care of patients and delegated medical tasks. Despite the recognition of the value of empirics, the caution that science alone was an inadequate practice guide appears frequently. A physician addressing a graduating class of diploma nurses told them that "the profession of nursing is an art depending upon science. . . . In nursing the art must always predominate though underlying science is important" (Worcester, 1902, p. 908).

THE EMERGENCE OF NURSING AS A SCIENCE

The shift toward a concept of nursing knowledge as predominantly scientific began in the 1950s and took a strong hold in the 1960s. This shift toward knowledge as science produced significant changes in what was considered important in nursing. Gradually, nursing shifted from a perspective that emphasized technical competence, duty, and womanly virtue to a perspective that focused more on effective nursing practice (Hardy, 1978). The shift toward science, in many ways, was a welcome change. However, this move was at the sacrifice of the development of ethics for individual and collective practice, the development of nurse character, the artistic and aesthetic dimensions of practice, and critical attention to injustices in health care practices. Development of knowledge in relation to other patterns of knowing, so necessary for practice and so evident in nursing's work historically, was largely neglected until the early 1990s.

The shift toward science as the basis for developing nursing knowledge was influenced by the involvement of nursing in the two world wars during the 1900s. The wars created social circumstances that brought about substantial shifts in roles for women and nurses. During the wars, with many men away from their homes, women were freed from constraints and learned to manage their responsibilities in accord with their own priorities and preferences. Many women entered the skilled or unskilled labor force during the years when men were away in battle. Women who were nurses were needed to support the war effort by providing care for the sick and wounded. War-related programs were instituted by the U.S. government to make nursing preparation available to women who agreed to serve in the war (Kalisch & Kalisch, 1995; Kelly & Joel, 2001).

Partly because of the greater demand for technically skilled nurses to serve the war effort, by the decade of World War II, women had begun to enter institutions of higher learning in greater numbers. The early nursing leaders' vision of nursing education within colleges and universities began to be realized. After the end of World War II, many educational programs were established within institutions of higher learning, and graduate programs for nurses began to appear. Academic institutions required faculty to hold advanced degrees and encouraged them to meet the standards of higher education with regard to service to community, teaching, and research. Research standards adhered to the more traditional objectivist criteria of scientific-empiric work, which limited the nature of credible scholarship among academic nurses. Nurse-scientist programs were established to enable nurses to earn doctoral degrees in other disciplines with the idea that research skills learned could then be applied in nursing. As academically based nurses gained skills in the methods of science, conceptual frameworks and other types of theoretic writings began to emerge.

In 1950 *Nursing Research,* the first nursing research journal, was established. Books on research methodologies and explicit conceptual frameworks, often called "theories of nursing," began to appear. Early research reports often focused on describing what nurses do, rather than clinical problems of patients. They were less sophisticated in method than those of today, but these writings changed and began to reflect qualities of serious empiric scholarship and investigative skill. Various schools of thought emerged about the nature of nursing practice and nursing's knowledge base, which provided a fresh flow of ideas that could be examined by members of the profession. These writings provided a stimulus for early efforts in developing theory and, eventually, to broader knowledge-development efforts.

By the 1960s doctoral programs in nursing were being established. By the end of the 1970s the number of doctorally prepared nurses in the United States had grown to nearly 2000. Approximately 20 doctoral programs in nursing had been established, and master's programs were maturing in academic stature and quality. Master's programs began focusing on preparing advanced practitioners in nursing rather than on preparing educators and administrators. With the development of advanced educational programs, nurses began to formally consider the processes for the development of nursing knowledge. Nurse scholars began to debate ideas, points of view, and methods in the light of nursing's traditions (Hardy, 1978; Leininger, 1976). These debates are reflected in the literature of the late 1960s and early 1970s (Dickoff & James, 1971; Dickoff, James, & Wiedenbach, 1968; Ellis, 1968, 1971; Folta, 1971; Walker, 1971; Wooldridge, 1971). Fundamental differences in viewpoints about nursing science provided nurse scholars the opportunity to learn, sharpen critical-thinking skills, and acquire knowledge about the processes and limitations of science.

As an overt and deliberative focus on knowledge development began to take shape in nursing, a prevailing view emerged of nursing as a service that required a strong base in science. Debates reflected various views of science and metatheory and the preferred methods for producing sound nursing knowledge. Despite the lively debates and substantive issues focused on scientific knowledge, the idea that nursing requires development of a broad knowledge base that includes all patterns of knowing has never been lost. Even when this broad view was not explicitly mentioned in the debates (as was common during the 1970s), the broad conceptualizations labeled theories implicitly required multiple ways of knowing. The persistent dominance of science can be attributed in part to academic nurses' need to gain legitimacy in their university communities and nurses' need to achieve political and personal legitimacy within medicine and society in general. Regardless of the societal context, the wholistic focus of nursing has endured.

EARLY TRENDS IN THE DEVELOPMENT OF NURSING SCIENCE

Throughout the second half of the 20th century, three major trends contributed to evolving directions in the development of nursing knowledge. These trends, as would be expected, centered on the scientific-empiric pattern. However, there are threads of continuity that reflect ethics, aesthetics, personal, and emancipatory knowing, as we show in the sections that follow. The three trends are (1) utilization of theories borrowed from other disciplines, (2) development of conceptual frameworks defining nursing, and (3) the development of middle-range theory linked to practice.

The Use of Theories Borrowed from Other Disciplines

As the educational preparation of nurses expanded, theories developed in other disciplines were recognized as important for nursing. Problems in nursing practice for which there had seemed no ready solution began to be viewed as resolvable if theories and approaches to theory development from other disciplines were applied. For example, nurses recognized that young children needed the continuing love and support of their parents and families during hospitalization. The strict rules of hospitals that severely restricted visitation interrupted these primary family ties. As psychologic theories of attachment and separation developed, nurses found an explanation for the problems experienced by hospitalized children and were able to change visitation practices to provide sustained contact between parents and children.

Although theories from other disciplines have been useful, nurses also have exercised caution in arbitrarily applying these theories. In some instances, the theories of other disciplines do not take into consideration significant factors that influence a nursing situation. For example, some theories of learning that are applicable to classroom learning do not adequately reflect the process of learning when an individual is faced with illness, nor do they deal with the ethical issues a nurse might face in disclosing sensitive information to a patient. Although borrowed theories may be useful, their usefulness cannot be assumed until they are examined from the perspective of nursing in nursing situations (Barnum, 1998; Walker & Avant, 2004). The trend to use theories within related disciplines may have been an outgrowth of pre- and postdoctoral fellowship funding for nurses that began in the mid-1950s. This funding nurtured a cadre of nurse scientists who studied research approaches in fields related to, but outside of, nursing. Once educated, these nurses would return to nursing and conduct research, thus strengthening nursing's knowledge base.

Development of Philosophies and Conceptual Frameworks Defining Nursing

As nurses began to reconsider the nature of nursing and the purposes for which nursing exists in light of science, they began to question many ideas that were taken for granted in nursing and the traditional basis on which nursing was practiced. They wrote and published idealized views about nursing and the type of knowledge, skills, and background needed for practice. As an ideal view of nursing, these frameworks and philosophies did not arise from practice per se but did reflect a reasonably attainable vision of what nursing could be. Writings of the 1960s and 1970s made significant contributions to the development of theoretic thinking in nursing. Many have been used as a basis for curricula and as guides for practice and research.

Many early nursing conceptual frameworks and philosophies include a description of the nursing process. This process, which is similar to both scientific methods of problem solving and research processes, is a framework for viewing nursing as a deliberate, reflective, critical, and self-correcting system. The nursing process replaced the rule- and principle-oriented approaches that were grounded in a medical model in which the nurse functions as a physician's assistant. The nursing process relied heavily on what could be assessed through observation. Before there was a focus on the nursing process, unexamined rules and principles were used to guide the nurse in routine hygienic care, performance of treatment procedures, and administration of medications to treat disease. Because a rule-oriented approach did not encourage reflective problem solving, nor was it consistent with education in institutions of higher education, the shift to the nursing process as a way to approach care encouraged nurses to cultivate basic inquiry skills. Nursing diagnosis, which evolved from the nursing process and began to move nursing away from theoretic dependence on a medical model, was one method for organizing the domain of nursing practice. The early literature concerning nursing diagnosis included both practical and theoretic ideas about developing a taxonomy of nursing diagnoses and testing their validity.

Conceptual frameworks for nursing education and practice proliferated in the 1960s and 1970s. The then current emphasis on systems theories is evident in the work of Callista Roy, Imogene King, Dorothy Johnson, and Betty Neuman. The movement of psychiatric care into community-based settings following the development of new drugs for management of psychiatric illness contributed to a theoretic focus on the importance of interpersonal communication—a focus notable in the work of Hildegard Peplau, Joyce Travelbee, and Ida Jean Orlando. The emergence of chronic disease with the control of communicable disease and a focus on wholism is reflected in Myra Levine's framework as well as in Dorothea Orem's theoretic writings on self-care. Many nurse scientists who benefited from early funding for doctoral education received training in fields such as sociology and anthropology where a focus on the development of broad, grand theories was prominent. This influence is notable in the work of Madeleine Leininger. The conceptual frameworks of Martha Rogers, Rosemarie Parse, and Margaret Newman reflect theoretic perspectives linked to developments in modern physics that moved beyond earlier system concepts of equilibrium.

There was considerable debate about whether the writings of leaders such as Callista Roy, Betty Neuman, Imogene King, and Dorothea Orem and others were to be called models, theories, or philosophies. This debate reflected an underlying acknowledgment that science alone was an inadequate metatheory for practice. How to name these theory-like constructions—theories? conceptual models? theoretical frameworks? conceptual frameworks?—remains a debatable subject, and various terminologies can be found in the contemporary theoretical literature. We have chosen to refer to these broad theory-like structures as conceptual or theoretic frameworks, and their authors we call theorists. Regardless of labels, nursing practice consistent with these (and other) conceptual frameworks was taught in educational institutions, integrated into practice, and used to guide research. The use of conceptual frameworks cultivated a tacit recognition of the significance of multiple patterns of nursing knowledge. As nurses began to integrate these ideas into practice settings, the actual and potential relationships between nursing's conceptual frameworks and

TABLE 2-1 Chronology and Key Emphasis of Early Conceptual Frameworks in Nursing: 1952–1989

Year of First Major Publication	Theorist	Key Emphasis
1952	Hildegard E. Peplau	Interpersonal process is maturing force for personality.
1960	Faye G. Abdellah, Irene L. Beland, Almeda Martin, and Ruth V. Matheney	Patient's problems determine nursing care.
1961	Ida Jean Orlando	Interpersonal process alleviates distress.
1964	Ernestine Wiedenbach	Helping process meets needs through art of individualizing care.
1966	Lydia E. Hall	Nursing care is person directed toward self-love.
1966	Virginia Henderson	Empathic understanding and the knowledge of the nurse helps people toward independence.
1966	Joyce Travelbee	Meaning in illness determines how people respond.
1967	Myra E. Levine	Wholism is maintained by conserving integrity.
1970	Martha E. Rogers	Person-environment are energy fields that evolve negentropically.
1971	Dorothea E. Orem	Self-care maintains wholeness.
1971	Imogene M. King	Transactions provide a frame of reference toward goal setting.
1976	Callista Roy	Stimuli disrupt an adaptive system.
1976	Josephine G. Paterson and Loretta T. Zderad	Nursing is an existential experience of nurturing.
1978	Madeleine M. Leininger	Caring is universal and varies transculturally.
1979	Jean Watson	Caring is a moral ideal: mind-body-soul engagement with another.
1979	Margaret A. Newman	Disease is a clue to pre-existing life patterns.
1980	Dorothy E. Johnson	Subsystems exist in dynamic stability.
1980	Betty Neuman	Individuals, as wholistic systems, interact with environmental stressors and resist disintegration by maintaining a normal line of defense.
1981	Rosemarie Rizzo Parse	Indivisible beings and environment co-create health.

TABLE 2-1 Chronology and Key Emphasis of Early Conceptual Frameworks in Nursing: 1952–1989—cont'd

Year of First Major Publication	Theorist	Key Emphasis
1982	Nola Pender	Health-promoting behavior is determined by individual characteristics and experiences as modulated by perceptions and interpersonal/situational factors.
1989	Patricia Benner and Judith Wrubel	Caring is central to the essence of nursing. It sets up what matters, enabling connection and concern. It creates possibility for mutual helpfulness.

nursing practice became clearer. Practicing nurses found a new sense of purpose and direction consistent with the basic values of nursing and a sense of the increasing effectiveness achieved through systematic and thoughtful forms of nursing practice. Transferring these ideals of practice into the health care setting also served to illuminate the difficulties of finding nursing opportunities in the increasingly competitive health care system. Table 2-1 is a historical chronology of nurse theorists' work during the latter half of the 20th century.

Many of these theorists are no longer alive, but their work is kept alive by nurses who use and continue to develop their models. Appendix A (available at http://evolve.elsevier.com/Chinn/knowledge) summarizes, from our perspective, the essential features of the early work of theorists listed in Table 2-1. Some of these theorists continue to develop their ideas and change their perspectives, but their work remains significant because their ideas have stood the test of time in forming fundamental values and perspectives of the discipline. Because conceptual frameworks change as they are linked to research findings, are used in education and practice, and are critiqued and expanded, users of Appendix A are cautioned that these summaries are historical in nature. There is a wealth of information about many of the nurse theorists listed in Table 2-1 available on the Internet that can provide perspectives on more current work for those theoretic frameworks that continue to evolve. Even for those theorists who continue to develop their ideas, their work remains true to the essential core of the conceptual model as originally proposed. Website resources and information can be accessed using key search terms or theorists' names. Applying the processes of description and critical reflection of theory as described in Chapter 8 will help to ensure your ability to appropriately evaluate the information available on theorist-related websites.

The conceptual frameworks developed in the 1960s and 1970s were important for broadly defining nursing and naming the phenomena central to nursing's domain of concern. These ideas were extremely valuable because they shifted nursing away from a medical model of practice characterized by correct performance of routine nursing and medical procedures and the administration of medication. They broadened nursing's role in society by describing how nursing functions to achieve a socially relevant purpose and delineating the contextual variables important to the practice of nursing. The philosophic values embedded in early nursing frameworks reflect central assumptions and value positions on which nursing rests. At the same time, these conceptual frameworks were characterized by a relatively functional view of nursing and health. They defined what nursing is, described the social purposes nursing serves, detailed how nurses should function to realize these purposes, and defined the parameters and variables influencing illness and health processes.

For example, Callista Roy, Dorothea Orem, Virginia Henderson, and Hildegard Peplau focused on descriptions of illness and health—what nurses do to assist the person to move toward health. These frameworks present explanations of how nursing actions function in practice to enhance health and well-being. The functions described are theoretic in nature, in that they are conceptualized at a relatively abstract level. Nursing is viewed as a set of roles or functions, not as concrete technical procedures. These abstract ideas about nursing functions are woven into explanations of relationships between the nurse's roles and function and the theorist's idea of a desired nursing outcome related to health and well-being.

In the later 1970s and the 1980s there was a noticeable qualitative shift in theoretic ideas developed for the purpose of broadly defining nursing practice. Rather than reflect a functional perspective of the role of nursing in society, later conceptual frameworks tended to move to qualitative dimensions that characterize nursing's role not as what nurses do but as the essence of what nursing is. This shift offered potential for moving nursing from a context-dependent reactive position to a context-interactive proactive stance. These approaches combined direct observations of nurses and their practice and systematized insights that were guided by existing conceptual and theoretic frameworks and philosophies of nursing as well as other literature sources. For example, both Jean Watson (1979) and Patricia Benner and Judith Wrubel (1989) grounded the essence of nursing in caring. They used theoretic reasoning derived from a deliberate philosophic stance that is explicit in their writings and from experience of the practice of nursing in many different contexts. The themes or patterns that characterize the essence of caring are those reflected in the actions, thoughts, values, and priorities of the practicing nurse.

Another early formal movement defined the discipline by locating the source of nursing theory in nursing practice and calling for the systematization of practice knowledge into theory. This approach was particularly influenced by the writings of Dickoff and James and their colleagues, who were well known for theorizing the nature of theory for a practice discipline (Dickoff & James, 1968; Dickoff, James, & Wiedenbach, 1968). The writings of Dickoff and James proposed a radically different view for developing theory that challenged the scientific metatheory prevailing in the 1960s. Dickoff and James described how theory is developed from the systematization of practice-based rules, guidelines, and nursing activities that were known to work. Theory was, in part, the systematization of practice-based variables and could exist at one of four levels: factor isolating, factor relating, situation relation, or situation producing.

Dickoff, James, and colleagues also recognized the value-laden nature of theory in nursing and called for an explicit recognition and naming of the values toward which theory development was proceeding—an aspect of theory they termed "goal-content." Their theory of theories proposed the formulation of prescriptions that would be used, in combination with a survey list, to reach the goal. The survey list was organized around six categories: agency, patiency, dynamics, structure, terminus, and procedure. The list was basically an enumeration of factors, not qualifying as prescriptions, that were recognized to affect movement toward the goal (Dickoff & James, 1968). The inclusion of values within the structure of theory and the recognition that theory was more like a flexible guide to practice, rather than a global framework to be systematically tested, provided a revolutionary view of empiric knowledge. The Dickoff and James approach to nursing metatheory, which was intensely discussed in the literature and at conferences, reflected a growing recognition that the nature and value of scientific-empiric theory for nursing was unclear. Dickoff and James asked the discipline to question the nature of theory and the value of objectivist prescriptions for practice theory, and to attempt to articulate a clearer concept of nursing practice.

METALANGUAGE OF NURSING CONCEPTUAL FRAMEWORKS

Central concepts, or shared images, can be described when the conceptual frameworks listed in Table 2-1 are grouped around common themes. Four concepts have been widely recognized as common to nursing's conceptual frameworks: nursing, the person, society and environment, and health. We have chosen the term *metalanguage,* rather than *metaparadigm,* to refer to these concepts. Although these four elements have been termed nursing's metaparadigm (Fawcett, 2004), our definition and use of the term *paradigm* is inconsistent with this terminology. The prefix "meta" means that which is encompassing or transcending. Thus, metalanguage is language that is used to describe or analyze (include or encompass) another language or system of symbols (*Encarta World English Dictionary,* 1999). The following sections provide a view of these four metalanguage concepts in early conceptual frameworks. Again, we consider only the first major publication of nurse theorists as dated in Table 2-1 in this analysis. It also merits mention that other early concepts of nursing that are not generally categorized as conceptual frameworks share this metalanguage.

Nursing

In nursing's theoretic writings, nursing generally is represented as a helping process with a primary focus on interpersonal interactions between a nurse and another individual. This general idea does not clearly distinguish nursing from other helping disciplines, but it provides an important focus for deciding what kind of knowledge is needed in nursing practice. The interpersonal nature of nursing practice distinguishes nursing from medicine, in that medicine focuses on surgical and pharmacologic interventions, with interpersonal interactions secondary to these interventions. Within a medical model of nursing, the nurse's primary functions relate to medical assessment, diagnosis and treatment, and medication administration as delegated medical tasks. Within a nursing framework, when interpersonal interactions are primary, technical and medical functions support the primary interpersonal interactions.

Although different nurse authors present conceptualizations of the nature of nursing that are consistent with the idea of interpersonal interactions as a primary focus, there are important differences in their definitions and conceptualizations. For some, the direction of the interaction and the specific actions that are taken in achieving the goals of the interaction are largely defined by the person with whom the nurse interacts. The nurse's role in the interaction primarily is one of facilitating. When this view of the nature of nursing is incorporated into a framework or model, nursing is viewed as enabling the will and behavior of the person receiving care.

Other theoretic models present a view of the interpersonal process as either shared or initiated by the nurse. In this view, nursing processes and actions rest primarily on the nurse's initiative, knowledge, and approaches.

The theoretic ideas that emerge from this view focus on nursing actions to reach the goal of the interaction.

Each of these perspectives is consistent with the practice of nursing in that nurses encounter some situations in which the patient primarily directs the interaction and other situations in which the nurse is the initiator, and some conceptual frameworks account for this diversity. The common significant thread is the primacy of human interaction in creating human health and wholeness. Table 2-2 describes the concept of nursing as reflected in the work of several nurse theorists.

TABLE 2-2 Theoretic Ideas About Nursing

Author	Concepts of Nursing
Hildegard E. Peplau (1952)	Nursing is a significant therapeutic interpersonal process. The interpersonal process is a maturing force and educative instrument for both nurse and patient. Self-knowledge in the context of the interpersonal interaction is essential to understanding the patient and reaching resolution of the problem. There are four sequential phases of the interpersonal process: (1) orientation, (2) identification, (3) exploitation, and (4) resolution.
Ida Jean Orlando (1961)	Nursing is a process of interaction with an ill individual to meet an immediate need. The nursing situation consists of (1) the person's behavior, (2) the nurse's reaction, and (3) nursing action appropriate to the person's need. The nurse is accountable to the individual receiving care.
Ernestine Wiedenbach (1964)	There are three components of nursing: (1) identification of a person's need for help, (2) ministration of the help needed, and (3) validation that the help provided was indeed helpful. The nursing process begins with an activating situation that arouses the nurse's consciousness. Clinical nursing has four components: philosophy, purpose, practice, and art.
Myra E. Levine (1967)	Nursing care is both supportive and therapeutic. Supportive interventions are designed to maintain a state of wholeness as consistently as possible with failing adaptation. Therapeutic interventions are designed to promote adaptation that contributes to health and restoration of health. All nursing actions are based on conservation of energy and structural, personal, and social integrity.
Jean Watson (1979)	Nursing is a human science and an art that is based on the moral ideal and value of caring. There are 10 carative factors that constitute the knowledge and practice of human-care nursing. The context of nursing is humanitarian and metaphysical; the goal of nursing is to gain a higher degree of harmony in mind, body, and soul, which leads to self-knowledge, self-reverence, self-healing, and self-care.

The Person

All conceptual frameworks include ideas about the general nature of human beings. The most consistent philosophic component of the idea of the person is the dimension of wholeness, or wholism. Although various conceptual frameworks may view the ill or diseased person as having problems with need fulfillment, integration, adaptation, role fulfillment, and so forth, the central impediment to health or healing is dealt with wholistically in various senses of the word.

The nature of wholism as a concept is difficult to address from the perspective of traditional Western philosophies that are grounded in reductionism. In the reductionist view of wholism, the whole is equal to the sum of the parts; interrelationships among parts are understood, and generalizations can be made about the whole (Newman, 1979). Western culture embraces this view, and nurses, like others in this culture, have learned to think about parts of lives, parts of bodies, and parts of human experiences.

In a purer sense more consistent with Eastern traditions, wholism means that the whole is greater than the sum of the parts. The whole cannot be reduced to parts without losing something in the process. Martha Rogers, Margaret Newman, Joyce Travelbee, and Patricia Benner are examples of nurse scholars whose work reflects a view that the individual is different from and greater than the sum of the parts. Other nursing theorists explicitly or implicitly hold that wholism is equal to the sum of parts, assuming the individual is a system with biologic, sociologic, and psychologic components. Although not consistent with wholism in its purest sense, there still is a strong commitment to the idea that all components of the individual need to be considered. Table 2-3 describes the concept of a person as reflected in the work of several nurse theorists.

Society and Environment

The concept of society and environment is central to the discipline of nursing and is reflected across conceptual frameworks, although these concepts are not addressed as explicitly in some writings as in others. Several nursing frameworks include a concept of society or culture and present these concepts as critical interacting forces that shape the individual (Table 2-4). Environment was central for Nightingale in formulating her concept of nursing. Nightingale believed the primary focus for nursing was to alter the physical environment to place the human body in the best possible condition for the reparative processes of nature to occur. More recent conceptual frameworks deemphasize environment or view it as encompassed within a concept of society, sometimes using the word *society*

TABLE 2-3   Theoretic Ideas About the Person

Author	Concepts of Person
Madeleine Leininger (1978)	Individuals and groups who require culturally sensitive care to improve human conditions.
Virginia Henderson (1966)	Mind and body are inseparable. No two individuals are alike; each is unique. The individual's basic needs are reflected in 14 components of basic nursing care.
Martha Rogers (1970)	Unitary human being is viewed as an energy field, the boundaries of which extend beyond the discernible mass of the human body. There are five unifying assumptions about the life process: (1) unified wholeness, (2) openness, (3) unidirectionality, (4) pattern and organization, and (5) sentience.
Dorothea E. Orem (1971)	The individual is an integrated whole composed of an internal physical, psychologic, and social nature with varying degrees of self-care ability.
Imogene M. King (1971)	Individuals are viewed as (1) reacting beings, (2) time-oriented beings, and (3) social beings, with the ability to perceive, think, feel, choose, set goals, and make decisions.
Patricia Benner and Judith Wrubel (1989)	The person is a self-interpreting being engaged in the world. Engagement is possible because of the human capacities of embodied intelligence, culturally acquired meanings, concern, and direct involvement in or grasp of a situation.

to include environment. However, the concept of environment remains a significant one. Martha Rogers and theorists who build on her ideas focus on a concept of environment as indistinguishable (except conceptually) from the concept of person. Most other conceptual frameworks separate person from environment, implying boundaries that separate the two. As with the concept of person, environmental concepts vary, but they appear across conceptual frameworks.

Health

The concept of health typically is identified as the goal of nursing. Nightingale stated that "the same laws of health or of nursing, for in reality they are the same, obtain among the well as among the sick" (1969, p. 9), implying health as a state of order within natural laws. Contemporary nursing models are remarkably congruent with this early conceptualization. Some frameworks are based on a conceptualization of a health-illness continuum, with the purpose of nursing to assist the ill patient to achieve the greatest possible

TABLE 2-4 Theoretic Ideas About Society and Environment

Author	Concepts of Society and Environment
Florence Nightingale (1969)	Environment is the central concept. It is viewed as all external conditions and influences that affect life and the development of the organism. The major emphasis is on warmth, effluvia (odors), noise, and light.
Joyce Travelbee (1966)	Environment is the context in which human-to-human relatedness or rapport is established.
Myra E. Levine (1967)	Society is viewed as the total environment of the individual, including family, significant others, and the nurse.
Callista Roy (1976)	Environment constantly interacts with the individual and determines, in part, adaptation level. Stimuli originate in the environment.
Dorothy Johnson (1980)	Environment is a source of factors that impinge upon and disturb the person's behavioral system.
Margaret A. Newman (1986)	Environment and person form a unitary pattern that is reflected in movement-space-time patterns of consciousness. Environment encompasses the total situation and is one with the person; environment includes the universe.

degree of health. Other nurse authors view the concept of health as something more than, or different from, the absence of disease. Health exists independently from illness or disease. In these views, it is a dynamic process that changes with time and varies with life circumstances. Some authors view the health process as interdependent with circumstances of the environment, whereas others view the health process as something that originates with the individual (Smith, 1983).

In an attempt to deal more specifically with ideas related to health, several nurse authors avoid using the terms *health* and *illness*. An example is Myra Levine's (1967) use of the term *conserving wholism*. This concept directs nurses to focus on the totality of a person's situation rather than on the typical parameters that have come to be commonly known as health. Table 2-5 identifies some of the terms that nurses have used in constructing their theoretic ideas about health. These terms suggest ideas that more specifically reflect nursing's concerns and deemphasize the focus on disease or illness.

THE DEVELOPMENT OF MIDDLE-RANGE PRACTICE-LINKED THEORY

During the 1980s, Meleis (1987) brought into clear focus the need for nurses to develop substantive theory that provides a meaningful foundation for the

TABLE 2-5 Theoretic Ideas About Health

Author	Terms Related to Health
Faye G. Abdellah, Irene L. Beland, Almeda Martin, and Ruth V. Matheney (1960)	Freedom from problems requiring nursing
Lydia E. Hall (1966)	Self-actualization, self-love
Virginia Henderson (1966)	Independent function
Myra E. Levine (1967)	Maintaining wholism/conservation
Josephine G. Paterson and Loretta T. Zderad (1976)	Authentic awareness
Betty Neuman (1980)	System stability
Rosemarie Parse (1981)	Open process of becoming
Nola Pender (1982)	Health resulting from health-promoting behavior

development of nursing practice in relation to specific practice concepts. In accord with the observation of many practicing nurses, Meleis acknowledged the value of broad-scope theories in defining general parameters on which nursing function is based but emphasized that theory of a different type was required to give more specific guidance for nursing practice, a form of theory that, it turns out, would more closely align with the scientific-empiric pattern of knowing and knowledge. Meleis' plea also reflected the need for nursing to move away from its long-term discussions and debates about the nature of theory, knowledge, and the proper functions of nursing. She called on nurses to focus on developing substance in theory—that is, a focus on substantive, more readily observable nursing concepts grounded in a practice context. Nursing theory of this type is developed in concert with research questions

TABLE 2-6 Researcher/Theorists and Focal Concepts in Selected Substantive Middle-Range Theories

Nurse Researcher	Substantive Theoretical Focus
Merle Mischel	Uncertainty
Afaf Meleis	Transitions
Cheryl Beck	Post-partum depression
Jean Johnson	Preoperative preparation
Kathryn Barnard	Infant-caregiver interaction
Katherine Kolcaba	Comfort
Ramona Mercer	Maternal role attainment
Kristin Swanson	Caring
Pamela Reed	Self transcendence

directly or indirectly linked to important practice issues. It avoids a focus on methodology for methodology's sake and shifts the focus to understanding nursing-related phenomena. Substantive middle-range theory can inform practice and lead to new practice approaches as well as investigate factors that influence the outcomes desired in nursing practice.

Im and Meleis (1999) introduced the idea of situation-specific theory. Situation-specific theory is a variant of middle-range theory that underscores the importance of considering the context in which theory will be utilized. Whereas middle-range theory narrows the conceptual focus of a theory, and substantive middle-range theory further defines the focus as clinically relevant concepts, situation-specific theory emphasizes the need to consider the unique context for which the theory is developed. Situation specificity is important because of variability within particular populations, fields of practice, and subsequent approaches to clinical phenomena. Unlike substantive middle-range theory, which is presumed to be more broadly generalizable across different populations, situation-specific theory addresses the particular and unique needs of a group of people in a specific context.

Substantive middle-range theory in nursing tends to cluster around a concept of interest, such as social support, uncertainty, grief, fatigue, or life transitions. Some examples of nurse researchers who have developed substantive middle-range theory are listed in Table 2-6. Several recent publications specifically focus on middle-range theory in nursing (Liehr & Smith, 1999; Peterson, 2007; Peterson & Bredow, 2003; Smith & Liehr, 2003).

TRENDS IN KNOWLEDGE DEVELOPMENT

What counts as knowledge does not remain static. Knowledge historically reflects the social, political, and professional climate in which knowledge development occurs. The context within which knowledge is developed determines and influences what counts as knowledge and how knowledge structures are valued and evaluated. After Carper (1978) first published her work on the knowing patterns and for several years thereafter, knowledge forms and development processes other than those associated with empirics were seen to be important to nursing and became more generally accepted. The adherence to a specific methodology or template for knowledge development is being replaced with a requirement for rigor and disclosure of methodology, versus following a formula "no matter what." Even though many knowledge developers in nursing remain firmly rooted in the assumptions and methodologies of empirics, knowledge structures are emerging that are not empiric in the sense that strict interpretation of the pattern of empirics assumes. These structures, although communicated and structured in language, are not grounded in objectivist assumptions and scientific notions of reliability and validity. It is possible to conceptualize empiric knowledge broadly, as we do, to include forms of interpretive work that culminate in the identification of themes (phenomenology) or detailed descriptions (ethnographies) as falling within the empiric pattern. However, some emerging knowledge forms and methods rest on different assumptions and methodologies and fall outside the realm of empirics. Several important trends in theory development and utilization are described in the following sections.

The Move from Methodolotry

Currently there is a trend to blend and use a variety of knowledge development processes to achieve a given research aim rather than adhering to strict methodologic imperatives. Many scholars are moving from a focus on method and technique to a focus on problem solution or achievement of study aims. As the methodologic process is tailored to accomplish the research objectives, various approaches to inquiry are modified and blended. The qualitative/quantitative dichotomy is being questioned as a way to categorize methodologic approaches. There is growing recognition that qualitative data may be important to obtain in primarily experimental designs and, conversely, that quantitative data may be useful in naturalistic inquiry. Rather than combining approaches (doing both a quantitative and qualitative study), the purpose of the research determines how findings are blended. Critical multiplism (Letourneau & Allen, 1999) and multivocality (Savage, 2000) are examples of terms used to denote these kinds of methods. This trend signals a maturity in nursing scholarship, wherein professional research purposes take precedence over methodologic loyalties.

Interpretive and Critical Approaches

In a classic article, Allen, Benner, and Diekelman (1986) suggested the following three categories for classification of research: empiric-analytic, interpretive-hermeneutic, and critical-social. Empiric-analytic work conforms to the traditions of empirics as conceptualized by Carper, meaning that the work relies on perceptually grounded and objective replication and validation research methods. Some forms of interpretive work remain faithful to this traditional objectivist assumption, but some forms of interpretive work fall outside the realm of traditional objectivist empirics. Interpretive approaches, such as grounded theory, phenomenology, analyses of language or discourse, and hermeneutic inquiry, assess truth value (reliability and validity) by consensus between the researcher and the participants. The assumption of an objective reality with meaning independent of the observer is not taken as a given. Grounded theory approaches, now applied in a variety of forms, are constructed out of shared understandings between researcher and participants (Crotty, 1998). Methodologies grounded in the philosophy of phenomenology seek to account for the nature of the experience from the experiencer's point of view. Even though they may be judged as "good" or "less than good" accounts, they clearly do not rest on objectivist assumptions about the existence and nature of a reality independent of the observer. As in empirics, however, their conclusions are drawn from interpretations that are fundamentally grounded in sensory perceptions, whereas truth value, or reliability and validity, rely on a consensus of meaning that is particular and situated. Noncritical forms of hermeneutic inquiry recognize context to be important in shaping knowledge. The researcher moves back and forth between what is being interpreted and an ever-enlarging context that accounts for the researcher's unique perspective within the situation to create a reasonable (loosely valid) understanding.

Critical approaches seek to illuminate structures of domination and in nursing are addressing health care structures that compromise the quality of care for people based on factors such as class, economics, race, age, gender, disability, or sexual orientation (Cowling & Chinn, 2001; Kramer, 2002; Maeve, 1999; Stevens, 1989; Thompson, 1987). Critical social theory is not theory in the sense of empiric theory, with the latter's focus on objectivity of observation that allows for a degree of generalizable description, explanation, and prediction. The primary purpose of critical theory is to create social and political change. Critical theory takes the form of narrative analyses that illuminate how social practices institutionalized in political or educational institutions, as examples, enable unjust practices for the benefit of a dominant group. Critical theory may have several foci. Critical feminist theory centers on issues of gender discrimination. Critical social theory focuses on class issues as they perpetuate unfair educational, political, and other social practices. The "critical" focus points to a need to undo and remake oppressive social structures.

Poststructuralist Approaches

Research consistent with the analytic methodology of poststructuralism are appearing with greater frequency within the nursing literature (Allen & Hardin, 2001; Arslanian-Engoren, 2002; Cloyes, 2006; Francis, 2000). Poststructuralism is an outgrowth of structuralism, terms originating in linguistics. Structuralism is the view that the meaning of words is given by context or the linguistic frame surrounding the word. The single word "duck," for example, has no stable referent, and whether this utterance is referring to a type of bird or is a directive to avoid hitting a low-hanging tree branch cannot be known without encountering the word in context. The poststructuralist movement moves language away from a representational view. That is, words do not "stand for" something that is either given objectively (as traditional forms of empirics assume) or known from a context of usage. Rather, language, or more broadly discourse, creates and determines possibilities. Discourses are whole systems of representations that include text, visuals, and behavioral actions surrounding, associated with, referencing, and/or creating experiences and understandings. Critical analyses that use language and systems of discourse as data uncover how language functions to perpetuate networks of oppression and domination add important new dimensions to nursing knowledge.

Deconstruction and Postmodernism

Deconstruction is a term that is elusive to define but generally means processes that take apart assumptions, ideologies, and frames of reference that are unnoticed yet buried in text. *Text* refers to what is written as well as other visual representations of situations and events such as advertisements, cartoons, and film. Often, deconstructive work focuses on text that is problematic in relation to sustaining inequities that disadvantage one group for the benefit of another. Yet, deconstruction is much more than analysis, even critical analysis. Deconstruction involves making explicit and coming to understand that features of text (e.g., implicit assumptions, ideologies, and frames of reference) cannot be warranted as a basis for truths. In this way, deconstruction is useful to undermine language and social contexts that promote inequities and injustices.

Postmodernism, on the other hand, is a term with broader meaning, but, like deconstruction, it has a variety of unclear meanings and usages. In a general sense, the postmodern is the era that followed the modern era. Modernism, as it relates to science, began with a move to account for natural phenomena using scientific approaches rather than an appeal to religious and metaphysical explanations. Thus, modernism signaled the end to religious authority as the basis for understanding the world. Modernism has become associated with the age of science and scientific inquiry. As discoveries in modern physics began to uncover the fallibility of scientific explanation, coupled with a failed social agenda of science, the move toward postmodernism was enabled. Postmodernism in relation to methods of inquiry is reflected in increasing use of nonscientific methodologies as well as the combining of multiple methods within a single research project. The reference to "anything goes" often is coupled with references to postmodernism. Although "anything goes" is reasonable in one sense, any notion of arbitrariness or relativism is unwarranted. The postmodern era has loosened the idea of what counts as legitimate knowledge, but it should not signal that sloppy approaches to knowledge development are acceptable. Even though various methods may be legitimate, they must be carried out carefully and rigorously to be useful.

Evidence-Based Practice

During the 1990s the idea of evidence-based nursing practice began to receive attention in the nursing literature. The idea of evidence-based practice originated in the medical literature and incorporated a variety of empiric and nonempiric knowledge forms that counted as evidence (Mazurek-Melnyk, Stone, Fincout-Overholt, & Ackerman, 2000). Evidence-based nursing practice focuses on the necessity to integrate quality research in practice decisions for clinical expertise that subsequently leads to high-level care. It is important to note that evidence-based nursing is not the application of single studies or even meta-analysis information in client care. Rather, evidence-based practice requires the integration of information about best research evidence, health care resources, clinical setting, state, and circumstances with patient preferences (DiCenso, Guyatt, & Ciliska, 2005). Models of research evidence are consistent with a hierarchy of evidences that generally accords randomized clinical trials and meta-analyses of randomized clinical trials as having the highest truth value. While counting as evidence, case analyses and qualitative studies have less credibility (Center for Evidence Based Medicine, 2006; Schunemann, Best, Vist, & Oxman, 2003). The nature of evidence-based nursing practice continues to evolve. We favor an approach that defines evidence-based practice as the integration of best research evidence with clinical expertise and patient values (DiCenso et al., 2005, p. 4). To characterize best research evidence as a highly empiric form of knowledge that evolves from data-based, experimental, and quasi-experimental research methodologies (Mowinski-Jennings & Loan, 2001; Rambur, 1999) has received criticism (Fullbrook, 2003; Holmes, Perron, & O'Byrne, 2006) and reflects the persistent predominance of empirics as a way of knowing in nursing. Models of evidence-based clinical decision making such as that proposed by DiCenso, Guyatt, and Ciliska (2005) require knowing in all knowing patterns. Empirics is well represented, to be sure, but the interpretation of patient preferences and actions, as well as the clinical circumstances in which clinical expertise occurs (DiCenso et al., 2005) requires aesthetic, ethical, and personal knowing. Understanding the politics of health care resources in relation to availability and client usage is grounded in emancipatory knowing. In short, clinical expertise, the core of the DiCenso, Guyatt, and Ciliska model, aligns well with the integration of all patterns of knowing.

Practice-Based Evidence and Translational Research

Two additional trends include a focus on practice-based evidence and translational research. References to practice-based evidence in the health care literature refers to the validation in practice of clinically used approaches and techniques known to be effective in promoting health-related goals. The call for practice-based evidence emphasizes a focus on investigating and validating what seems to be effective in practice as a way to generate research evidence for integration into evidence-based decision making (Fox, 2003, Margison et al., 2000; Simons, Kushner, Jones, & James, 2003). Proponents of practice-based evidence suggest that the top-down approach (research to practice) currently valued in hierarchies of research evidence use methodologies to generate outcomes that may not be workable in the practice arena. For example, randomized clinical trials—taken to be highly valuable sources of empirical evidence—control for variables that are operating in the clinical environment. Proponents of practice-based evidence suggest that the stripping away of situational variables and control necessary for many experimental studies produces a knowledge structure that is too decontextualized to be useful and will not be used to guide practice. Rather, evidence must be generated out of, or situated in, the context from which it is generated in order to be useful to practitioners (Simons et al., 2003).

Translational research, on the other hand, reflects on a more "research to practice" approach. Translational research initiatives are now part of the United States National Institutes of Health roadmap. Interest in promoting translational research has been prominent in clinical practices where there is interest in moving basic research studies into practice as quickly as possible (NIH Roadmap for Clinical Research, http://nihroadmap.nih.gov/clinical-research/overview-translational.asp). Simply stated, translational research is designed to take evidence a step further by validating it in the practice setting. Thus, translational research promotes the utilization of research discoveries in clinical settings.

In summary, the grip of traditional empirics in nursing seems to be moderating, perhaps signaling a return to our history of wholism in knowing and knowledge development. During the 1960s a scientific metatheory dominated the literature, but never really took hold. Gradually nursing moved from a metatheoretical focus on empirics as expressed in objectivist research approaches that are descriptive, correlational, quasi-experimental, or experimental. Naturalistic and qualitative approaches to practice began to appear with greater frequency in the 1980s. More recently, the importance of language for determining what counts as knowledge is being recognized, and critical research that undermines unjust and inequitable social conditions is being conducted. Ongoing emphases on evidence-based nursing practice that require integration of broad forms of knowledge formally acknowledge that empirical evidence is only part of what it takes to make good clinical decisions. A focus on practice evidence and translational research reemphasizes moving evidence into practice in a way that benefits the patient/client.

THE CONTEXTS OF KNOWLEDGE DEVELOPMENT

As illustrated in this chapter, specific circumstances and contexts affect the development of knowledge. What knowledge is, the sources of best knowledge, and how nurses use and construct knowledge is greatly influenced, if not determined, by the interrelationship between values and resources at multiple levels. These levels can be categorized as individual, professional, and societal. Table 2-7 identifies some of the values and resources that have influenced and continue to influence the development of knowledge in nursing. As you review the table, identify additional values and resources and reflect on how you see your own circumstances. Some questions are provided to help you understand the table and its meaning, but we are confident that you can think of many more examples to illustrate how the interrelationship of values and resources affects knowledge in nursing.

Values

Individual values include an individual nurse's commitment, personal philosophy, motives, beliefs, and priorities. Think about what sorts of research approaches you might find more valuable than others, and even whether you believe research is an important area to study. If you value research, what is your motive for learning about it? A 9-to-5 job in an academic setting? Making a difference in people's lives? Both? Is uncovering research evidence something you attend to because you have to? Want to? Something you do after you have practiced technical skills?

Professional values are beliefs and attitudes about what is good and right that generally are held in common by members of the profession and are used to guide professional action. They are expressed in formal statements issued by professional groups in the form of codes, standards of practice, and ethical

TABLE 2-7 Values and Resources That Influence Theory Development

Source of Influence	Examples of Specific Factors
Values	
Individual	Commitment to the discipline
	Philosophy of nursing
	Motives
	Worldview or philosophy of life
	Priorities for action
Professional	Commitment to development of knowledge
	Code of ethics
	Standards for practice
	Standards for protecting research participants
	Willingness to challenge social traditions
	Priorities for allocating resources
Society	Cultural mores and sanction
	Ethical codes
	Normative values
	Priorities for allocating resources
Resources	
Individual	Cognitive style
	Intellectual ability
	Personality
	Lifestyle and setting
	Educational background
	Life experience
	Economic power and wealth
Professional	Educational requirements for members
	Body of literature and communication style
	Methodologies and instrumentation
	Practice traditions
	Educational, economic, and political group profile
	Settings for practice, education, and research
	Funding for the discipline's activities
	Material resources
Society	Settings for practice, education, and research
	Funding for the discipline's activities
	Material resources
	Support for other cultures and societies

principles and also are reflected in repeated themes that occur in the literature and in the collective actions taken by professional organizations. The current interest in development of the professional doctorate and the move toward evidence-based nursing practice reflect professional values that are being expressed today. How has the professional valuing of evidence-based practice, for example, influenced your learning? The practice of nurses you come in contact with? Has the move toward the professional doctorate energized your thinking about pursuing such education?

Societal values are expressed through societal choices, sanctions, and moral behavior during a given period in history. The focus on national and international security in the wake of terrorist activities and the use of monetary resources to promote security reflects its value for society. Has the valuing of national security affected financial resources available to you as a student? How have societal values affected the faculty's ability to compete for grant funding? Determined what you focus a research proposal for funding on? Has the valuing of capitalism, corporate structures, and the consolidation of hospital services into large entities changed your and others' ability to enact evidence-based clinical decision making?

Resources

Resources also can also be viewed as individual, professional, and societal. Individual resources include the natural and acquired talents shared among members of the discipline, including cognitive style, intellectual abilities, life circumstances, and educational preparation. The nature of your educational preparation—what you are exposed to and learn as a student—is a resource you will bring to nursing. Will an ability to think in a linear fashion mean you will bring expertise in quantitative methods to the profession? Might the gift of a nonlinear cognitive style signal your contribution to aesthetic knowing and practice? What talents will you share that evolve from those life experiences and interests that are unique to you? Did you grow up in another country and thus can contribute a unique understanding of how to effectively study the health care needs of your country's citizens? How might the financial and other resources you have to support additional education determine the resources you bring to nursing?

Professional resources reflect the collective resources of the discipline for knowledge development. Examples of professional resources include a growing body of literature and practice traditions, the ability to communicate these among members of the profession, the educational attainments of members of the profession, and the nature of their education, as well as methodologies and instrumentation available for knowledge development. That is, what you bring to nursing and develop as a practitioner added to the contributions of hosts of other nurses will constitute nursing's professional resources. As practitioners and students are exposed to the techniques and meanings of evidence-based practice (which is likely the case), will knowledge resources of the discipline change? Might you and others embrace critical theory or the tenets of practice-based evidence as a way to better integrate research into clinical decisions? If you are interested in knowledge development related to aesthetic knowing, are there professional resources to assist you in learning how to do this? Do available information systems ease or deter the retrieval of evidence to be integrated into clinical decision making? Has nursing made use of the Internet in such a way that it is a valuable resource for care? Are there professional practice traditions you must obey that you think are counterproductive? Will nursing pay enough to sustain a reasonably comfortable lifestyle? Will nursing services where you work have the political clout to advocate for improved client and patient care?

Societal resources affect the nature of material and nonmaterial resources available to support knowledge development in nursing. Acquisition of societal resources depends on features of both society and the profession. For example, political influence is required to obtain funds, materials, and space to carry out the activities of the discipline. If the political system of society reflects priorities other than those that concern nursing, societal resources are less available to nursing than to other groups that reflect those priorities. How, for example, has the societal interest in national and international security affected resource allocation for nursing in your practice area? If you are a student, what trends are affecting your financial aid possibilities? Have you or someone you know been relocated out of your space or lost your job because of special funding initiatives? How successful will nursing be in securing resources to develop a broad conceptualization of knowing if scientific knowledge still is largely held to be most valuable? Has the tax base available for health care been deflected into other arenas, changing the way you counsel an elderly person about how to obtain prescription medications?

The relationships between and among values and resources are intertwined, and in some cases it is difficult to determine how a given factor affecting knowledge development should be categorized. Categorization is never the goal—rather, what is important is understanding how factors in a broad array of contexts interrelate to determine health care needs, how those needs are approached, and who provides care.

In addition, when individual, professional, and societal values are basically congruent, there is relative stability, and new insights tend to build on what already is established as knowledge in the discipline. When individual, professional, or societal values change, the potential exists for creating fundamental change in knowledge and practice. For example, political decisions made by government entities require value decisions about who does and does not deserve the resources of society. If, as the course of history shows, women scientists are consistently provided limited or no societal resources, the ability of women to influence value decisions about how money should be allocated is lessened. The fact that nursing is a group composed mostly of women (a professional resource) within a societal context that devalues women scientists influences the profession's ability to exert influence on society to gain access to resources. The contemporary women's movement has created a stimulus for recognizing societal restrictions on nursing as a sex-segregated occupation and the effects of systematic oppression on nurses and nursing (Group & Roberts, 2001; Roberts, 1983). Feminist theory, which shares many of the traits of nursing theory, provides a perspective for changing social values and shifting social resources. Feminism places on society an urgent demand for a values transformation that is consistent with nursing's vision of health, the health care system, and nursing (Chinn & Wheeler, 1985; Roberts & Group, 1995). As women's experience is increasingly valued as a resource for developing knowledge, the resulting values conflict with traditional views and the new values will open avenues for change.

REFLECTION AND DISCUSSION

In this chapter, we surveyed the history from which our nursing knowledge has evolved and outlined current trends in knowledge development. Values and resources that influence knowledge development and determine the nature of knowledge in nursing were outlined. The centrally important message of this chapter is: An understanding of nursing's history and current state with regard to knowledge development is critically important. Without an understanding of where we have been, we run the risk of repeating mistakes that impede knowledge development. Linking events of today with our history helps the profession shape knowledge development in ways that will promote high-level nursing care.

To deepen your appreciation of history, consider the following questions related to the content of this chapter:

1. Do early writings of nurses in relation to a nursing situation you are experiencing offer a perspective that you had not considered? Was it useful or not?
2. How are Nightingale's *Notes on Nursing* helpful, or not, in relation to contemporary problems in nursing?
3. How are some of the events, trends, and issues alive in nursing today related to, or dependent on, past events?
4. What "mistakes" do you think we are making today with regard to knowledge development, and how will they affect future nursing

care? What current events and trends are definitely "not mistakes" in relation to knowledge development, and why?

5. If you could, how would you change nursing's values and resources to promote knowledge development?

6. How will historians writing in the year 2060 characterize nursing during the first few years of the 21st century? What will history remember us for, and why will we be proud of that history?

Reference List

Abdellah, F. G. (1969). The nature of nursing science. *Nursing Research, 18*(5), 390–393.

Abdellah, F. G., Beland, I., Martin, A., & Matheney, R. V. (1960). *Patient-centered approacher to nursing.* New York: Macmillan.

Achterberg, J. (1991). *Woman as healer.* Boston: Shambhala.

Aikins, C. A. (1915). Teaching ethics in hospital schools. *Trained Nurse and Hospital Review, 54,* 135–137.

Allen, D., Benner, P., & Diekelman, N. Three paradigms for nursing research: Methodological implications. In P. L. Chinn (Ed.), *Nursing research methodology: Issues and implementation* (pp. 23–28) Rockville, MD: Aspen.

Allen, D., & Hardin, P. K. (2001). Discourse analysis and the epidemiology of meaning. *Nursing Philosophy, 2*(2), 163–176.

Arslanian-Engoren, C. (2002). Feminist poststructuralism: A methodological paradigm for examining clinical decision-making. *Journal of Advanced Nursing, 37*(6), 512–517.

Ashley, J. (1976). *Hospitals, paternalism, and the role of the nurse.* New York: Teachers College Press.

Barnum, B. J. S. (1998). *Nursing theory* (5th ed.). Boston: Lippincott-Raven.

Benner, P. A., & Wrubel, J. (1989). *The primacy of caring: Stress and coping in health and illness.* Menlo Park, CA: Addison-Wesley.

Bixler, G. K., Bixler, R. W. (1945). The professional status of nursing. *American Journal of Nursing, 45*(9), 730–735.

Brigh, S. M. (1944). We cannot afford to hurry: Training within industry applied to nursing. *American Journal of Nursing, 44*(3), 223–226.

Burgess, M. E. (1941). A plan for nursing care. *American Journal of Nursing, 41*(2), 215–218.

Carper, B. A. (1978). Fundamental patterns of knowing in nursing. *ANS. Advances in Nursing Science, 1*(1), 13–23.

Center for Evidence Based Medicine. (2006). *Levels of evidence and grades of recommendation.* Retrieved September 2006 from www.cebm.net/levels_of_evidence.asp.

Changes in nursing practice. (1947). *American Journal of Nursing, 47*(10), 665.

Chinn, P. L., Wheeler, C. E. (1985). Feminism and nursing. *Nursing Outlook, 33*(2), 74–77.

Christy, T. E. (1969). Portrait of a leader. *Nursing Outlook, 6*(6), 72–75.

Cloyes, K. G. (2006). An ethic of analysis: An argument for critical analysis of research interviews as an ethical practice. *ANS. Advances in Nursing Science, 29*(2), 84–97.

Cohen, I. B. (1984). Florence Nightingale. *Scientific American, 250*(3), 128–137.

Conrad, M. E. (1947). What is expert nursing care? *American Journal of Nursing, 47*(3), 655.

Cowling, W. R., & Chinn, P. L. (2001). Conversation across paradigms: Unitary-transformative and critical feminist perspectives. *Scholarly Inquiry for Nursing Practice, 15*(4), 347–365.

Crotty, M. (1998). *The foundations of social research: Meaning and perspective in the research process.* London: Sage.

De Witt, K. (1901). Specialties in nursing. *American Journal of Nursing, 1,* 14–15.

Dennis, K. E., & Prescott, P. A. (1985). Florence Nightingale: Yesterday, today, and tomorrow. *ANS. Advances in Nursing Science, 7*(2), 66–81.

DiCenso, A., Guyatt, G., Ciliska, D. (2005). *Evidence based nursing: A guide to clinical practice.* St. Louis: Mosby.

Dickoff, J., & James, P. (1968). A theory of theories: A position paper. *Nursing Research, 17*(3), 197–203.

Dickoff, J., & James, P. (1971). Clarity to what end? *Nursing Research, 20*(6), 499–502.

Dickoff, J., James, P., & Wiedenbach, E. (1968). Theory in a practice discipline. Part 1: Practice-oriented theory. *Nursing Research, 17*(5), 415–435.

Dock, L. L. (1902–1903). Sanitary inspection: A new field for nurses. *American Journal of Nursing, 3,* 529–532.

Donahue, P. M. (1995). *Nursing, the finest art: An illustrated history* (2nd ed.). St. Louis: Mosby.

Dossey, B. M. (1999). *Florence Nightingale: Mystic, visionary, healer.* Philadelphia: Lippincott Williams & Wilkins.

Drake, A. (1934). How the patient judges nursing. *Trained Nurse and Hospital Review, 93,* 135–138.

Ehrenreich, B., & English, D. (1983). *Witches, midwives and nurses: A history of women healers.* New York: Feminist Press.

Ellis, R. (1968). Characteristics of significant theories. *Nursing Research, 17*(3), 217–222.

Ellis, R. (1971). Commentary on "Toward a clearer understanding of the concept of nursing theory." *Nursing Research, 20*493.

Encarta World English Dictionary. (1999). Microsoft Corporation. Avaliable at http://encarta.msn.com.

Faber, M. J. (1927). The education of the self. *American Journal of Nursing, 27*(12), 1047–1050.

Fawcett, J. (2004). *Contemporary nursing knowledge: Analysis and evaluation of nursing models and theories.* Philadelphia: FA Davis.

Folta, J. R. (1971). Obfuscation or clarification: A reaction to Walker's concept of nursing theory. *Nursing Research, 20*(6), 196–199.

Fox, N. J. (2003). Practice-based evidence: Toward collaborative and transgressive research. *Sociology, 37*(1), 81–102.

Francis, B. (2000). Poststructuralism and nursing: Uncomfortable bedfellows? *Nursing Inquiry, 7*(1), 20–28.

Fullbrook, P. (2003). Developing best practice in critical care nursing: Knowledge, evidence and practice. *Nursing in Critical Care, 8*(3), 96–102.

Garesche, E. F. (1927). Professional honor. *American Journal of Nursing, 27*(11), 901–904.

Geister, J. M. (1937). Strength at the roots. *Trained Nurse and Hospital Review, 37*(9), 260–263.

Goostray, S., & Brown, E. L. (1954). American nursing: History and interpretation. *American Journal of Nursing, 54*(6), 719–721.

Gregg, A. (1940). An independent estimate of nursing in our times. *American Journal of Nursing, 40*(7), 735–737.

Group, T. M., & Roberts, J. I. (2001). *Nursing, physician control and the medical monopoly.* Westport, CT: Praeger.

Hall, L. E. (1964). Nursing: What is it? *The Canadian Nurse, 60*(2), 150–154.

Hall, L. E. (1966). Another view of nursing care and quality. In K. M. Straub & K. S. Parker (Eds.), *Continuity in patient care: The role of nursing.* Washington, DC: Catholic University Press.

Hardy, M. E. (1978). Perspectives on nursing theory. *ANS. Advances in Nursing Science, 1*(1), 37–48.

Henderson, V. (1964). The nature of nursing. *American Journal of Nursing, 64*(8), 62–68.

Henderson, V. (1966). *The nature of nursing.* New York: Macmillan.

Holmes, D., Perron, A., & O'Byrne, P. (2006). Evidence, virulence, and the disappearance of nursing knowledge: A critique of the evidence based dogma. *Worldviews on Evidence Based Nursing, 3*(3), 95–102.

Hughes, L. (1980). The public image of the nurse. *ANS. Advances in Nursing Science, 2*(3), 55–72.

Im, E.-O., & Meleis, A. I. (1999). Situation-specific theories: Philosophical roots, properties, and approach. *ANS. Advances in Nursing Science, 22*(2), 11–24.

Johnson, D. E. (1980). The behavioral system model for nursing. In J. P. Riehl & S. C. Roy (Eds.), *Conceptual models for nursing practice* (2nd ed.). New York: Appleton-Century-Crofts.

Johnson, P. E. (1928). What should ethics teach? *American Journal of Nursing, 28*(11), 1084–1090.

Kalisch, P. A., Kalisch, B. J. (1995). *The advance of American nursing* (3rd ed.). BostonLippincott-Raven.

Kelly, L. Y., Joel, L. A. (2001). *The nursing experience: Trends, challenges and transitions* (4th ed.). New York: McGraw-Hill).

Kilpatrick, W. H. (1921–1922). The basis of professional ethics in nursing. *American Journal of Nursing, 22,* 790–798.

King, I. M. (1971). *Toward a theory for nursing: General concepts of human behavior.* New York: Wiley.

Kinloch, J. P. (1932). The science of life. *Trained Nurse and Hospital Review, 88,* 710–718.

Kramer, M. (2002). Academic talk about dementia caregiving: A critical comment on language. *Research and Theory for Nursing Practice, 16*(4), 263–280.

Leininger, M. M. (1976). Doctoral programs for nurses: Trends, questions, and projected plans. *Nursing Research, 25*(3), 201–210.

Leininger, M. M. (1978). *Transcultural nursing: Concepts, Theories and practices.* New York: Wiley.

Letourneau, N., & Allen, M. (1999). Post-positivistic critical multiplism: A beginning dialogue. *Journal of Advanced Nursing, 20*(3), 623–630.

Levine, M. E. (1967). The four conservation principles of nursing. *Nursing Forum, 6*(1), 93–98.

Levine, M. E. (1999). On the humanities in nursing. *Canadian Journal of Nursing Research, 30*(4), 213–217.

Liehr, P. R., & Smith, M. J. (1999). Middle range theory: Spinning research and practice to create knowledge for new millennium. *ANS. Advances in Nursing Science, 21*(4), 81–91.

Lovell, M. C. (1980). The politics of medical deception: Challenging the trajectory of history. *ANS. Advances in Nursing Science, 2*(3), 73–86.

Maeve, K. (1999). The social construction of love and sexuality in a women's prison. *ANS. Advances in Nursing Science, 21*(3), 46–65.

Margison, F. R., McGrath, G., Barkham, M., Clark, J., Audin, K., Connell, J., et al. (2000). Evidence-based practice and practice based evidence. *British Journal of Psychiatry, 177,* 123–130.

Mazurek-Melnyk, B., Stone, P., Fincout-Overholt, E., & Ackerman, M. (2000). Evidence-based practice: The past, the present and recommendations for the millennium. *Pediatric Nursing, 26*(1), 77–80.

McClure, K. (1951). Ingredients of gracious nursing. *Nursing World, 125*221–224.

Mead, M. (1956). Nursing—primitive and civilized. *American Journal of Nursing, 56*(9), 1001–1004.

Meade, A. B. (1936). Training the senses in clinical observation. *Trained Nurse and Hospital Review, 97,* 540–544.

Meleis, A. I. (1997). ReVisions in knowledge development: A passion for substance. In L. H. Nicoll (Ed.), *Perspectives on nursing theory* (3rd ed., pp. 122–123, Ch. 110). Philadelphia: Lippincott.

Melosh, B. (1982). *The physician's hand: Work culture and conflict in American nursing.* Philadelphia: Temple University Press.

Mossman, L. C. (1923). The place of beauty in life. *Trained Nurse and Hospital Review, 81,* 318–319.

Mountin, J. W. (1943). Nursing: A critical analysis. *American Journal of Nursing, 43*(1), 29–34.

Mowinski-Jennings, B., & Loan, L. A. (2001). Misconceptions among nurses about evidence-based practice. *Image: Journal of Nursing Scholarship, 33*(2), 121–127.

Neuman, B. (1980). The Betty Neuman health care systems model: A total person approach to patient problems. In J. P. Riehl & Sr. C. Roy (Eds.), *Conceptual models for nursing practice* (2nd ed.). New YorkAppleton-Century-Crofts.

Newman, M. A. (1979). *Theory development in nursing.* Philadelphia: FA Davis.

Newman, M. A. (1986). *Health as expanding consciousness.* St. Louis: Mosby.

Nightingale, F. (1859). *Notes on Hospitals.* London: John W. Parker and Sons.

Nightingale, F. (1969). *Notes on nursing: What it is and what it is not.* New York: Dover Publications, Inc. (Original work published 1860.)

Nightingale, F. (1979). *Cassandra.* New York: Feminist Press.

NIH roadmap for clinical research. (2006). Retrieved October 6, 2006, from http://nihroadmap.nih.gov/clinicalresearch/overview-translational.asp.

Noble, G. E. (1940). The spirit of nursing. *American Journal of Nursing, 40*(2), 161–162.

Oettinger, K. B. (1939). Toward inner freedom. *American Journal of Nursing, 39*(11), 1224–1229.

Orem, D. E. (1971). *Nursing: Concepts of practice.* New York: McGraw-Hill.

Orlando, I. J. (1961). *The dynamic nurse-patient relationship: Function, process, and principles.* New York: G. P. Putnam's Sons.

Parse, R. R. (1981). *Man-living-health: A theory of nursing.* New York: Wiley.

Paterson, J. G., & Zderad, L. T. (1976). *Humanistic nursing.* New York: Wiley.

Pender, N. J. (1982). *Health promotion in nursing practice* (1st ed.). New York: Appleton-Century-Crofts).

Pender, N. J. (1987). *Health promotion in nursing practice* (2nd ed.). Norwalk, CT: Appleton-Lange).

Peplau, H. E. (1952). *Interpersonal relations in nursing.* New York: G. P. Putnam's Sons.

Peterson, S. J. (2007). *Middle range theories: Application to nursing research.* Philadelphia: Lippincott Williams & Wilkins.

Peterson, S. J., & Bredow, T. S. (2003). *Middle range theories: Application to nursing research.* Philadelphia: Lippincott Williams & Wilkins.

Pfefferkorn, F. (1933). What of nursing field studies? *American Journal of Nursing, 33*(3), 258–261.

Porter, E. K. (1953). What it means to be a professional nurse. *American Journal of Nursing, 55*(8), 948–950.

Rambur, B. (1999). Fostering evidence-based practice in nursing education. *Journal of Professional Nursing, 15*(5), 270–274.

Reverby, S. M. (1987). *Ordered to care: The dilemma of American nursing, 1850–1945.* Cambridge, UK: Cambridge University Press.

Riddles, A. R. (1928). The force of example. *Trained Nurse and Hospital Review, 80*(1), 27–30.

Roberts, J. I., & Group, T. M. (1995). *Feminism and nursing: An historical perspective on power, status, and political activism in the nursing profession.* Westport, CT: Praeger.

Roberts, S. J. (1983). Oppressed group behavior: Implications for nursing. *ANS. Advances in Nursing Science, 5*(4), 21–30.

Rogers, M. E. (1970). *An introduction to the theoretical basis of nursing.* Philadelphia: FA Davis.

Roy, S. C. (1976). *Introduction to nursing: An adaptation model.* Englewood Cliffs, NJ: Prentice-Hall.

Sanger, M. (1971). *Margaret Sanger, an autobiography.* New York: Dover.

Savage, J. (2000). One voice, different tunes: Issues raised by dual analysis of a segment of qualitative data. *Journal of Advanced Nursing, 31*(6), 1493–1500.

Schunemann, H. J., Best, D., Vist, G., & Oxman, A. D., for the Grade Working Group. (2003). Letters, numbers, symbols and words: How to communicate grades of evidence and recommendations. *Canadian Medical Association Journal, 169*, 677–680.

Silverstein, N. G. (1985). Lillian Wald at Henry Street, 1893–1895. *ANS. Advances in Nursing Science, 7*(2), 1–12.

Simons, H., Kushner, S., Jones, K., & James, D. (2003). From evidence-based practice to practice-based evidence: The idea of situated generalization. *Research Papers in Education, 18*(4), 347–364.

Simpson, L. F. (1914). The psychology of nursing. *Trained Nurse and Hospital Review, 52–53*, 133–137.

Smith, J. A. (1983). *The idea of health: Implications for the nursing professional.* New York: Teachers College Press.

Smith, M. J., & Liehr, P. R. (Eds.). (2003). *Middle range theory for nursing.* New York: Springer.

Staupers, M. (2006). Retrieved September 23, 2006, from www.workingworld.com/magazine/viewarticle.asp?articleno=392&wn=1.

Staupers, M. (2006). Retrieved September 2006 from www.ana.org/hof/stauperm.htm.

Stevens, P. E. (1989). A critical social reconceptualization of environment in nursing: Implications for methodology. *ANS. Advances in Nursing Science, 11*(4), 56–68.

Stewart, I. M. (1921–1922). Some fundamental principles in the teaching of ethics. *American Journal of Nursing, 22*, 906–913.

Taylor, E. J. (1934). Of what is the nature of nursing? *American Journal of Nursing, 34*(5), 473–476.

Thompson, J. L. (1987). Critical scholarship: The critique of domination in nursing. *ANS. Advances in Nursing Science, 10*(1), 27–38.

Thoms, A. (2006). Retrieved September 2006 from www.ana.org/hof/thomab.htm.

Thoms, A. (2006). Retrieved September 2006 from http://tjsworldforreal.blogspot.com/2006_02_01_tjsworldforreal_archive.html.

Tooley, S. A. (1905). *The life of Florence Nightingale.* New York: Macmillan.

Travelbee, J. (1966). *Interpersonal aspects of nursing.* Philadelphia: FA Davis.

Wald, L. (1971). *The house on Henry Street.* New York: Dover.

Walker, L. O. (1971). Toward a clearer understanding of the concept of nursing theory. *Nursing Research, 20*(5), 428–435.

Walker, L. O., Avant, K. C. (2004). *Strategies for theory construction nursing* (4th ed.). Upper Saddle River, NJ: Prentice-Hall.

Warnshius, F. C. (1926). The future of medicine and nursing: The ideal to be sought. *American Journal of Nursing, 26*(2), 123–126.

Watson, J. (1979). *Nursing: The philosophy and science of caring.* Boston: Little, Brown & Co.

Wheeler, C. E. (1985). The American Journal of Nursing and the socialization of a profession. *ANS. Advances in Nursing Science, 7*(2), 20–33.

Wiedenbach, E. (1964). *Clinical nursing: A helping art.* New York: Springer Publishing.

Woodham-Smith, C. (1983). *Florence Nightingale: 1820–1910.* New York: Atheneum.

Wooldridge, P. J. (1971). Meta-theories of nursing: A commentary on Dr. Walker's article. *Nursing Research, 20*(6), 494–495.

Worcester, A. (1902). Is nursing really a profession? *American Journal of Nursing, 2*, 908–917.

Wright, E. U. (1953). *Interpersonal Relations in Nursing, 1*(8), 451.

Yellowtail, Susie Walking-Bear. (2006). Retrieved September 2006 from www.ana.org/hof/yellowtail.htm.

Yellowtail, Susie Walking-Bear. (2006). Retrieved September 2006 from www.missoulian.com/specials/100montanans/list/062.html.

Young, A. D. (1913). The nurse's duty to herself. *Trained Nurse and Hospital Review, 51*(5), 265–270.

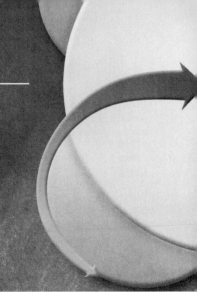

CHAPTER 3

Emancipatory Knowledge Development

Why have women passion, intellect, moral activity—these three—and a place in society where no one of the three can be exercised?

Florence Nightingale (1979, p. 25)

After one has worked for a time in healing wounds which should never have been inflicted, tending ailments which should never have developed, sending patients to hospitals who need not have gone if their homes were habitable, bringing charitable aid to persons who would not have needed charity if health had not been ruined by unwholesome conditions, one loses heart and longs for preventive work, constructive work ... something that will make it less easy for so many illnesses and accidents to occur; that will help to bring better homes and workshops, better conditions of life.

L. L. Dock (1902–1903, p. 531)

Specifically, there is a need to further explore the political, economic, and social forces in communities around the country that influenced the growth of both nursing and medicine during this century. The rigidities and inflexibilities of mythical conceptions about the roles of men and women in health care and the resulting responses of community members need examination also.

J. Ashley (1976, p. x)

The women who wrote these opening quotes represent a long tradition of emancipatory knowing in nursing. They, and many others over the decades, spoke and wrote passionately about the social, economic, and political conditions that create barriers to health and health care for all people. They recognized that these conditions are beyond the control of any individual. They worked to understand how social inequities and injustices come to be and why, what needs to change, and how to go about creating the changes that are needed.

Emancipatory knowing makes social and structural change possible. It is the human ability to recognize social and political problems of injustice or inequity, to realize things could be different, and to piece together complex elements of experience and context in order to change a situation as it is, to a situation that improves people's lives. It leads to realization of ways in which problematic conditions converge, reproduce, and remain in place to sustain a status quo that is unfair for some groups within society. Realization of the problem leads to imagining a more just and equitable situation, to action to change the situation, and ongoing awareness of injustices that persist even as change occurs. This constant reflection and action to transform the world is *praxis*—the process of emancipatory knowing (Chinn, 2004, p. 8; Freire, 1972, p. 36).

In this chapter we provide a description of the concept of emancipatory knowing, an overview of the background and foundations from which emancipatory knowing in nursing has developed, and a summary of significant literature in nursing that has reflected emancipatory perspectives. We then present explanations of the processes for emancipatory knowing that are represented in Figure 3-1, which we introduced in Chapter 1. As represented in the figure, the processes of emancipatory knowing surround and connect with the four fundamental patterns of knowing in nursing, placing a critical lens on nursing's knowledge development activities, on the practice of nursing, and on the social and political contexts within which nursing functions. This chapter provides many examples of approaches that are used to address the critical questions posed from an emancipatory perspective: "What are the barriers to freedom?" "What is invisible?" "Who benefits?" and "What is wrong with this picture?" The creative development processes of critiquing and imagining are explained, drawing on distinct grassroots and academic methods. We use many examples of these processes and describe ways in which formal expressions of emancipatory knowledge are presented and authenticated. Throughout this chapter we build explanations that will deepen your understanding of praxis, the fundamental process of emancipatory knowing.

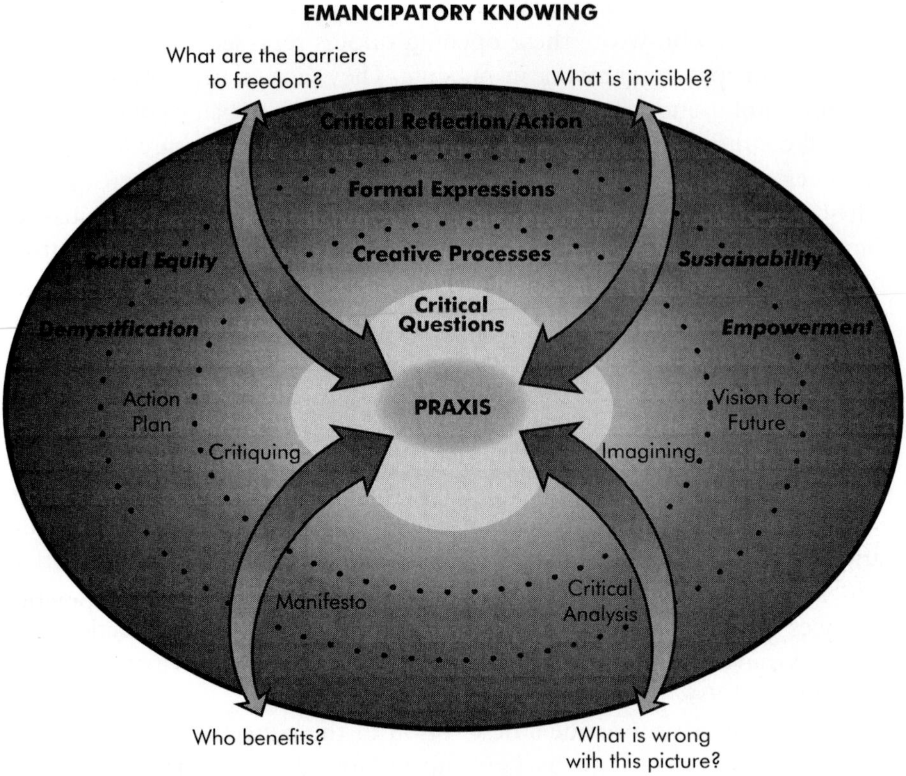

EMANCIPATORY KNOWING

FIGURE 3-1 Processes for developing emancipatory knowledge.

THE CONCEPT OF EMANCIPATORY KNOWING

Emancipatory knowing is the capacity not only to notice injustices in a social order, but also to critically examine why injustices seem not to be noticed or remain invisible, and to identify social and structural changes that are required to right social and institutional wrongs. This kind of knowing also examines the nature of knowledge and the ways in which knowledge itself, or what is taken to be knowledge, contributes to larger social problems. It takes into account the power dynamics that create knowledge, and the social and political contexts that shape and influence knowledge and knowing. It seeks freedom from institutional and institutionalized social and political contexts that sustain that which is unjust, and that perpetuate advantage for some and disadvantage for others.

From an emancipatory perspective, knowledge is constructed by language and patterns of thinking that are reflected in hegemonic mental images, or assumptions about "the way things are." Hegemony is the dominance of certain ideologies, beliefs, values, or views of the world over other possible viewpoints; these dominant perspectives privilege certain groups over others and are taken for granted as fact, or as the only possibility. For example, a dominant assumption in nursing is the view that nurses practice as employees of an agency or a corporation, and not as independent practitioners. Institutionalized reimbursement practices of insurance companies and licensure laws are powerful social and political structures that keep in place this view of how nurses can and should practice. Policies that govern how nurses are paid for their services make it difficult to secure reimbursement for independent nursing services. Even when reimbursement is possible, it is more difficult for nurses to receive reimbursement than it is for other health care workers, or they have to receive reimbursement indirectly. A few nurses have refused to accept the hegemonic assumption that they cannot or should not practice independently, and most nurses are aware that there is such a thing as being self-employed, or practicing independently. However, the prevailing hegemonic view is that the "norm" is to be an employee and work within the structures of an agency or corporation, and that it would not be feasible to practice any other way.

Language systems, ideologies, and hegemonic patterns of thinking are created and re-created out of dominant practices within a culture or society, where the leaders and spokespersons in power practice and verbalize how the world is and how it should function, and where people learn to conform to the practices and values that are professed by those who dominate. Often people are not aware that they are trapped within a system that disadvantages them, and they remain unaware of alternatives or see the alternatives as not possible. It is the human capacity for emancipatory knowing that gives rise to a realization that there is something wrong with the way things are, and that it is possible to change for the better. This realization can happen when things become intolerable, or when someone comes along and challenges or questions the status quo. When people come to understand situations as unjust and challenge the way things are, they are exercising an emancipatory human interest that redefines what is problematic about their situation from their own point of view. They begin to recognize that there are others who share their experience of the situation. Together with others in similar circumstances, they begin to speak about and make visible the structures and dynamics that sustain that which is problematic, and develop actions, insights, and knowledge concerning the problem and what is required to correct the problem or change their situation for the better.

The emergence of the women's movement in the latter half of the 20th century provides an example. During the decades of the world wars in the early part of the 20th century, the hegemonic view of women that dominated public discourse included ideas about the ideal wife and mother who remains a subservient homemaker, devoted to her family. This discourse was reflected in the media, in government policies, business practices, religious beliefs—in virtually every aspect of public life. In the United States and many other countries around the world, small groups of women began to examine the circumstances of their lives in consciousness-raising groups, sharing their experiences and feelings about their lives, and formed ideas about how their lives could and should be. Many of their ideas became formalized as feminist theory. Those who spoke publicly were often derided by men and women who were threatened by the social and cultural changes that feminist ideas suggested. But despite widespread resistance, feminist ideas began to make sense to more and more people, and many significant social and cultural changes started to happen. One of the first changes that feminist leaders called for was a shift to gender-neutral language, and widespread shifts began to occur. Newspaper classified ads, for example, ceased publishing "Help Wanted—Male" and "Help Wanted—Female" columns; instead these ads became simply "Help Wanted." In this example, emancipatory knowing was awakened for some women by their distress with the restrictions that the hegemonic ideals of womanhood imposed on their lives. For others, emancipatory knowing emerged as they began to hear about and comprehend the challenges and alternatives that feminist perspectives offered. These realizations came about gradually for some, whereas others experienced "lightbulb" moments of new awareness.

Emancipatory knowing is different from, but related to, the ideas of problem solving, critical thinking, and reflective practice. It is much more than problem solving in that it defines what is problematic in relation to fundamental social and structural contexts. Unlike problem solving, which usually focuses on a single, discrete instance, emancipatory knowing requires seeing the larger picture, detecting patterns and structures reflected in day-to-day situations that are problematic, and seeking solutions that correct fundamental social inequities and injustices. As an example, prior to the social changes that came about with the women's movement in Western societies, some women who wanted to be employed in a "man's" job (such as medicine or operating heavy machinery) solved the problem by dressing and posing as a man. They may have been aware that the policies and practices of their culture were unjust, but rather than pursuing a critical, emancipatory approach to changing societal rules and policies, they solved the problem by accommodating to a fundamentally unfair practice—an individual and temporary, rather than a long-term, solution.

Emancipatory knowing differs from critical thinking in that it does not simply seek to improve one's thinking ability, judgment, and problem-solving skills. Instead, the emphasis is on seeing what lies beneath issues and problems and redefining those issues and problems to reveal linkages among and between complex social and political contexts that create how people think about and act in the world. For example, a critical thinking approach to hiring practices based on gender would focus on gathering the evidence and examining the rationale for restricting hiring in some jobs to women only, and others to men only. The soundness and logic of each explanation for the practice would be examined, and conclusions would be drawn about the practice. Even though critical thinking approaches would probably reveal injustices and inequities, critical thinking alone would not examine the underlying network of social practices that kept the injustice of gender-specific hiring in place or challenge the status quo in a way that would demand change.

Praxis, the process of emancipatory knowing, is akin to reflective practice, in that action and reflection are constantly interacting to shape and improve what is done and how it is done. However, praxis requires more than personal reflection; it requires deliberately cultivating the ability to see what is unfair and unjust, envision how it could be different, understand how it came to be, and then uncover alternate explanations and possibilities for change coming from a range of perspectives much broader than that of the individual alone. Praxis requires a new lens with which to view the world—a lens that reveals something that is not perceived because it may "seem natural" or because it is difficult to see beyond those things that are assumed to be "true." Once this new lens reveals what has not been perceived before, it becomes "perfectly obvious" and the situation begins to make sense. Praxis requires both inward and outward reflection—critically examining your own experience, assumptions, and actions, and critically examining the contexts within which your experience is situated. Praxis is critical reflection and action that occur in synchrony toward transforming the world (Chinn, 2004, p. 8; Freire, 1970, p. 36). As an example, many women find a great deal of satisfaction and personal joy in their roles as mothers and homemakers. From a reflective practice perspective, they might recognize that their experience fits a hegemonic view of ideal womanhood that could be restrictive in certain ways, but their personal experience is satisfying and rewarding and therefore requires no change. Praxis, on the other hand, would call for looking beyond personal experience alone to reflect on the broader social and cultural implications, taking in the political as well as personal implications of the situation. The personal satisfactions and rewards of homemaking for some women are not negated, but the focus shifts to broader issues and the outcomes for women and society in general when homemaking and motherhood is prescribed as a primary role of women in society. Praxis involves recognizing the political and social outcomes of prescriptions and restrictions placed on women by hegemonic practices.

Emancipatory knowing does not just attempt to think critically about a problem, or solve it, but asks, "Why do we have this problem in the first place?" Emancipatory knowing addresses underlying problems that are deeper than the problem on the surface. For example, when approached from an emancipatory perspective, you not only ask, "How can we create opportunities for women in the workplace?" but also ask, "Why are women excluded from full access to employment in the first place?" As a nurse, you not only ask, "How can we overcome the stigma of HIV/AIDS" but also ask, "Why is this stigmatized in the first place?" Or, not only "How do we create tolerance for transgendered persons?" but also "Why does intolerance persist?" Or, not only "How can we end the unfair policy of mandatory overtime for nurses?" but also "Why has this practice emerged" and "Who benefits from this policy?"

NURSING'S EMANCIPATORY LEGACY

In the discipline of nursing, a foundational perspective that grounds emancipatory knowing is what is commonly termed "critical theory." The term *critical theory* is confusing in that it does not reflect the usual connotation of theory in nursing. The concept of "critical" has a range of negative common meanings that are not relevant in the context of critical theory. "Critical" in this context implies a deep analysis that moves beyond the surface, beyond that which is usually assumed. Generally, *critical theory* is a broad term used to describe both the process and the product of work that takes a historically situated and sociopolitical perspective and challenges social inequities and injustices. It is critical in the sense that it analyzes the roots and consequences of social inequities and injustices that privilege one group over another.

As a method, critical theory has roots in the classical sociological traditions of Karl Marx, Max Weber, and Emile Durkheim (Morrow, 1994). These early philosophic traditions were quite unfavorable to capitalist governments such as that of the United States and were viewed in the United States as allied with communist ideology. The extreme anti-communist sentiments that prevailed in the United States in the 20th century made it difficult for U.S. scholars to engage in the discourses of early critical theory and philosophy. Scholars in countries that have strong social welfare policies and values have generally been more open and accepting of critical theory. As the political structures of the world began to change and the 40-year Cold War that began in the late 1940s abated, scholars in the United States gradually assumed more open reception and responses to critical theory. This circumstance illustrates the tremendous influence of context on people's thinking, either creating barriers to understanding or supporting openness to possibilities.

Critical theory began to emerge as a specific approach to the study of society through the work of scholars exiled from Germany by Adolf Hitler in 1932. These scholars became known as the "Frankfort School" and established the term *critical theory* to designate a form of sociological theory that recognized society as evolving historically and that assumed a deliberate engagement with the problems of society and the processes of social transformation. Typically, but not always, when the term *critical theory* is capitalized, it refers specifically to the work of the Frankfort School (Morrow, 1994). We use the lowercase format throughout our discussion to indicate a perspective that encompasses a broad range of philosophies, methods, and approaches that share in common a fundamental engagement with problems of society.

In the 1960s Jürgen Habermas assumed a prominent position in shaping new conceptions of critical theory with broad interdisciplinary connections between the human sciences and philosophy (Morrow, 1994). Habermas' critical social theory posited three fundamental human interests, each demanding its own method. Technical interests require empirical methods, practical (communicative) interests require interpretive/philosophic methods, and emancipatory interests require critical/reflective methods. Each of these interests define what it means to be human, and each is necessary for human survival (Habermas, 1973, 1979). Although nurse scholars have grounded their thinking in a number of notable critical scholars and philosophers, the influence of Habermas is significant.

Paulo Freire's ideas have also had a significant influence among nursing scholars and activists. Freire was a Brazilian educator who initiated the movement for critical approaches to education. Freire's work is grounded philosophically in the ideas of Karl Marx and Friedrich Engels, Georg Hegel, Gyorgy Lukacs, Herbert Marcuse, and Erich Fromm (Freire, 1970). Freire's work grew out of a project to teach peasants to read. His ideas include specific approaches not only to teaching, but also to any grassroots project of human liberation. Education traditionally is based on the assumption that its primary purpose is to pass along the existing knowledge and values of the culture. Freire questioned this assumption, and in doing so formalized a view of education as a means of challenging the existing knowledge and values of the culture (Freire, 1970; hooks, 1993; Weiler, 1991). Because of the broad significance of his philosophy as well as the practical action-oriented perspective that he articulated, his ideas have had a widespread influence, beyond the scope of education.

Michel Foucault's poststructural philosophy has also had a major influence on nurse scholars because of his insights concerning power imbalances embedded in and sustained by verbal and symbolic social discourses—human interactions and the systems of discourse that make them visible. Verbal and symbolic discourses are powerful because they interconnect to create and limit what is socially acceptable to be known. Discourses are whole systems of representation—writing, images, advertisements, artwork, and everyday verbal and nonverbal language that create social "reality." As an example, discourses of beauty for young women suggest that a flawless face is more beautiful than a normally flawed, plainer face. Discourse also reinforces that "beauty" of a certain type (that attained by cosmetics and airbrushing) is attainable and a normal way to be. Since these messages appear everywhere, young women may only understand what is constructed as "beauty" as it is prescribed by systems of discourse. Such discourses are powerful because they create barriers to societal resources for some, and opportunity for others. Young women who cannot, or choose not to, achieve the popular standard of "beauty" run the risk of being denied social resources such as popularity among peers and social interactions that most young people yearn for. This same example could be applied to young men for whom popular discourses prescribe that which is considered handsome, standards of muscular development, and clothing that is considered "cool," as opposed to that which is considered "nerdy"—being thin, wearing glasses, plaid short-sleeved shirts, and white socks. It is in this way that discourses construct "realities" that create power imbalances—in our example, between young women and men who are "beautiful" or "handsome" and those who are not.

Emancipatory knowledge can develop in resistance to the limitations imposed by the exercise of power by discourse and language. For example, a current television commercial shown in some areas of the United States depicts how "beauty" was created in a young woman's face using cosmetics, airbrushing, and computerized image editing techniques. This commercial raises awareness that "beauty" as marketed to young women is unattainable. As alternative discourses begin to undermine dominate discourses around beauty (as they seem to be currently doing), dominant discourses begin to lose their power to control how young women spend their money and time.

As a poststructuralist, Foucault viewed language and discourse, including theory, as systems of representation that are necessary in the social order in that they produce meaning, or ways to comprehend the world. But, as the examples of discourses related to beauty illustrate, these systems of language and discourse also limit what is understood, known, or perceived. According to Foucault, we can only know things as they have meaning, and it is systems of discourse that produce, or construct, meaning (Hall, 2001). Poststructuralism addresses how language and systems of discourse create normative views. Critical poststructuralism analyzes how discourse functions to create imbalances that disadvantage whole classes of persons and illuminates possibilities for change (Doering, 1992; Dzurec, 1989; Foucault, 1980, 1984).

Early Literature Related to Emancipatory Knowing in Nursing

Despite nursing's history of subservience and servitude, nursing has always had courageous workers, leaders, and scholars who have spoken out against the prevailing conditions under which nurses work, and against deplorable conditions of society that prevent people from living full and healthy lives. In the latter half of the 20th century, a growing number of nurse scholars and activists began to connect their ideas with larger philosophic, theoretic, and social movements and to develop disciplinary perspectives that are clearly connected to an emancipatory pattern of knowing.

In the 1960s, Lydia Hall, declaring there is no "shortage of nurses" but rather a "shortage of nursing," established the Loeb Center for Nursing and Rehabilitation at Montefiore Hospital in the Bronx, New York. Her ideas and the actions that flowed from them are notable examples of emancipatory knowing in nursing. Believing that nursing was the chief therapy for those recovering from chronic illness, Hall organized the Loeb Center as a place where nursing, rather than medicine, could be practiced and physicians were under the direction of nurses (Hall, 1966). Hall established Loeb when she saw nurses taking on medical tasks and becoming physician extenders rather than providing bodily care and nurturing the core of persons in need of care subsequent to medicine's curative role. Hall's model of nursing at Loeb was revolutionary because it differentiated nursing from medicine and allowed nurses to practice in an environment that did not require performance of curative tasks associated with the growth of medical technology in the 1960s.

Early literature in nursing that reflected an emancipatory perspective also reflected feminist perspectives. As reluctant as nurses in general were to accept feminist ideas and to align themselves with the women's movement of the 1960s and 1970s in the United States, there were those who spoke out and published ideas that challenged the status quo (Chinn, 1995).

One of the earliest publications that reflected an emancipatory perspective was an article by Wilma Scott Heide published in the *American Journal of Nursing*, in which Heide explained the importance of the feminist movement for nursing (Heide, 1973). Three years later, JoAnn Ashley's book titled *Hospitals, Paternalism, and the Role of the Nurse* was published (Ashley, 1976). Basing her argument on historical evidence, Ashley contended that the apprenticeship system of education that prevailed in nursing situated nurses and nursing in a context that not only exploited the labor of women in hospitals, but also undermined the fundamental values of nursing related to health and health care. Her feminist analysis drew the essential connection between a misogynist (woman-hating) society and the resulting health policies and practices that constricted the role of nurses in the delivery of health care (Kagan, 2006).

Another major publication to influence nursing's development of emancipatory perspectives was the 1983 publication of Susan Jo Roberts' article titled "Oppressed Group Behavior: Implications for Nursing" (Roberts, 1983). Drawing on Freire's work and literature on colonized Africans, Latin Americans, African Americans, Jews, and women, Roberts made the claim that nurses also can be viewed as an oppressed group. Emphasizing that this insight can lead to substantive action to change nursing and health care, she concluded:

> Nurses are an oppressed group with characteristics similar to those of [other oppressed] groups. It is hoped that with this understanding nurses can learn from the experience of others to liberate themselves and develop an autonomous profession that can greatly contribute to the improvement of health care. (p. 30)

In 1982, in the same decade that Roberts' article appeared, Cassandra: Radical Feminist Nurses Network was founded by a group of nurses gathered at the American Nurses Association convention in Washington, DC, coinciding with June 30, 1982, the expiration date for ratification of the Equal Rights Amendment to the United States Constitution. The Cassandra founders present at the convention were astonished that they saw no acknowledgment at the convention of the political significance of the date and the major events being held through the District of Columbia to commemorate the death of this amendment to the United States Constitution. The women who formed Cassandra divided their time between various convention activities and events throughout the city celebrating a renewal of commitment to continue the struggle for women's full equality in U.S. society. They formed Cassandra to bring critical and feminist insights to the forefront in nursing, and to use critical feminist insights as a basis for change in nursing. They chose the name from Nightingale's essay titled

"Cassandra," in which she asked the question that opens this chapter: "Why have women passion, intellect, moral activity—these three—and a place in society where no one of the three can be exercised?" (Nightingale, 1979, p. 25). The network's newsjournal (*Cassandra: Radical Feminist Nurses Newsjournal*, 1982–1989) was published until 1989 and, although not widely distributed, provided a significant source of affirmation for many practicing nurses and nurse scholars who were beginning to develop an emancipatory perspective.

By the close of the 1980s and the beginning of the 1990s nursing litera-ture was beginning to reflect a strong presence of works informed by eman-cipatory perspectives, including critical, feminist, and poststructuralist theory (Allan & Hall, 1988; Allen, 1985, 1986, 1987; Allen, Allman, & Powers, 1991; Bunting & Campbell, 1990; Campbell & Bunting, 1991; Charleston Faculty Practice Conference Group, 1986; Chinn, 1989; Chinn & Wheeler, 1985; Doering, 1992; Dzurec, 1989; Hedin, 1986; Kleffel, 1991; MacPherson, 1985, 1989; Muller & Dzurec, 1993; Poslusny, 1989; Thompson, 1987, 1991; Webb, 1993). These early writings remain impor-tant foundations for nursing's emancipatory scholarship. They explained the particular critical perspectives from which they drew, and offered critiques of nursing and nursing knowledge, along with proposals for shifts in nursing, health care, and society that could address persistent and seem-ingly intractable problems in nursing and health care.

Growth of Contemporary Emancipatory Thought in Nursing

By the mid-1990s, emancipatory perspectives appeared more frequently in nursing literature, and although these perspectives remained on the mar-gins of dominant scholarly discourses in nursing, they gradually gained depth and quality that was increasingly recognized as noteworthy. White (1995) offered a critique of Carper's (1978) conceptualization of empiric, ethical, personal, and aesthetic patterns of knowing, and the first published proposal to identify a fifth pattern of knowing that addressed the social and political context of nursing knowledge. She developed her proposal for a "sociopolitical" pattern of knowing from her critical analysis of Carper's original conceptualization and our 1988 extensions of nursing's funda-mental patterns of knowing (Jacobs-Kramer & Chinn, 1988). White's description of this fifth pattern of knowing is background for our current thinking related to emancipatory knowing, particularly concerning the need to focus attention on the "wherein" of nursing practice, and viewing sociopolitical knowing as one that is all-encompassing of the four funda-mental patterns of knowing. Our choice of the term *emancipatory* knowing is meant to embrace a wide range of historical and contextual considerations, and to also emphasize the fundamental intent to seek freedom from conditions, largely hidden, that restrict the realization of full human potential.

Examples of more recent critical scholarship in nursing are summarized in Table 3-1. These examples illustrate the nature of problems that are identified from an emancipatory perspective, and the kinds of actions that are identified to create the change that is envisioned. The *critical perspective* challenges prevailing hegemonies; the *critical problem* typically involves seeing something as problematic that more generally is taken as simply the way

TABLE 3-1   Examples of Turn-of-the-21st-Century Critical Scholarship in Nursing

Author/Year	Perspective(s)	Critical Problem	Envisioned Change
Boutain (1999)	Critical social theory	Nursing knowledge has not accommodated multiple representations of social identity and does not directly challenge negative and degrading stereotypes of African Americans	Critical interpretations and analyses of nursing theory must be informed by the perspectives of African American scholars in order to develop research that is relevant to the concerns of African Americans
Browne (2001)	Critical	Liberal political philosophy embedded in nursing theories has diverted attention away from structures and practices that create inequities in health and health care	Political philosophies embedded in nursing knowledge need to be critiqued and new knowledge developed to address social and political inequities
Butterfield (2002)	Critical ecological	Nursing has not played a significant role in developing knowledge concerning the etiology of disease and has overlooked nursing approaches to reduce environmental health risk	Nurses take responsibility for reducing environmental health risk by systematically obtaining clinical and research data concerning environmental etiologies of disease and taking strategic action to reduce risk and place citizen health as top priority

TABLE 3-1 Examples of Turn-of-the-21st-Century Critical Scholarship in Nursing—cont'd

Author/Year	Perspective(s)	Critical Problem	Envisioned Change
Hardin (2003)	Critical poststructuralist	An individualized approach to the study of recovery from anorexia nervosa has resulted in conflicting and incomplete understanding	Theorizing that focuses on social and cultural discourses is needed to understand the process of recovery, individualism, and women's experience of the body
Georges (2005)	Critical feminist	Nurses' failure to recognize and oppose political realities that oppress and cause suffering renders us active participants in sustaining the suffering of others	Theory, research, and practice related to suffering needs to change to reflect awareness of the global realities of political conditions that sustain human suffering.
Falk-Rafael (2006)	Critical postcolonial	Economic globalization is a new form of colonialism that sustains poverty and disease	Nurses take political action at the local, national, and international levels to reform the global economic order and move toward health and well-being for all
Cloyes (2006)	Critical poststructuralist	Analysis of research interviews is a mystified process that often sustains disadvantage of marginalized and vulnerable people	Political discourse analysis is needed as an ethical practice to overcome research practices that sustain injustice
Mohammed (2006)	Postcolonial	Traditional views of culture have contributed to stereotyping and unjust practices that sustain white privilege and disadvantage other groups	Postcolonial approaches are needed that view the interplay among health beliefs, practices and culture as fluid, historically situated and discursively constructed; these approaches engage a concern for scientific integrity and social justice

the world is. This involves extensive critical analyses of how the problem came to be, who is advantaged and who is disadvantaged, and how social practices intersect to keep it in place. Emancipatory scholarship also includes the *change that is envisioned* and the action needed to reach what is envisioned.

EMANCIPATORY CREATIVE DEVELOPMENT PROCESSES: CRITIQUING AND IMAGINING

Emancipatory creative development processes grow from the critical questions of emancipatory knowing such as "What is wrong with this picture?" "What is hidden from view or invisible?" "Whose voice is not heard?" "What are the barriers to freedoms, and where do they occur?" and "Who benefits from the status quo?" These questions are rooted in the assumption that all people seek and deserve freedom and opportunity to develop or exercise their full human potential. They are also rooted in the assumption that developing and exercising one's potential is not solely a matter of individual will or desire, but that culture and society create conditions and structures within which people can thrive or fail to thrive. From an emancipatory perspective, any conditions that limit people from developing their full human potential become problematic and must be changed. Emancipatory knowing assumes that injustices can be made visible, that what is imagined can become real, and that humans have the innate capacity to bring about changes to improve the human condition.

Asking a critical question such as "What is wrong with this picture?" requires noticing that someone is benefiting to the detriment of another; or that some people are being denied something that others have and that every person deserves. Addressing this critical question requires a lens that sees beyond the obvious and beyond one's own personal experience—that sees beyond what is presented to us as being "true," because often what people need to see is hidden or difficult to perceive. Whereas people may notice the obvious, emancipatory knowing requires a deep sort of awareness that recognizes how social processes and institutions create and recreate inequities. This kind of awareness is not easy, and typically it creates a major personal and professional dilemma. Most people are socialized to accept an unfair status quo as the "way things are" (hegemony) and not to question the uncomfortable fact that some people are privileged and others disadvantaged. To bring this kind of awareness to the surface and to act on this awareness requires a great deal of courage, persistence, and the support of colleagues and allies who remain committed to action (Giddings, 2005a).

The creative processes that are used to develop emancipatory knowing are:

- Critiquing the status quo from every possible point of view (e.g., the lenses of race, ethnicity, class, gender, sexual orientation)
- Imagining what might be different to create a better world—one that is more equitable for all

The creative development processes of critiquing and imagining occur in complementary and often intersecting or overlapping approaches: grassroots activism and academic analysis. Each calls forth unique creative development methods. Grassroots activism brings together those most directly affected to discuss, identify, and define what is problematic from their perspective, and to imagine ways to create sustainable change. Academic analysis relies on scholarly approaches that have all too often been used as tools of oppression, but that can be put to use in an emancipatory context to liberate. The Internet provides a powerful avenue to bring together grassroots nurses and academic scholars who are concerned about pressing issues of social injustices in nursing and health care, and to communicate their emancipatory analyses to a broad audience. The Nurse Manifest Project ("Nurse Manifest Project," 2002) is an example that brings together nurses from all walks of life to examine issues vital to the practice of nursing. The purpose of the Center for Nursing Advocacy ("Center for Nursing Advocacy," 2003–2006) is to increase public understanding of nursing. The Center brings together diverse groups of nurses and focuses on a media-watch campaign that critiques public discourses and images of nursing and takes action calling for accurate and positive portrayals of nursing in the media.

Grassroots activism and academic analysis can both be used by people directly affected by an injustice, as well as by allies who are not directly affected, but who witness the plight of those who are. Allies join those directly affected to change the status quo and develop knowledge that will contribute to the fundamental social changes that are required. Allies who join the struggle for liberation have a responsibility to remain fully loyal to the perspectives and perceptions of those who are directly affected, in order to work toward effective solutions and develop useful knowledge. From a critical perspective, those who are directly affected are responsible to define what is problematic and to enact that which is required to achieve emancipation. The problem, and solutions or desired changes, must be grounded in grassroots experience.

Allies engage in grassroots activism and use academic analysis, not as experts or leaders, but as partners in the shared struggle to understand

and change unjust conditions. Allies recognize their relative privilege, and are obligated to carefully refrain from any action that would distort or diminish the experience of those directly affected by injustice. Allies rely on those who are directly affected, place utter trust in their judgments and perceptions, and remain loyal to their goals (Freire, 1970). Allies probe for possibilities that might not yet have entered full awareness, suggest alternative explanations that may or may not fit, share information that can contribute to understanding, and assist in applying methods for knowledge development that are needed in the project for change.

Emancipatory knowing can draw on any of the creative knowledge development processes used for empiric, ethical, personal, and aesthetic knowing. However, it assumes a deeper look into the problem, because praxis requires seeing what people are conditioned not to see. This "deeper look" typically emerges for individuals interacting in groups of people committed to addressing one or more of the critical questions of emancipatory knowing. Once an emancipatory critical question is posed and the problems begin to be defined in a new light, awareness begins to take shape concerning the circumstances that sustain what is problematic.

Empiric methods can be used to document the extent of the problem or the nature of the structures that sustain the status quo (see Chapter 9). For example, in a critical study to understand girls' experience of menarche and to create change toward a more healthy experience, the adolescent participants used a survey method to determine what menarche education approaches were being used in schools throughout their district. They also examined corporate reports to uncover the extent of profit being made by menstrual care products manufacturers that also produced the educational materials used in the schools. The participants used this information to affirm what they suspected—that menarche education was not adequate to meet the girls' real needs, but rather served the interests of powerful corporate entities (Hagedorn, 1995). In this study, the grassroots context was a high school setting where adolescent girls came together to explore their experiences of menarche and the meaning of their experience of menarche as constructed by larger social and political circumstances. The study also relied on academic support that placed the adolescent's insights and knowledge into a larger realm of knowledge development for nursing.

The methods used for developing ethical knowledge—valuing and clarifying—can be used to better understand dimensions of injustice (see Chapter 4). The manifesto of the Nurse Manifest Project was developed primarily from the extensive values clarification, dialogue, and justification work of the three authors (Cowling, Chinn, & Hagedorn, 2000). Their discussion raised awareness of a deep conflict between the values that nurses typically hold dear, and the values that are enacted by the systems in which they are employed. This underlying conflict of values was identified as the problem that was fundamental to the shortage of nursing. The manifesto project led the authors to imagine ways in which nursing values could be more fully realized, or manifested, in the practice of nursing. This project began with an academic analysis of ethical dimensions of nursing's core values and the exercise of those values in practice. Subsequently, grassroots nurses became centrally involved in studies to reveal more completely the actual experience of practicing nursing in the context of an acute nursing shortage.

The personal knowing processes of opening and centering are vital to the development of emancipatory knowing, in that the experience of those most deeply affected provides the substance required to define the problem (see Chapter 5). As an example, in a critical feminist study of the experience of practicing nursing today, nurses brought to their first group meeting an object or symbol that represented their personal experience of practicing nursing (codification). They shared the personal meanings embedded in their symbolic object and discussed the connections that their personal experience revealed. A food strainer brought to the group by a participant represented for her a feeling of loss of control of nursing practice, a personal sense that the other nurses in the group shared. As they shared personal meanings of feeling loss of control, they came to realize that this problem was not personal failure, but rather came from systematic structural problems in the ways nursing was institutionalized and practiced. They formed realizations of personal and collective actions that they could take to change the circumstances of practicing nursing (Jacobs, Fontana, Kehoe, Matarese, & Chinn, 2005).

The aesthetic methods of envisioning and rehearsing can be used in a wide range of art forms to reflect the depth of human suffering that the status quo sustains (see Chapter 6). Aesthetic methods are also crucial in portraying the social ideal that is sought. The codifications used by the nurses in the Jacobs study illustrate how simple objects can be used to symbolize a complex human experience (Jacobs et al., 2005). In the Nurse Manifest Project, the research team developed fictionalized "metastories" of nursing practice from stories told by practicing nurses of experiences in nursing, and Cowling created artistic representations to synthesize the powerful human experiences reflected in the collection of nurse stories ("Nurse Manifest 2002 Research Study Report," 2002). The grassroots stories were contributed by nurses throughout the world. The metastories and artwork were developed by the academic research team with the commitment to remain fully loyal to the full meaning as expressed by grassroots nurses. The stories and artwork bring into vivid focus the distress of practicing nursing, and in doing so project broad systematic changes that are needed to address what nurses need in order to form practice based on human caring values.

Grassroots and academic approaches can be used in any one project to develop emancipatory knowing/knowledge. Both approaches provide for critique of existing conditions that remain embedded in the experience of those who are disadvantaged. Both approaches also remain faithful to the emancipatory purpose of creating change that removes structural obstacles to equity and justice for all. However, each approach has unique characteristics, which we describe in the sections that follow.

Grassroots Approaches to Creative Development Processes

Grassroots creative development processes occur in small groups (face-to-face or virtual) where the focus is discussion of the experience and circumstances of those who are most directly disadvantaged—those who feel most acutely the disadvantage of their current social and political situation. Significant social change can arise from spontaneous discussions that center around growing awareness of something that is not right among a group of people. For example, the mid–20th-century women's movement in the United States grew out of spontaneously formed "consciousness-raising" groups, informally conducted in women's homes. From the early consciousness-raising groups grew dramatic theoretical insights, action plans for changing the conditions of women's lives, artistic expressions of women's experience, research that revealed vital knowledge concerning the extent and complexity of the problems, and fundamental social and political change.

The grassroots group process forms an emancipatory context in which people can openly and safely reveal the circumstances of inequity or suffering in their lives and seek to know that which is not yet known in order to transform the conditions of their lives. This context is created using a dialectic process of reflection and action that is embodied in dialogue, an essential element of which is critical reflection. In this context, critical reflection is: (Freire, 1970, p. 81)

- Discerning an indivisible solidarity between social and political conditions and the circumstances of the individual.
- Perceiving experience as process, potential and transformational, rather than as a static entity.
- Moving constantly from reflection to action, action to reflection without fear of the risks involved.

Members of the group share a mutual interest in changing the status quo and using discussion to raise everyone's awareness of the conditions that are sustaining the status quo. Simultaneously, the group analyzes that which limits full human potential and identifies what needs to change to create a more equitable, just, and nurturing future for all.

Emancipatory group process is grounded in Freire's (1970) approach; the specific approaches described here were developed by Chinn (2001). The group comes together out of a shared recognition that something is awry with the conditions of their lives. Often they do not have a clear idea as to exactly what is wrong, and typically they are not aware that others share similar experiences. Emancipatory group process is characterized by each person respectfully hearing and respecting the views of all participants, raising questions and suggesting possibilities to assist in discovering "background awareness" of the complexities of the situation, the contradictions between and among their various perspectives, and the most creative (sometimes outrageous) changes that might be made.

At the outset, the group considers codifications (pictures, stories, images) that represent their focal concern, or the problem or issue that has brought them together. Through discussion in which every voice is heard, the group members come to clarify and identify in new ways what is wrong with this picture (problematization) and begin to imagine what might be instead (untested feasibilities). The group also begins to imagine how they might bring about various possible alternatives (testing untested feasibilities). Based on these insights, actions begin to happen. Early actions are often changes that individuals begin to make in their own lives, followed by collective actions that the group pursues as a group or as individuals. Freire called this process in its entirety *conscientizacao,* a Portuguese term that "refers to learning to perceive social, political, and economic contradictions, and to take action against the oppressive element of reality" (Freire, 1970, p. 19). This emergent pattern is not orchestrated or in any way controlled or directed by any one member of the group. Rather, it is a process that emerges spontaneously in the group, arising from an innate human emancipatory interest (Freire, 1970; Habermas, 1979; Hagedorn, 1995). When leadership is needed, it arises from individuals in the group able and willing to assume leadership for the task at hand, not from socially prescribed roles that privilege some individuals above others.

Typically, group participants come together several times over a period of weeks or months. Individuals may or may not attend every meeting, and new members can join the group at any time. Continuity from time to time is maintained by a process of summarizing the insights at the end of each group meeting, and bringing that summary forward at the beginning of the next meeting. The process is circular rather than linear, which means that despite who is present, a constant process of reflection, reconsidering, and rethinking issues is valued, with new insights coming from each circular "turn" that is made in the process of discussion and analysis. All participants can make notations and personal journal entries to retain ideas and insights during the discussion as well as to provide a point of reference for reflection between the group meetings. Participants continue their critical dialogue around the codifications, engaging also in a process of "decoding" that involves considering all possible circumstances that create and sustain the situation as it is, and forming ideas about what could be instead.

As discussion progresses, participants begin to explore meaningful themes and links between themes. They begin to pose the themes as problems, to situate the problems in their historical, cultural, political, and socioeconomic context. From the themes, the participants also explore the circumstances that maintain the status quo—the existence of persons or circumstances that are directly or indirectly served by the status quo and persons or circumstances that are negated and disadvantaged by the status quo. Out of this analysis, actions that would be required to change the status quo are identified, and the feasibility of taking action is explored.

Academic Approaches to Creative Development Processes

Academic creative development processes must grow out of an alliance with grassroots experience. In some circumstances, people who directly experience disadvantage can pursue academic processes. In others, such as the projects of liberation (literacy education) that Freire (1970) described in his early work, the disadvantage of those directly affected requires the support and participation of those who are educationally advantaged. Allies who have the skills to pursue academic development processes remain with the people but are not the people. Allies provide insights and knowledge that might not otherwise be possible and that can be crucial in creating the social changes that are required. Allies remain acutely aware that people who are oppressed are typically not heard and are very often silenced by those who do not share their experience. Allies are constantly self-reflective and open to the criticisms of others to ensure that they remain loyal to grassroots perspectives and that they do not take any path that would distort or diminish the experience of those who are disadvantaged. As Freire explains, allies are obligated to enter into the project of liberation with full love and trust of those who are oppressed (Freire, 1970).

Various academic disciplines have developed approaches for creating emancipatory knowledge, such as critical feminist and critical social analysis, as well poststructuralist analysis. The data for analysis can be drawn from any variety of images such as art, popular culture, advertisements, interview data or data from persons gathered in any number of ways, or written accounts that reflect the status quo. Regardless of data source or method, emancipatory approaches cross disciplinary lines that have falsely fragmented knowing and knowledge and have not served the best interests of society. Disciplinary lines have also sustained the academic heritage of the "ivory tower," which distances academic thinking and processes from the grassroots experiences of people in society. Without denying the valuable contributions of various disciplines to society and human welfare, the realization remains that disciplinary lines have tended to limit the creative development process, resulting in limited explanations for many of the world's most persistent social problems.

Regardless of the specific methods used, academic emancipatory processes are characterized by a fundamental critical perspective—a perspective that: (Fontana, 2004; Freire, 1970; Morrow, 1994)

- Uncovers hidden ideologic premises embedded in social structures
- Examines that which is assumed, or is presupposed in that which is taken as knowledge or truth, revealing assumptions that are false
- Unveils conventions of language and symbols that are used to represent the situation
- Challenges current institutionalized power relations
- Trusts and remains loyal to grassroots experience, to the perspectives of the people, without assuming the right to speak for the people
- Projects actions and processes that are envisioned to change the status quo and create equitable social relationships
- Calls forth a self-reflexive attitude that constantly challenges one's own understandings

Taken together, these traits of a critical perspective reveal its explicitly political and value-laden stance, while maintaining the highest standards of academic rigor. From a critical perspective, all academic processes used to develop knowledge are inherently value-laden despite traditional scientific claims to the contrary. Traditional approaches that claim to be value-free are in fact viewed as compromising the scientific standards of rigor that call for full disclosure of the limitations of the work, the particular perspective that is assumed, and the ultimate goals that the work serves. For example, most academic products come from a Eurocentric, male, heterosexual, economically privileged perspective; however, this perspective is very rarely acknowledged as a limitation of the knowledge claims that are published. Critical perspectives require that those participating in the work bring to conscious awareness and disclose their own personal perspectives, and that they share their intentions related to their work. By making their perspective clear, the values that underpin the work are made accessible for challenge, discussion, and debate. The overriding intention is to deepen explicit ethical commitments to full human health and well-being for all, and to act upon those commitments (Fontana, 2004; Freire, 1970; Thomas, 1993).

Discourse and Language. Fundamental to academic emancipatory process is a concern for the language used to talk and write about a concern or a situation. Once assumed to be a neutral representation of observations and experiences, language has come to be recognized as mediating and creating meanings (Hardin, 2001; Muller & Dzurec, 1993; van Dijk, 1997). In other words, how people write, speak, or communicate is shaped by and shapes the larger social, cultural, and political context within which they live their personal and professional lives.

There are many approaches to the academic study of language (Hardin, 2001; van Dijk, 1997). Early approaches reflected the prevailing scientific paradigm of the mid–20th century and focused on understanding language as a stable system with a uniform, decontextualized meaning and order (Kress, 2001). Eventually the meanings of words were seen to be dependent on context. For example, consider the multiple meanings of the word "patient" and how, without seeing or hearing the word used in a sentence, you do not know if it is to be taken as a personal characteristic ("being a patient person") or as a term for a person who is hospitalized. The idea of uniform meanings for "speech utterances" gave way to an understanding that the intentions of the user, voice inflections, gestures, and how words were linked together and embedded in a language system were important for conveying and understanding meaning (de Beaugrande, 1997). As the role of context for understanding meaning became clearer, the search for "rules" governing language began to give way and a structuralist understanding of language emerged. Structuralism acknowledged that language practices are structured by a context of use that reflects the broader social, cultural, and political situation in which language is used.

With the influence of Foucault and Derrida, the study of language began a transition from structuralist understandings into poststructuralism. From a poststructuralist perspective, language does not merely reflect a contextually embedded meaning, but rather is constructive of meaning. For poststructuralists, nothing "is" prior to its manifestation in language (Hall, 2001). In other words, language creates meanings; we do not "have language," but rather "language has us." Commonly language is assumed to be something that follows from experience and is named. In contrast, from a poststructuralist point of view, language and systems of discourse create perceptions of the world and how it is understood. When language, symbolic representations, and systems of discourse consistently represent experience in a given way (e.g., thin women are more beautiful than heavy women), those representations are taken as the norm. Eventually normative representations become understood as "truth"; a truth that is not often or easily questioned and people's behavior becomes consistent with the "constructed truths."

Poststructuralist theory deals with how language and discourses tune people in to what is going on around them. When people have no language or discourse expressions for what is going on, it simply does not exist for them. For example, when the word "man" was used as a generic term to include women and other gender configurations, the subjugation of women as an outcome of this language practice was simply not recognized or perceived and was often denied as a possibility. In cultures where there is no language for lesbian, gay, bisexual, or transgendered experience, these experiences are not perceived as existing or possible. When the term *nurse* is taken to mean "female nurse," the possibility of a man who is a nurse is not perceived, and the qualifier "male" is required to bring this particular instance to awareness.

Critical poststructuralist analysis, with its emphasis on how systems of language and discourse create and reinscribe beliefs and values, is a valuable approach to uncovering representations that maintain oppressive boundaries. Analyzing what is not said, what is not represented, and how representations intersect and converge to maintain what is constructed as "truth" can allow ideas for changing the status quo to emerge.

FORMAL EXPRESSIONS OF EMANCIPATORY KNOWLEDGE

Out of the creative processes emerge the communicable products of emancipatory knowing (emancipatory knowledge), which can take a number of forms. Manifestoes are action-oriented and impassioned portrayals of that which is problematic, actions required to effect change, and descriptions of the ideals that are envisioned. Formal expressions include a critical analysis of what is, how it came to be, and who is disadvantaged, as well as a detailed description of what is envisioned for the future and what is required to reach that which is envisioned.

Some grassroots projects do not immediately result in formal expression because of the primary commitment to act, to move emancipatory insights directly into action that can alleviate suffering and remove barriers to human freedom. Formal expressions, regardless of specific form, remain grounded in a critical perspective that reveals false assumptions, critiques representations of what is, challenges the status quo, unveils hidden and systematic practices that sustain the status quo, and explains what could be in place of the status quo. Critical expressions or writings are deliberately value-laden. They reveal explicit political agendas grounded in the intention to free people from constraints that disadvantage their development of full human potential. They include critiques that originate in emancipatory knowledge development processes and, from those critiques, project a vision of the changes that are needed to create social equity and justice.

Formal expressions can take any imaginable form, including drawings, sculptures, fictionalized stories, or poems, which portray the distress of disadvantage, a vision for the future, or both. Action plans, blueprints for the future, and manifestoes are typically written works that draw on theoretical reasoning as well as grassroots experience. The expressions explain critical insights concerning the situation as it is and how it came about, as well as visions for what could be in the future and how it is possible to move in that direction—based on explicit values and goals for human well-being. Chinn's (2007) "Challenge to Action" is an example of a critical analysis based on theoretical analysis and on critical reflection of personal experience in nursing, and includes a call for action to create a future for nursing that is grounded in emancipatory insights.

The Nurse Manifest Project provides an example of an alliance between grassroots nurses and academic nurses who have joined together "to raise awareness, to inspire action, and to open discussion of issues that are vital to nursing and health care around the globe" (Cowling et al., 2000; Jarrin, 2006). This project also combined grassroots approaches and academic approaches in creating emancipatory knowledge. The project began with the web-based publication of a manifesto that opens with an explicit statement of the concerns and values from which the project began:

> As nurses, we reach for meaningful expressions of our values, too often finding overwhelming constraint and resistance, sometimes within ourselves and sometimes imposed from without. We are calling for a movement to awaken those precious and powerful ideals that are rooted in nursing's worldwide historical traditions. We call forth the written and spoken voice of nursing to be claimed and reclaimed. We seek to inspire the fullest expression of the heart of nursing through individual and collective acts. We believe there are profound possibilities in claiming our individual and professional sovereignty. (www.nursemanifest.com/manifesto.htm)

The first major study of the project, completed in 2002, engaged the participation of nurses worldwide to tell their stories of what it was like to practice nursing. From their stories, the research team developed metastories and artwork to express the meanings conveyed in nurses' accounts of their practice. The works from this study can be viewed at www.nursemanifest.com/2002studyreport.htm ("Nurse Manifest 2002 Research Study Report," 2002).

Formal theoretical analyses tend to be labeled with the term *critical* to specify the critical perspective that informs the work and to suggest the methodological tradition from which the creative processes for development were drawn. The phrase *critical social theory* suggests a sociological approach. *Critical ethnography* suggests an anthropological approach that examines structures and practices that sustain social inequities within a culture. *Critical feminist theory* examines the conditions and outcomes of inequities that affect women. *Critical poststructural* approaches analyze how language and systems of discourse construct particular meanings as "truth"—a "truth" that can be shown to reinscribe injustices and inequities.

Giddings' (2005a) model of social consciousness is an example of a formal theoretical outcome of a critical feminist research study (Giddings, 2005b). Giddings interviewed nurses in the United States and New Zealand who identified with the dominant Eurocentric culture, the experience of being lesbian, or the experience of being a racial minority (African American in the United States or Maori in New Zealand). The nurses were invited to participate in the study because of their reputations as people who actively engaged in advocating for others who were disadvantaged. The purpose of the study was to explore how they became aware of the plight of those who were disadvantaged, how they came to speak up and act on their behalf, and what their experience of doing so in nursing had been. Based on their life stories, Giddings developed a model of social consciousness that provides explanations of the challenges and barriers to nurses acting from their awareness of injustices in health care (Giddings, 2005a).

PRAXIS AND PROCESSES OF AUTHENTICATION

The disciplinary processes for authenticating emancipatory knowing/knowledge involve affirming the sustainability of real change and transformation, empowerment for all, social equity, and demystification of that which was previously hidden. The authentication processes require ongoing engagement of thoughtful reflection and action—the processes of praxis.

Methods for authenticating emancipatory knowledge can be drawn from any of the fundamental patterns of knowing. Analyses, action plans, statements of future visions, and manifestoes can be examined using processes of dialogue and justification, validation and confirmation, response and reflection, and inspiration and appreciation. However, the process of praxis itself, when engaged in a collective sense, is the most important form of authentication. When authentication processes are used with an eye toward uncovering, understanding, and rectifying injustices and unfair social practices, praxis is enabled. Praxis, collectively engaged, ensures a constant process of engagement in thoughtful reflection and action to transform the world. With each turn of reflection and action, at least four ideals are used as a benchmark for determining the worth and validity of emancipatory knowing/knowledge:

Sustainability refers to how well the envisioned social change survives and thrives.

Social equity refers to a demonstrable elimination or reduction of conditions that create disadvantage for some and advantage for others.

Empowerment refers to the growing ability of individuals and groups to exercise their will, to have their voices heard, and to claim their full human potential.

Demystification refers to making things that were formerly hidden from understanding visible and openly disclosed.

REFLECTION AND DISCUSSION

In this chapter we have presented our conceptualization of an emancipatory pattern of knowing in nursing—a pattern of knowing that challenges existing social and political circumstances that limit human potential and creates structural shifts toward social justice for all. This pattern of knowing has longstanding roots in nursing, but has not been generally recognized as inherent and essential for nurses and nursing. The central message of this chapter is that emancipatory knowing is foundational to nursing's commitment to develop knowledge that will lead to the fulfillment of full human potential for all, and to high-level wellness for individuals, families, and societies.

To deepen your appreciation of emancipatory knowing, consider the following questions related to the content of this chapter:

1. Recall a situation in which you recognized that someone was being treated unfairly. How did others in the situation react? Did anyone speak up at the time? If they did, how did others respond? What could have happened to change the situation? What needs to happen differently in other similar circumstances? What could prevent this from happening in the future? What was at the root of this unfair treatment?

2. What do you know of the experience and perspective of others who would identify as having a different sexual orientation or identity?

A different gender? A different racial or ethnic heritage? Any other imaginable difference? Think about some ways that you might gain a fuller appreciation and respect for those who would speak from these different perspectives. Why is it necessary for anyone to gain a fuller appreciation and respect in the first place?

3. Do you have a language for the experience of taking into account preferences or points of view that do not coincide with your own, and working to achieve a solution to a problem that addresses all points of view? Consider a situation where three nurses working together have very different ideas about caring for people who refuse treatment on the basis of their religion. What language possibilities can you think of to describe reaching a point of understanding among the three nurses that respects each nurse's point of view? What actions would each term imply?

4. Divide a sheet of paper into two columns. In one column list all the ways in which you are relatively privileged. In the other list all the way in which you are disadvantaged. Which of your lists is longer? What are the circumstances that contribute to your various privileges, and what are the circumstances that contribute to your disadvantages? What would it take to change any of these circumstances? Are any of the circumstances things you alone can change? Whose privilege are your disadvantages contributing to? What maintains, or has maintained, your position of privilege? Who benefits?

5. Go into a group—a meeting, a classroom, or an informal social gathering—and place yourself in a position to observe what happens in the group. Who dominates or leads? Who is left out or ignored? What characteristics are typical of those who dominate or lead? What characteristics are typical of those who are left out or ignored? Does anyone make attempts to participate that are ignored or disregarded? Does anyone in the group speak up or act on behalf of a person who is ignored or disregarded? What cultural or social traditions or rituals contribute to the power dynamics in the group?

6. Select an object or picture that is symbolic of a difficult situation you are experiencing. Place this object in front of you and write a brief explanation of the connection between this object and your experience. If possible, share this exercise with a few others who are also experiencing the same or a similar situation, and discuss your various symbolic objects and what they mean. What do you learn?

7. Identify some situation you believe is unjust, or unfair to a group of persons. Who or what is benefiting from this situation? Do you benefit and how?

8. Leaf through a popular magazine marketed to some group, such as *Ladies Home Journal, Family Circle, Gentlemen's Quarterly, Men's Health, Modern Maturity*—pick something of interest. How does the magazine maintain or undo stereotypes? Why is either (maintaining or undoing) necessary?

9. Identify some situation of personal privilege. Who or what contributed to your privilege? Would you give up your privilege so others could benefit?

10. Identify some situations that are, or that you believe are, "closed" to you but available to others like you. What is the basis for your feelings of exclusion? Do you believe this is fair? Necessary?

11. In what ways do mass media perpetuate unfair and unjust beliefs about a group of people? Why is this happening?

12. How is the typical hospital an oppressive place? What would you change about it and why? How would you go about changing it?

13. Talk with a classmate (or another person) who is not "like you" in some significant way—if you are healthy, perhaps someone who has a disability, or someone who is much older, or much younger, has a different sexual orientation or identity, is from a different country, etc. How is their experience of the world different from yours, or is it? Why?

Reference List

Allan, J. D., & Hall, B. A. (1988). Challenging the focus on technology: A critique of the medical model in a changing health care system. *ANS. Advances In Nursing Science, 10*(3), 22–34.

Allen, D. (1985). Nursing research and social control: Alternative models of science that emphasize understanding and emancipation. *Image—The Journal of Nursing Scholarship, 17*(2), 58–74.

Allen, D. (1986). Nursing and oppression: "The family" in nursing texts. *Feminist Teacher, 2*(1), 15–20.

Allen, D. (1987). Professionalism, occupational segregation by gender and control of nursing. *Women and Politics, 6*(3), 1–24.

Allen, D., Allman, K. K. M., & Powers, P. (1991). Feminist nursing research without gender. *ANS. Advances in Nursing Science, 13*(3), 49–58.

Ashley, J. (1976). *Hospitals, paternalism, and the role of the nurse.* New York: Teachers College Press.

Boutain, D. M. (1999). Critical nursing scholarship: Exploring critical social theory with African American studies. *ANS. Advances in Nursing Science, 21*(4), 37–47.

Browne, A. J. (2001). The influence of liberal political ideology on nursing science. *Nursing Inquiry, 8*(2), 118–129.

Bunting, S., & Campbell, J. C. (1990). Feminism and nursing: Historical perspectives. *ANS. Advances in Nursing Science, 12*(4), 11–24.

Butterfield, P. G. (2002). Upstream reflections on environmental health: An abbreviated history and framework for action. *ANS. Advances in Nursing Science, 25*(1), 32–49.

Campbell, J. C., & Bunting, S. (1991). Voices and paradigms: Perspectives on critical and feminist theory in nursing. *ANS. Advances in Nursing Science, 13*(3), 1–15.

Carper, B. A. (1978). Fundamental patterns of knowing in nursing. *ANS. Advances in Nursing Science, 1*(1), 13–23.

Cassandra: Radical Feminist Nurses Newsjournal. (1982–1989). Available at http://ans-info.net/PLC.htm#Cassandra.

Center for Nursing Advocacy: Increasing public understanding of nursing. (2003–2006). Retrieved October 11, 2006, www.nursingadvocacy.org/news/news.html.

Charleston Faculty Practice Conference Group. (1986). Nursing faculty collaboration viewed through feminist process. *ANS. Advances in Nursing Science, 8*(2), 29–38.

Chinn, P. L. (1989). Nursing patterns of knowing and feminist thought. *Nursing and Health Care, 10*(2), 71–75.

Chinn, P. L. (1995). Feminism and nursing. In J. J. Fitzpatrick & J. S. Stevenson (Eds.), *Annual review of nursing research* (Vol. 13, pp. 267–289). New York: Springer Publishing.

Chinn, P. L. (2001). *Peace & power: Building communities for the future* (5th ed.). Sudbury, MA: Jones & Bartlett.

Chinn, P. L. (2004). *Peace & power: Creative leadership for building communities* (6th ed.). Boston: Jones & Bartlett.

Chinn, P. L. (2007). Challenge to action. In S. C. Roy & D. A. Jones (Eds.), *Nursing knowledge development and clinical practice* (pp. 93–101). New York: Springer Publishing.

Chinn, P. L., & Wheeler, C. E. (1985). Feminism and nursing. *Nursing Outlook, 33*(2), 74–77.

Cloyes, K. G. (2006). An ethic of analysis: An argument for critical analysis of research interviews as an ethical practice. *ANS. Advances in Nursing Science, 29*(2), 84–97.

Cowling, W. R., Chinn, P. L., & Hagedorn, S. (2000). *The Nurse Manifesto.* Retrieved September 28, 2006, from www.nursemanifest.com.

de Beaugrande, R. (1997). The story of discourse analysis. In T. A. van Dijk (Ed.), *Discourse as structure and process: Discourse studies: A multidisciplinary introduction* (Vol. 1, pp. 35–62). London: Sage.

Dock, L. L. (1902–1903). Sanitary inspection: a new field for nurses. *American Journal of Nursing, 3,* 529–532.

Doering, L. (1992). Power and knowledge in nursing: A feminist poststructuralist view. *ANS. Advances in Nursing Science, 14*(4), 24–33.

Dzurec, L. C. (1989). The necessity for and evolution of multiple paradigms for nursing research: A poststructuralist perspective. *ANS. Advances in Nursing Science, 11*(4), 69–77.

Falk-Rafael, A. R. (2006). Globalization and global health: Toward nursing praxis in the global community. *ANS. Advances in Nursing Science, 29*(1), 2–14.

Fontana, J. S. (2004). A methodology for critical science in nursing. *ANS. Advances in Nursing Science, 27*(2), 93–101.

Foucault, M. (1980). *Power/knowledge: Selected interviews and other writing 1972–1977.* New York: Pantheon.

Foucault, M. (1984). *The Foucault reader.* New York: Pantheon.

Freire, P. (1972). *Pedagogy of the oppressed.* (M.B. Ramos, Trans.). New York: Herder and Herder.

Georges, J. M. (2005). The politics of suffering: Implications for nursing science. *ANS. Advances in Nursing Science, 27*(4), 250–256.

Giddings, L. S. (2005a). A theoretical model of social consciousness. *ANS. Advances in Nursing Science, 28*(3), 224–239.

Giddings, L. S. (2005b). Health disparities, social injustice, and the culture of nursing. *Nursing Research, 54*(5), 304–312.

Habermas, J. (1973). *Theory and practice* (J. Viertel, Trans.). Boston: Beacon.

Habermas, J. (1979). *Communication and the evolution of society.* (T. McCarthy, Trans.). Boston: Beacon.

Hagedorn, S. (1995). The politics of caring: The role of activism in primary care. *ANS. Advances in Nursing Science, 17*(4), 1–11.

Hall, L. E. (1966). Another view of nursing care and quality. In K. M. Straub & K. S. Parker (Eds.), *Continuity in patient care: The role of nursing.* Washington, DC: Catholic University Press.

Hall, S. (2001). Foucault: Power, knowledge and discourse. In M. Wetherell, S. Taylor & S. J. Yates (Eds.), *Discourse theory and practice* (pp. 72–81). Thousand Oaks, CA: Sage.

Hardin, P. K. (2001). Theory and language: Locating agency between free will and discursive marionettes. *Nursing Inquiry, 8*(1), 11–18.

Hardin, P. K. (2003). Social and cultural considerations in recovery from anorexia nervosa: A critical poststructural analysis. *ANS. Advances in Nursing Science, 26*(1), 7–18.

Hedin, B. A. (1986). A case study of oppressed group behavior in nurses. *Image—The Journal of Nursing Scholarship, 18*(2), 53–57.

Heide, W. S. (1973). Nursing and women's liberation. *American Journal of Nursing, 73*(5), 824–827.

hooks, b. (1993). Bell hooks speaking about Paulo Freire—The man, his work. In P. McLaren & P. Leonard (Eds.), *Paulo Freire: A critical encounter* (pp. 146–154). London: Routledge.

Jacobs, B. B., Fontana, J. S., Kehoe, M. H., Matarese, C., & Chinn, P. L. (2005). An emancipatory study of contemporary nursing practice. *Nursing Outlook, 53*, 6–14.

Jacobs-Kramer, M., & Chinn, P. L. (1988). Perspectives on knowing: A model of nursing knowledge. *Scholarly Inquiry for Nursing Practice, 2*(2), 129–139.

Jarrin, O. F. (2006). Results from the Nurse Manifest 2003 study: Nurses' perspectives on nursing. *ANS. Advances in Nursing Science, 29*(2), E74–E85.

Kagan, P. N. (2006). JoAnn Ashley 30 years later: Legacy for practice. *Nursing Science Quarterly, 19*(4), 317–327.

Kleffel, D. (1991). Rethinking the environment as a domain of nursing knowledge. *ANS. Advances in Nursing Science, 14*(1), 40–51.

Kress, G. (2001). From Saussure to critical sociolinguistics: The turn towards a social view of language. In M. Wetherell, S. Taylor & S. J. Yeats (Eds.), *Discourse theory and practice* (pp. 29–38). London: Sage.

MacPherson, K. I. (1985). Osteoporosis and menopause: A feminist analysis of the social construction of a syndrome. *ANS. Advances in Nursing Science, 7*(4), 11–22.

MacPherson, K. I. (1989). A new perspective on nursing and caring in a corporate context. *ANS. Advances in Nursing Science, 11*(4), 32–39.

Mohammed, S. A. (2006). Moving beyond the "exotic": Applying postcolonial theory in health research. *ANS. Advances in Nursing Science, 29*(2), 98–109.

Morrow, R. A. (1994). *Critical theory and methodology* (Vol. 3). Thousand Oaks, CA: Sage.

Muller, M. E., & Dzurec, L. C. (1993). The power of the name. *ANS. Advances in Nursing Science, 15*(3), 15–22.

Nightingale, F. (1979). *Cassandra.* New York: Feminist Press.

Nurse Manifest 2002 research study report. (2002). Retrieved September 30, 2006, from www.nursemanifest.com/2002studyreport.htm.

Nurse Manifest Project. (2002). Retrieved December 4, 2006, from www.nursemanifest.com.

Poslusny, S. M. (1989). Feminist friendship: Isabel Hampton Robb, Lavinia Lloyd Dock, and Mary Adelaide Nutting. *Image—The Journal of Nursing Scholarship, 21*(2), 64–68.

Roberts, S. J. (1983). Oppressed group behavior: Implications for nursing. *ANS. Advances in Nursing Science, 5*(4), 21–30.

Thomas, J. (1993). *Doing critical ethnography.* Newbury Park, CA: Sage.

Thompson, J. L. (1987). Critical scholarship: The critique of domination in nursing. *ANS. Advances in Nursing Science, 10*(1), 27–38.

Thompson, J. L. (1991). Exploring gender and culture with Khmer refugee women: Reflections on participatory feminist research. *ANS. Advances in Nursing Science, 13*(3), 30–48.

van Dijk, T. A. (1997). The study of discourse. In T. A. van Dijk (Ed.), *Discourse as structure and process: Discourse studies: A multidisciplinary introduction* (Vol. 1, pp. 1–34). London: Sage.

Webb, C. (1993). Feminist research: Definitions, methodology, methods and evaluation. *Journal of Advanced Nursing, 18*(4), 416–423.

Weiler, K. (1991). Freire and a feminist pedagogy of difference. *Harvard Educational Review, 61* (4), 449–474.

White, J. (1995). Patterns of knowing: Review, critique, and update. *ANS. Advances in Nursing Science, 17*(4), 73–86.

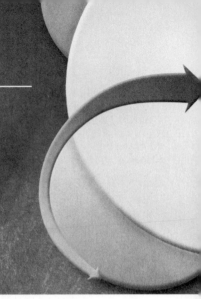

CHAPTER 4

Ethical Knowledge Development

Certain fundamental ethical principles are universal and unchangeable, but the interpretation and application of truth changes and different people arrive at truth by widely different methods.... Adults who are dominated by the opinions of the herd may be morally retarded. We do not act morally unless we act from a sense of conviction and reason, guided by our own conscience.

Isabel Stewart (1922, pp. 906, 909)

In this chapter we focus on methods for creating ethical knowledge. Figure 4-1 shows the quadrant of our model pertaining to the development of this pattern of nursing knowledge. The figure highlights the creative processes of valuing and clarifying as central for the generation of ethical knowledge forms for nursing, shown in the figure as principles and codes. Other forms of ethical knowledge are possible—for example, ethical theories—but we have chosen the forms shown in the model for their central importance to practice.

Like the other patterns, ethical knowledge development begins with ethical knowing. Nurses, regardless of setting, bring to practice the heritage of their own moral development and understandings. With this background, nurses reflect on their practice and begin to ask the following questions, "Is this right?" and "Is this responsible?" These questions set into motion

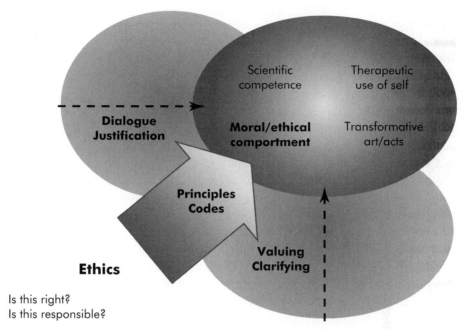

FIGURE 4-1   Valuing and clarifying ethical situations to create formal expressions of ethical knowledge that provide a foundation for moral/ethical comportment.

the processes of valuing and clarifying. As these questions are answered, knowledge that can be shared is developed. Through the collective disciplinary processes of dialogue and justification, ethical knowledge is evaluated and understood in relation to practice.

According to our model, nurses who practice using ethical knowledge that has been strengthened through disciplinary processes of dialogue and justification can be expected to increasingly practice with moral/ethical comportment. Moral/ethical comportment, expressed in practice as integrated knowing, can undergo further questioning: Is this right? Is this responsible? As this occurs, the stage is set for the ongoing processes of valuing and clarifying.

In this chapter we begin with a discussion about the nature of ethical and moral knowledge in nursing. Then we consider the processes and forms of ethical knowledge development in nursing that are shown in the model.

ETHICS, MORALITY, AND NURSING

Clearly nursing is a profession that requires ethical knowledge to guide practice. Whether a seasoned nurse or a beginning student, whether working in a high-tech intensive care environment or in a rural, isolated elementary school, the outcomes depend on the nurse's ethical knowing and morality. According to Levine (1989), all nursing actions are moral statements. We would add that all nursing actions also are ethical statements. But what constitutes ethical behavior? And how is morality determined? These are difficult questions to answer, and even when every effort is made to address ethical issues fully and appropriately, there is no guarantee that the right decision will be made. Whether the business of ethics really is more complex today than it was historically is questionable, but certainly the need to make ethical decisions has always been part of the modern nurse's role. Ethics is receiving renewed emphasis today and nursing organizations are deliberately focusing on the need to attend to ethical issues. Certainly, the complexity of today's health care arena has raised questions about what is ethical behavior. Advances in technology, concerns over the proper care of marginalized groups, laws regulating disclosure in health care and research practices, and a focus on the rights of individuals in the health care system are but a few factors that have contributed to the unbelievable complexity of ethical decisions, creating confusion about what is the morally right thing to do.

Ethics and *morality* are commonly interchanged and used synonymously in the nursing literature. We see ethics and morality as meshed and use both terms together in this chapter and elsewhere in this book. The distinction between ethics and morality reflects the tension between epistemology and ontology and the difficulty of separating what we know from who we are. In general, ethics relates to matters of epistemology, or knowledge, whereas morality focuses on ontology, or being. Ethics is a discipline that structures knowledge, a branch of inquiry that tries to make sense of what is right or wrong. Ethics, then, is more like head work, the products of which are things such as ethical principles, theories, rules, codes, and laws; lists of obligations or duties; and descriptions of ethical/moral behavior.

There are two branches of ethics—descriptive and prescriptive. Descriptive ethics is an empiric endeavor that systematizes what people believe ethically and how they behave in relation to those beliefs. For example, suppose you conducted a survey of your student peers and asked the following: (1) "Is it wrong to use purchased term papers about nurse theorists and their work to fulfill course requirements?" and (2) "Have you ever done this?" Collating and reporting their answers would be in the realm of descriptive ethics. Prescriptive, or normative, ethics is concerned with the "oughts" of behavior. Using cognitive reasoning processes that incorporate emotional and other nonrational sources of behavior, prescriptions for ethical behavior are put into language and set forth as theories, codes, duties, principles, and so forth. Using the student peer survey example, you might reason how and why it is not permissible to purchase term papers to meet college course requirements by invoking a rule that deception is wrong. In this example, such a practice could be understood as deceiving faculty who expect you to do your own work. It also might be understood as self-deceit because thoroughly learning about a theorist's work is short-circuited by simply reading a paper, rather than composing it. You might, as a result of your logical thought processes, propose an addition to the student code of ethical behavior in your school. In our example, then, the use of descriptive ethics (what is, with regard to beliefs and actions about term paper purchase) might reveal that prescriptions for ethical behavior need clarification because they are being violated (such practices are deceitful and therefore wrong). Notice that in this example that the need for ethical directives around purchasing papers on the Internet would not have been necessary, or even seen as a possibility, 50 years ago. In this text our focus is on prescriptive ethics, but it is important to recognize the value of descriptive ethics for examining the nature of ethical knowledge in nursing.

Morality, by contrast, is expressed in behavior and grounded in values. If ethics is head work, you might think of morality as heart work that is expressed in doing. Morality refers to our day-to-day living expressions of what we believe to be good, beliefs that are firmly embedded in our character. When people consistently behave in concert with their values, moral integrity is shown. When moral behavior is blocked by situational factors in a way that matters to persons, moral distress results. For example, if ethically you believe it important to obey Provision 1 of the American Nurses Association Code of Ethics for Nurses, which states that you should practice with compassion and respect for the dignity and worth of every individual (www.nursingworld.org/ethics/ecode.htm), and time constraints due to a heavy patient load prohibit you from doing this in ways that really matter to you, you will experience moral distress.

Morality is determined largely by situational and background experiences. Although people can appeal to ethical codes or principles to justify their actions, more often morality is shown on a less deliberative and conscious level. Daily expressions of belief about the right, the good, and the decent are filtered through lenses that are influenced by family, friends, religion, gender, and developmental stage. Thus, what constitutes moral behavior can vary, and what is important in one society, for example being on time out of respect for others, may be unimportant in another. A religious affiliation associated with one community may provide a lens that justifies war; another affiliation may offer a lens that justifies pacifism.

Morality and ethics interrelate in that ethical knowledge can provide a basis, or template, for judging and evaluating moral standards and behavior. Consider the example of the Patients' Bill of Rights in Medicare and Medicaid that was finalized in 1999 (www.hhs.gov/news/press/1999pres/990412.html). One of eight directives states, in part, that patients have the right to have the confidentiality of their individually identifiable health care information protected. Suppose one day as you worked your shift in a long-term care facility you overheard a well-meaning social worker talking with a nursing attendant in a hallway. The social worker was helping the attendant understand the nature of a resident's dementia while visitors and other residents walked by. Because the resident was identified by name in the conversation, this activity clearly constituted a breach of right to privacy as guaranteed in the Patients' Bill of Rights. Because right to privacy (the ethical directive) was breached, the behavior of the social worker and attendant could be judged as immoral. Within some systems of ethical reasoning, *intent* of the participants is important in ethical decision making. In this instance, the social worker had good intentions of helping the attendant better care for the resident. Might the extent to which the social worker's actions would be judged immoral change if the participants "knew better" but "just didn't care"? Regardless of how an incident such as this breach of confidentiality would be judged in relation to morality, it does violate a justifiable ethical directive. Several courses of action might be appropriate, including posting the Patients' Bill of Rights in a public space as a reminder of its meaning, or approaching the social worker and aide and bringing to their attention the inappropriateness of their behavior in reference to privacy protections.

Not only can ethical directives be used to judge the morality of behavior, but the converse is true. Moral or immoral behavior can provide a template for judging ethical knowledge. Using another example from the Medicare–Medicaid Bill of Rights, another ethical directive states that patients must take greater responsibility for maintaining good health. On your same shift in the long-term care facility, you notice that a newly employed nursing attendant has taken this directive to heart and is encouraging a resident with compromised cognitive function to take more responsibility for his self-care. Given the resident's cognitive state, you understand that the attendant is asking the resident to do things that are physiologically impossible, and, as a result, the resident's health is being compromised. In this example, the attendant attempts to behave morally in light of the directive, but is unknowingly compromising other ethical principles generally accepted in health care, for example the prescription to "do no harm." In this instance, the attendant's moral expression of the ethical directive is helpful in realizing that the directive needs to be changed or clarified for persons whose cognitive function is not intact.

Although the foregoing examples are fairly obvious and straightforward, not all knowing related to ethics is that clear cut. Rather, much moral behavior is fluid, occurs in the moment without time for contemplation, and depends on situational understandings and circumstances. As an example, suppose you felt justified in providing information to a patient who asked you about alternative health care practices when you knew the primary physician was not willing to supply any information about their use. When the physician discovers you have provided this information, she asks to talk with you about it. It turns out that both you and the physician felt that your respective actions were morally right. You "felt the patient had the right to know" and thus used precepts around a patient's right to information to justify your action. The physician, on the other hand, provided reasons that indicated her intent was to "do no harm." The physician stated that in the past she had given the same information to the patient, who had not acted on the information and subsequently became extremely anxious about making treatment choices. In short, your action of providing information based on the patient's right to know (autonomy) was judged as the right thing, whereas the physician, by withholding information, was doing the right thing by protecting the patient's vulnerabilities (doing no harm) based on reasonable knowledge about the patient's condition. In this instance, the physician provided you with a perspective about the right thing to do that you can draw on in the future.

Sometimes when moral positions of physician and nurse collide, both positions are reasonable and both parties to the moral positions hold strong beliefs about their correctness. In these instances there may be no clear answers about how to proceed, and it becomes important to identify the political processes that are operating. If the client's welfare is the concern for both parties, then the nurse and physician should be successful in engaging in dialogue that questions how right and responsible any decision is. Through this process, both physician and nurse (and client when feasible) can come to more fully understand the nature of the decision to be made and its potential outcomes. If the nurse's or physician's attitude reflects more of a power-over, controlling, or paternalistic position in relation to the client, other strategies may be warranted. In this instance the nurse and physician should recognize the nature of power imbalances and how they are sustained and seek avenues related to emancipatory knowing that fundamentally will undermine or circumvent paternalistic patterns of control.

Legal requirements may also create moral distress and ethical conflict. Although appeals to ethical knowledge can be used to challenge and justify morality, they do not supersede the law. For example, if you have a strong moral disposition toward counseling an underage woman about her options for birth control but such information is prohibited by state statute, an appeal to ethical knowledge, such as a code of rights, will not get you off the hook in a court of law. In these instances you have the choice to break the law, engage in deliberate civil disobedience to make a political statement, or work within professional organizations and local political circles to change oppressive laws. What is important here is to understand that you, as a nurse, may act morally in relation to strong ethical precepts and end up in a court of law because your actions were illegal. Historically, changes in ethical and moral traditions have been made because people were willing to risk their lives and their personal freedom and security to ensure a broad base of human rights for others. Taking such a risk to make a political statement and to press a community to consider ethical and moral alternatives requires courage and strong moral conviction. It is also the case that ethical principles, held historically, may eventually become law. A recent example is the Health Insurance Portability and Accountability Act (HIPAA), which passed into law directives that protect the privacy of personal health information (www.hhs.gov/ocr/hipaa/). With regard to HIPAA, doing what was once only the right thing to do is now legally required.

Ideally, whatever constitutes moral behavior in nursing (elusive though that may be) needs to be in place and understood, grounded in ethical knowledge that supports and justifies yet challenges that morality. Nursing, like other professions, has a unique set of values, a particular culture and practice that affects the ethical decision-making processes. The goal to be approached by nurses is moral and ethical coherence that is supported by laws and other societal contexts that do not prohibit, but allow for, the expression of nursing's highest moral and ethical ideals.

Figure 4-1 depicts those elements of both morality and ethics that are embedded within the ethical pattern of knowing in nursing. We have retained the pattern name, *ethics,* after Carper's (1978) original terminology because our primary focus is on knowledge development, or the ethics of nursing. In this pattern, the expressions of ethical knowledge are principles and codes, which reflect the normative or prescriptive focus of ethics. Principles and codes represent and include the intellectual work of nurses who develop ethical knowledge. The processes whereby such knowledge generates and regenerates involve examining the behavior and claims of nurses—the examination of individual and collective morality.

OVERVIEW OF ETHICAL PERSPECTIVES

Within philosophic ethics, various theoretic perspectives have emerged that attempt to set forth the foundation on which to base ethical action. These approaches to ethics have been important for nursing as it attempts to create an ethical perspective on practice. The following four perspectives that appear commonly in nursing literature are briefly examined here: teleology, deontology, relativism, and virtue ethics.

Teleology and Deontology

Teleology and *deontology* are two common labels that refer to ethical systems based on the expected outcome of human actions. Most ethical codes and principles, as well as systems of ethical reasoning or decision making, can be broadly classified into one of these two types. In teleology, what is right produces good. Teleological systems look toward the ends produced by a course of action as the measure that determines the action's goodness. What a right course of action yields is expressed in the familiar phrase "the greatest good for the greatest number of people." Taken to extremes, teleological systems could be used to justify behavior deemed harmful to a societal group if the harm that was done produced good for the rest of society. Using teleology, one could justify stripping a wealthy person of personal assets for redistribution to those who are poor and thereby producing a greater good for greater numbers of people.

In deontology, what is right may not necessarily produce a good outcome—that is, deontological systems separate right from good. In deontological systems, ethically right actions may have a bad outcome, as expressed in the phrase "the end does not justify the means." In deontological frameworks for ethical decision making, knowledge forms such as external rules or codes determine what is right, regardless of the outcome produced. An extreme view of deontology is exemplified by someone who, required by rule or precept to tell the truth, does the morally right thing and tells the truth, causing great emotional distress to a client and family (a bad outcome). Deontological systems suggest that the rules and the makers of rules are in charge of ethical decision making, whereas teleological systems assign decision-making authority to persons making reasoned calculations and judgments about what constitutes the greatest good. Both deontological and teleological systems focus on the individual as a decision maker who is autonomous in action. How the social context imparts meaning and how emotional content and other nonrational forms of behavior affect decision making are not formally considered.

Relativism

Relativism exists in many varieties and basically is the claim that what is morally and ethically correct varies across cultures and societies. In relation to ethical systems of reasoning, relativists would argue that universal generalities about what constitutes moral action cannot be made. In relativism, ethical behavior and moral viewpoints are justified by, or relative to, any one of many viewpoints or standards—that is, what is moral behavior and ethical knowledge is determined by the framework used in making a judgment, and no standard or viewpoint is privileged over any other. In relativism any one standard of morality is as good as the other, and all ethical precepts are equally true—assuming, of course, that they can be justified using one acceptable framework or the other (Blackburn, 2005). A relativist position might argue that an ethical system grounded in deontology is just as good as one grounded in teleology. For relativists, ethical systems and morality depend on historical timing, the culture and language within which the justification system is embedded, and the particular group and individual subjects involved in decision making (Bandman & Bandman, 2001; Mappes & DeGrazia, 2006).

Relativism may be a comfortable position to take because it circumvents a responsibility to know how to behave with some degree of certainty in the face of moral and ethical dilemmas. Under the extreme relativist view, incorporating any idea of moral/ethical comportment into a knowledge development model becomes something of a nonissue. This is because moral/ethical comportment would be relative to every possible ethical situation and standards for behavior could not be generalized to all nurses. Relativist claims also preclude the advancement of ethical knowledge because no standpoint for judging behavior is taken to be better than any other. Then again, some dimensions of relativism are useful and seem necessary in that nurses often face tremendous clinical complexities in ethical decision making that prevent knowing with much certainty what the best course of action is. Despite the fact that moral/ethical decision making involves uncertainties for action that cannot be solved by a priori knowledge of what is moral/ethical, we believe we can move toward a shared idea of what constitutes moral/ethical comportment for nursing.

Virtue Ethics

Virtue ethics introduces the character of the person as an important determiner of moral/ethical decision making. Virtue or individual character is unimportant within the frame of reference provided by deontology and teleology. If ethical behavior can be reduced to application of rules or calculations of good, then character would be irrelevant. Character, however, determines how we perceive or frame situations, so a focus on the virtues of the nurse is critically important. Virtue ethics also offers a structure for moral/ethical comportment that can balance relativism by suggesting that a virtuous person will behave in a moral/ethical way. Virtue ethics allows flexibility in approaching moral/ethical situations that deontological and teleological systems alone do not offer.

However, virtue ethics can be a particularly dangerous ethical system for a profession that is gendered in traditional female roles. Some focus on the cultivation of virtuous behavior seems important to ethical knowledge and knowing. However, historically for women, to be virtuous meant to embrace a feminine ethic of being submissive, obedient, and self-sacrificing. It is important to question who defines what is virtuous and who benefits from the particular way in which *virtuous* is defined (Tong, 1998).

Our system for knowledge development includes aspects of both teleological and deontological perspectives. It also includes a dimension of relativism. Although the knowledge forms include principles and codes, they are not taken to be infallible or to be adhered to at all costs. Processes of valuing and clarifying can help elucidate the situational contexts and decision-making frameworks that are important considerations for modification of principles and codes. The disciplinary processes of dialogue and justification can function to temper rules and precepts and sensitize them for different contexts. Also, as the nurse acts, moral behavior and ethical knowledge are integrated with the other knowing patterns to create the best possible decision. This can, in turn, be further examined by questioning whether, rather than assuming that, the action is right and responsible. Our model incorporates a focus on virtues through the pattern of personal knowing, which grants the individual nurse the responsibility to examine what is virtuous. Emancipatory knowing suggests a focus on how and why particular virtues of nurses (caring and being on the job for patients despite heavy patient loads) might operate to maintain a problematic status quo (inadequate staffing that maximizes profits for hospital corporations rather than for caring nurses). The processes within the ethical knowledge quadrant help ensure that within the discipline individual practitioners reflect on, discuss, and debate that which is virtuous in the context of nursing. As moral/ethical comportment is integrated with other knowing patterns and then subsequently examined by the questions "Is this right?" and "Is this responsible?" we expect that growth of the discipline toward action and reflection consistent with praxis will evolve.

NURSING'S FOCUS ON ETHICS AND MORALITY

The virtues of a dutiful nurse were the focus of much literature on ethics during the first half of the 19th century, as noted in Chapter 2. Reverby's (1987) historical work underscores the nature of the nurse's duty to care while being denied the means to effect or create an environment in which caring is valued and possible. In more recent nursing literature there has been increasing interest in the concept of caring as a centrally important focus for the development of both empiric and ethical theory. Much of the literature on ethics of care centers around the relative merits of an ethic of caring versus an ethic of justice and how moral behavior relates to both.

Nursing's focus on the caring perspective owes much to work that evolved from Carol Gilligan's (1982) critique and challenge of Kohlberg's (1976) theory of moral development. Kohlberg's work staged moral development using male research subjects, and Gilligan challenged its validity as a normative template for judging moral development in women. Gilligan found that women tended to care about relational concerns that focused on the needs and feelings of major players involved in the dilemma. Autonomy in decision making, by contrast, was a central feature of Kohlberg's theory. This theory supported a morality in which actors could remain detached from the situation and appeal to rules or calculations of good as a guide to action. An approach that emphasizes detachment and objectivity in ethical decision making has been linked to traditional medical ethics approaches and critiqued as inappropriate for nursing. Fry (1989), for example, has suggested that the context of nursing practice requires a moral view of the person rather than a theory of moral action or a system of moral justification. For Fry, caring as a moral value ought to be central to any theory of ethics. Others have pointed out that concerns for autonomy and justice that are central to biomedical ethics traditionally have been male-gendered traits. Not only do these imply a separate-from or autonomous stance toward ethical challenges, but they also may be inappropriate for nursing, where gendered traits typically are female (Condon, 1992). Crowley (1994) outlined how Noddings' (1984) ethics of care might be used as a guide to transforming curriculum and subsequently approaches to moral comportment in practice.

Feminists (Hoagland, 1990; Houston, 1990; Liaschenko, 1993; Tong, 1999) have cautioned nurses about the alignment of moral decision making in women with care perspectives because of its potential to further entrench oppressive values. These authors point out the political reality of caring and urge caution lest we embrace a feminine, not a feminist, ethic (Liaschenko, 1993). Although it can become difficult to differentiate feminine and feminist ethics, writers such as Liaschenko suggest that a feminine ethic reflects the uncritical acceptance and embracing, often unknowingly, of traditionally feminine values around caring. Embracing a feminine ethic of caring means promoting as ethical the enactment of virtues associated with caring—altruism, acceptance, loving unconditionally, and a host of other stereotypical feminine traits. Although this type of caring may seem a perfectly good thing to do, and a very good way to be, such feminine virtues associated with caring may preclude nurses from understanding how this type of caring benefits the health care industry to the detriment of nurses' salaries, working conditions, and social value. Whereas a feminine ethic is associated with uncritical acceptance of stereotypical female caring as a template for judging moral behavior, a feminist ethic is associated with critically understanding the sociopolitical contexts that have gendered caring as feminine and why and how this is problematic in relation to changing the situation of nurses within the health care system. In short, a feminine ethic of caring proclaims the importance of caring consistent with female-gendered virtues. A feminist ethic would recognize that morality and social lives are interconnected and that nursing's lack of power shapes our morality, determining whose ethical vision is authoritative (Tong, 1999). Feminist ethics require critical analyses that help nurses understand how to create contexts that would, in fact, allow nurses to care. The caution to embrace a feminist rather than a feminine ethic, for feminist writers such as Liaschenko (1993), is a plea to understand how blind adherence to the feminine virtues of caring can, in fact, preclude caring by allowing the continuance of conditions that exploit those who care.

We believe that nurses must be concerned with issues of both care and justice if nursing's purposes are to be realized. Walker (1993) suggests that nurses' moral expertise is not a question of mastering codes and laws, but a matter of being architects of moral space within the health care setting and mediators in the conversations taking place. To do this requires attention to the vulnerabilities of an ethic of care as well as the vulnerabilities of an ethic of justice. As Cooper (1991) explains, we must take seriously the moral demands of care in the development of ethics. Doing so requires radical responses and moral courage as well as political astuteness. Ethical choices should be guided not only by rules and principles but also by thoughtful analysis of feelings, intuitions, and experiences (Cooper, 1991).

PROCESSES FOR ETHICAL KNOWLEDGE DEVELOPMENT

Our view of ethics is in concert with Carper's original conceptualization of the ethical pattern, which included dimensions of both morality and ethics intersecting with legally prescribed duties. Moreover, no one ethical or moral view is embraced, but there is a constant need to be vigilant about the sociopolitical context within which nurses function.

> The ethical component of nursing is focused on matters of obligation or what ought to be done. Knowledge of morality goes beyond simply knowing the norms or ethical codes of the discipline. It includes voluntary actions that can be judged as deliberately right and wrong. (Carper, 1978, p. 20)

In examining the nature of ethical knowing and knowledge, the following questions naturally arise: Toward what end should ethical knowledge be developed? What ought to be done in practice to earn the label *ethical* or *moral*? What values support nursing's ethics and morality? Toward what clinical ends should ethical theories reason and ethical principles move us? What sort of moral development perspective should we embrace and encourage? In the context of teleology we might ask the following: How do we know what the greatest good is? In the context of deontology: How do we know which rules are good and which are not? For virtue ethics: Which virtues are worthwhile for us to cultivate? Such questions relate to the final value from which no others can be derived and which centers our knowledge development efforts and professional activities. Although we will not answer these questions, we do provide some guidelines for ways to create answers in your own situation. Because our model combines aspects of each of these positions, these are central questions that require thoughtful consideration.

As the products and processes within this quadrant of the model are discussed in the next sections, some answers will be provided, but additional questions will be raised. For us the merit of ethical knowledge will be judged on the basis of the extent to which ethical codes and principles contribute to our collective ability to thoughtfully reflect and act in such a way that what we think and know is fully consistent with what we do. This implies increasing the reflective awareness or consciousness on the part of nurses as nursing is practiced. It implies a move toward action grounded in an open awareness and choice for client and nurse—a move toward health. It implies a move to reduce the moral distress nurses face as they encounter and negotiate ethical and moral dilemmas.

The pattern of ethics includes nurses' usual day-to-day moral decision making. Ethics goes beyond what many tend to think of as ethics—the weighty, dramatic decisions often involving end-of-life contexts or controversial political and social issues. Important ethical knowing is used and created in everyday incidents. Ethical knowing is reflected in the decision to ignore a comment or attend to it, what to say, what not to say, or whether to keep information to ourselves or reveal it. Ethical decisions that are made around a conference table by an ethics committee, although important, are not our major focus or the major domain of nursing's morality and ethics. Rather, ethics arises from the work that nurses do and is about everyday uses of morality and ethical knowledge as expressed in ethical comportment in typical practice settings. Nursing's morality is, in large measure, an everyday ontology.

Ethical knowledge development fundamentally comes from the questioning of moral/ethical comportment—that is, who we are as ethical and moral beings and what we believe is good and right. We assume that nurses bring to their work some base set of values that guide their ethical decisions and moral behavior. As they work within the everyday world, their moral/ethical selves are challenged daily. For example, a nurse might wonder the following: Should I reveal to an elderly woman that her family is cleaning out her apartment and don't intend to allow her to return home? Should I share my views about what is responsible childbearing with a young couple who discovers they both have diabetes? Would this cause more harm than good? What would be gained? Who would gain? If you reflect for a moment, several instances in which you have faced such ordinary decisions should come to mind. You probably will notice that your decisions were made relatively quickly without obvious reference to ethical codes or principles.

We begin the discussions of knowledge development for ethics with the following questions: "Is (was) this right?" and "Is (was) this responsible?" As you work as a nurse, this type of questioning is in the background whether you realize it or not, for without such questioning you would be unable to make day-to-day moral/ethical moves. When this sort of question becomes deliberative, it leads to the creation and re-creation of shared knowledge.

As you or others inquire about how right and responsible your decisions are within your particular context, different perspectives on ethical decision making will become apparent. Valuing and clarifying are the system processes used to answer these questions. Simply stated, as you consider whether your moral/ethical behavior was right and responsible, you are making your values clearer for yourself and others and you gradually are internalizing your values more fully.

Values Clarification

Values clarification processes deliberatively question the moral/ethical correctness or "rightness" of a decision. The specific values that give rise to a nurse's moral/ethical decisions and actions (and subsequently ethical knowledge expressions) often are hidden. Values can be thought of as the assumptions or background information that create moral/ethical questions and moral/ethical moves. Values provide a lens that brings into focus certain aspects of a moral problem, while distancing or blurring others. Values vary among individuals and reflect the contexts of our experiences with family, friends, social institutions, gender boundaries, and age. The questioning of values by using formal techniques of clarification assumes that values may not always be "good." It also assumes a disjunction between values we believe are important in influencing our actions and those that actually do influence what we do and say.

There are various techniques for values clarification (Bandman & Bandman, 2001; Catalano, 2000; Davis, 1997; Simon, Howe, & Kirschenbaum, 1992; Steele, 1983; Sweeting, 1990; Wilderding, 1992), but fundamentally the processes involve the use of rational thought and emotional awareness to understand, examine, and actualize values. Approaches can use real or contrived dilemmas, group or individual work, self-analyses or interview, or any number of other methods that free individuals to examine and embrace their values. Clarification of values often is an emotionally charged activity involving deeply held personal beliefs. Individuals or groups undertaking values clarification processes need an environment that allows for freedom of value choices and affirmation of the values clarified. Regardless of the technique used, values clarification is an individual process that seeks to challenge and understand inculcated values. Values clarification is an important part of the valuing-clarifying processes within the ethics quadrant because it emphasizes affective thinking and behavior-motivated choice and allows one to question how responsible one's moral/ethical decisions are.

Various approaches for values clarification can be adapted to a specific situation. Some general guidelines are useful. First, it is important to select or create an moral/ethical dilemma that participants will emotionally relate to and will not see as fictitious to their practice. Although commonly used approaches such as "which person to throw from the sinking boat" may suffice, we believe more benefit is gained if the situations relate to actual or potential nursing practice. Second, focus on clarifying individual values that should emerge from the process, regardless of the process used for clarification. In values clarification there may be a tendency to avoid what is difficult. Lively discussions about what should be done do not substitute for a deliberative focus on one's personal values. A third guideline emphasizes writing about or listing personal values that emerge. Journaling about your values helps to make values explicit, clarifying what the values are, and also provides a forum for examining how and why values change. Because it is difficult to provide a public forum where learners can freely explicate and examine values, journaling becomes important—especially when the moral/ethical dilemmas that are the focus for deliberation arise from practice situations the participants are likely to encounter.

Values Analysis

Another important process for questioning the moral/ethical correctness of a decision is values analysis. Unlike values clarification, which is an attempt to emotionally understand, clarify, and embrace individually held values, values analysis seeks to more objectively understand and analyze the values operating in a situation. In values analysis, participants examine the processes involved in deciding on a course of action for an ethical problem. They are required to recognize and stand apart from their own values as much as possible and view value structures, their own or others', objectively and critically. In values analysis the participants strive to gain clarity on an issue, examine various points of view factually and logically, and examine different approaches to resolving the dilemma for empiric consistency and inconsistency.

If factual evidence for one point of view is provided, it is questioned for accuracy. The ethical decision is arrived at logically, and then the decision is tested in some manner—for example, by looking at its consistency with a principle or code for ethical behavior. Values analysis is important because it points out the relativism and subjectivity, as well as congruence among individual points of view. As with values clarification, the situations chosen for values analysis should arise from practice. Although explication of personal values is important in clarification, in analysis one looks at the values and justification processes that are operative in the situation. Rather than clarifying what you would do in a given situation, in values analysis you examine what is occurring and the underlying issues involved in the process. Box 4-1 lists questions that may be asked to accomplish values clarification and analysis.

Values Clarification and Analyses Using Ethical Decision Trees

A number of sources suggest the use of decision trees as an approach to ethical decision making (Burkhardt & Nathaniel, 2002; Ellis & Hartley, 2004; Frame & Williams, 2005; Hall, 1999; Johnstone, 1999; Overshok, 2002; Storl, DuBois, & Seline, 1999). Although the elements that constitute ethical decision-making trees vary somewhat, fundamentally they are depicted as flow charts or a series of ordered questions that begin with the identification of the ethical issue or problem. Once the problem is identified, the user is guided linearly through a number of steps that, when followed, suggest an ethically correct decision. Ethical decision trees call for the gathering of facts about the situation in relation to the ethical framework that is being used. Options are considered, situational factors are identified, and evaluation of various courses of action is required before a decision is proposed. Some decision trees prescribe, at least in part, the ethical framework to be used, whereas others expect the user to designate or choose the framework relevant to the situation. Ethical decision trees are particularly useful when there is enough time to effectively think about and spell out the requisite details within the elements of the tree prior to

---

Box 4-1
Questions for Clarification and Analysis of Values

VALUES CLARIFICATION

- What outcome would I like to see?
- What would I do?
- How do I feel about this? How strongly do I feel?
- What is guiding my potential actions? Feelings?
- What would need to change about the context for me to act or feel differently?
- Are there any alternatives in this situation, and how viable are they?
- How proud do I feel about my choices?
- Would I affirm them to others?
- Does there seem to be a hierarchy of choices?
- What is the central value that seems to be operating in my choices?
- What values do I not embrace or believe in? Can I imagine a situation where a value I do not embrace might be important to hold?

VALUES ANALYSIS

- What are the moral/ethical issues in this situation?
- What moral/ethical decisions are being made?
- What moral/ethical bases are operating to guide those decisions?
- How strong are the arguments? The counterarguments?
- Are the intentions of the decision makers important?
- Is more evidence needed to justify a decision? What sort?
- Are there any inconsistencies related to ethical decisions being made?
- What evidence do we need to know whether the decisions are moral/ethical?
- What are the social and political contexts of the decision, and how are they affecting outcomes?

---

making the decision. Ethical decision-making trees reflect what Liaschenko and Peter (2004) identify as a disciplinary ethics: an ethics suggesting that professional activities of nurses that are understood in a certain way are inherently moral. These authors suggest that approaches that limit what counts as a moral or ethical concern and authorize how these concerns are resolved, as decision trees do, incompletely reflect the complexity of contemporary health care (Liaschenko & Peter, 2004).

Decision trees, however, are useful as a learning tool. Like the nursing process, ethical decision trees offer a system that, once learned, helps nurses more quickly integrate details involved in ethical situations and make an appropriate decision. They also make less opaque the factors and processes involved in ethical decisions and help learners understand what is and is not ethically justifiable.

Completing decision trees can be useful for values analyses and values clarification processes. Case studies of ethical problems can be organized into decision trees rather than being discussed directly. Decision trees can be completed by individual participants and then examined using the questions for values clarification in Box 4-1. Also, as participants individually complete trees, details important to consider within various elements required by the tree, for example detail about the consequences of an action, will not be self-evident. When placing details of an ethical situation within a decision tree, noticing which details require deliberation before making a choice and which go unquestioned is important, as individual values tend to emerge at these points. Values are also clarified when groups attempt to complete decision trees in relation to an ethical problem. As different members of the group suggest what must be included as relevant, the validity of various views within the group is likely to be challenged. Some group members may notice that certain details were omitted that, in their view, should have been included. Others may not even have thought about certain details as relevant, whereas still others in the group may offer reasons for omissions as well as inclusions. As discussion and disagreements occur, underlying values are made more visible to individual participants within the group. Also, when individuals separately or groups collectively reflect on the extent, and conditions, of their agreement with a completed decision tree, values are clarified. Finally, changing the details entered in elements of a decision tree and noticing how it affects both the processes and outcomes of decision making is a useful clarification technique. Similar processes can be used for values analyses using completed decision trees. Elements required within the trees, as well as the details within completed trees, can be questioned for underlying assumptions and conditions of context that have precluded the possibility of making some decisions. As participants notice the details within various elements, as well as the elements themselves, the underlying values and how they are operating come to light.

Both values clarification and values analysis are important processes for understanding the nature of right and responsible moral/ethical decisions in relation to the knowledge form that is generated. The juxtaposition of personally cherished, but problematic, values (from values clarification) and objectively required values (from value analysis) deepens understanding of what is possible and what is necessary for nursing practice. When problematic value positions are challenged by an objective stance, they can change. As the more objective value decisions are approached, we can understand the limitations objectivism has in determining what constitutes moral/ethical decision making.

The processes of values clarification and analysis include, whether recognized or not, reference to justice and care perspectives on ethical decision making, as well as reference to ethical principles and codes consistent with the deontological and teleological perspectives. Within our model, then, valuing and clarifying processes—primarily values analysis and clarification—occur when questions are raised about what is right and what is responsible behavior.

ETHICAL KNOWLEDGE FORMS

The model we have created identifies principles and codes as ethical knowledge forms; however, other forms exist. Ethical knowledge may take the format of sets of rules; statements of duties, rights, or obligations; theory; or laws. The Nightingale Pledge (not created by Nightingale, we might add) and Hippocratic Oath also are forms of ethical knowledge. An individual nurse or group of nurses setting forth an ethical position for disciplinary use and critique that flows from values clarification and analysis processes could put it in the form of an article, a case analysis, or even poetry. We have chosen principles and codes as generic forms of ethical knowledge because they are attainable and common forms of ethical knowledge in nursing. The American Nurses Association, for example, has created a code of ethics for nurses. Nurses also are taught to operate within common forms of ethical knowledge such as principles of autonomy and beneficence. We also prefer to avoid associating ethical knowledge forms with "theory" to prevent confusion of the differences between ethical and empirical theories. Regardless of form of ethical knowledge, we suggest that eventually it can be reduced to principles and codes, which are shorthand ways of expressing ethical knowing.

DIALOGUE AND JUSTIFICATION

The disciplinary processes of dialogue and justification, like valuing and clarifying, require the collective and open examination of both behavior and knowledge. The model's central focus of moral/ethical comportment clearly suggests that the morality of practice and disciplinary ethical knowledge must be brought together. Notions of what is right and what is responsible not only question the moral/ethical dimensions of practice knowledge but also consider legal ramifications of practice as expressed in the language of rights and duty. In short, the ethics pattern embodies both epistemology and ontology through its focus on both ethics and morality.

It is within the model's processes of dialogue and justification that knowledge is more deliberatively examined with reference to established principles and codes and the perspectives of justice and care. Through these processes ethical knowledge is examined and refined and becomes part of the disciplinary heritage that individual nurses subsequently carry into practice and revisit and challenge, with the use of the valuing and clarifying processes previously described.

Dialogue implies a community of askers who use established ethical perspectives, principles, and codes to accept, reject, or modify the knowledge form. Traditionally ethical knowledge forms have been examined for an internal logic as a standard of validity. Although internal logic is important for coherence, it is an insufficient standard for establishing the value of ethical knowledge. Dialogue implies an ideal that multiple voices, over time, will be integrated into justification processes, whereas the choice of the word "justification" itself suggests no particular framework for establishing the value of an ethical knowledge form.

Justification processes for ethical knowledge forms in nursing can appeal to the authority of historical values associated with nursing, existing moral/ethical knowledge, and currently held values, as well as values and moral knowing consistent with an envisioned future—to name but a few. For example, the value of caring might be cited as an important historical factor that can be used to justify caring in nursing—that is, caring as a historically embedded duty justifies caring as a contemporary value. Principles of nonmaleficence or autonomy, which baccalaureate students are generally exposed to, might be called up to justify ethical knowledge. Also, an envisioned future may form a critical template against which to reflect ethical knowledge. This occurs when we question whether caring is an ethic that will help us achieve professional autonomy and identity. It is assumed that the collective voice of nursing will be the best hope for the emergence of appropriate and productive justification frameworks as the basis for re-visioning the form of ethical knowledge.

We have chosen an eclectic approach to form and justify ethical principles because we believe no one perspective is entirely useful for all situations. Rather, the more likely scenario is that multiple justification perspectives will be used. Care must be balanced with a concern for justice; rules must be used in the context of doing the least harm.

As an example of how care and justice might emerge as important using the processes of dialogue and justification, suppose you and your peers are examining a situation beginning with a deontological perspective that provides a rule for ethical action. The situation involves a mother who is suspected of inflicting physical harm on her young child.

The 2-year-old girl, currently hospitalized for an emergency appendectomy, has bruises and marks you believe are due to being struck, but the mother attributes them to the caregiver, who, you subsequently learn, is the child's grandmother. Although there are old and new bruises, there are no broken bones, and otherwise the child appears to be quite healthy.

Assume the rule being discussed is the rule of nonmaleficence—of doing no harm. This is a principle that is generally followed by you and the professional group you work with. You and others initially suggest that doing no harm in this case means establishing the source of the child's bruises and subsequently protecting the child from further injury. As the dialogue proceeds about how to report concerns to child protective services or ask the mother more pointedly about the bruises and their source, the dialogue and justification processes take an unexpected turn, and you begin to realize that doing no harm in this instance is becoming fairly complex.

The social worker on your team reveals that the mother is unmarried, must work outside the home to support herself, and out of necessity is leaving the child in the care of the child's grandmother to minimize child-care expenses. The mother, it turns out, cannot afford paid child care because she needs her income to meet expenses, including renting an apartment that keeps her whereabouts hidden from a former partner who has abused both her and the child in the past.

A staff nurse states he has talked with the grandmother during a recent visit. He offers that although the child's grandmother is well-meaning and loving, she was recently confined to a wheelchair with the progression of a long-term debilitating muscular disease. The staff nurse believes it possible that the grandmother bruises the child inadvertently by bumping her against the wheelchair as she provides care. An intern on the team shares that the grandmother had voluntarily offered in a conversation with her that on occasion the child slips from her arms to the floor, and the grandmother "hopes this did not cause the child's appendicitis." The intern, from talking with the grandmother, believes that generally she manages to care for the child properly, and certainly she intends to be a good caregiver to help her daughter out.

Given the ongoing dialogue, it is becoming apparent that it might actually be harmful to the young child not to allow the grandmother to provide care during the day if it means the child's return to the mother's care, the loss of the mother's income, the discovery of the mother and child by the abusive partner, and the risk of harm to both. Though contrived, the point of the example is that dialogue and justification has led the team to question the initial thinking about what was right, in that unconsidered approaches to protecting the young child from harm could quite likely result in unintended consequences of harm.

Justification and dialogue have raised the question of what should prevail. What about the rule of doing no harm? Should the rule be violated to produce a greater good? The answers are never totally clear, but open, reasoned, and knowledgeable dialogue seems an effective approach to making the best decision. In the example, perhaps the best decision might be—assuming the bruises are unintended, are not seriously life threatening, and are occurring because of the grandmother's physical condition—to let the grandmother continue to care for the child, and teaching her care techniques that minimize physical harm to the child. As the situation changes, for example, if the child is, or has potential to be, seriously injured while in the grandmother's care, then a different decision would emerge from the justification and dialogue processes. In this example, it is ethical knowledge for praxis, that is, knowledge within the pattern of emancipatory knowing, that would be a core solution. Such knowing would require critical analysis and action around, for example, the sociopolitical context that contributed to the situation of a single parent with no options for financial support or safe child care.

The justification and dialogue processes that are envisioned to evolve ethical knowledge are carried out over time, by multiple groups, with a variety of justification perspectives. Ethical knowledge often is communicated in a vacuum, and we know little about how it actually is used or applied. Arguments for one type of approach versus another are academically interesting, but there is much blurring about positions, and the conditions within the work environment of nurses are often ignored. As analyses and understandings subsequent to the process of dialogue and justification find their way into the disciplinary literature and other venues where dialogue can occur, ethical knowledge forms will achieve legitimacy in relation to practice. It is unlikely that anything that could be considered final will ever evolve since the context for usage changes. However, the ideal of generating ethical knowledge from practice and refining that knowledge with the intent that it will be returned to practice needs to be the goal. It is through dialogue and justification that a breadth of voices can be brought to bear on ethical knowledge. It is that open questioning and dialogue that considers the context of working nurses that is nursing's best hope for usable, effective ethical knowledge and moral behavior. It is through justification processes that an understanding of ethics and morality in nursing will be approached and knowledgeable, committed action that is requisite for praxis will emerge.

REFLECTION AND DISCUSSION

In this chapter we have considered the nature of ethics and morality, provided an overview of major approaches to ethical decision making, and detailed processes for the development of disciplinary knowledge within the pattern of ethics. The centrally important message of this chapter is that nursing ethics is complex and must take into account the health care environment where moral behavior is enacted. Although the formalized approaches for developing ethical knowledge that we described are useful for creating knowledge, it is critical that in using these processes you consider how ethical knowing is integrated in everyday practice.

To deepen your appreciation of ethics, consider the following questions related to the content of this chapter:

1. How have you integrated the patterns of knowing in making ethical decisions? Describe the situation and how the various patterns were reflected in it.
2. Consider a situation where you experienced moral distress, that is, you were unable, through no fault of your own, to do the right thing. What needs to happen so "next time" you will not experience moral distress?
3. Think of an ethical decision you have made in the past. Would you make the same decision today? If so, why? Or why not?
4. What is it about the environment you work in—patterns of control, rules, prohibitions—that affects, positively or negatively, your ethical decision making?
5. Reflect on a situation where you deliberately did not do what you felt was morally right. Why did this situation occur?
6. When you are in the clinical area (or if you are not working clinically, in any public space such as a supermarket, movie line, or sporting event), identify some examples of moral behavior that exemplify nurses' (or others') everyday practice of moral and ethical behavior.
7. Consider a time you had a disagreement with a colleague about an ethical problem. How might you use the processes of values clarification and analysis to come to a better mutual understanding of the ethical principles involved?

Reference List

American Nurses Association. (2005). *Code of professional ethics.* Retrieved September 2006 from www.nursingworld.org/ethics/ecode.htm.

Bandman, E. L., & Bandman, B. (2001). *Nursing ethics through the life span* (4th ed.). Upper Saddle River, NJ: Prentice-Hall.

Blackburn, S. (2005). *Truth: A guide.* New York: Oxford University Press.

Burkhardt, M. A., & Nathaniel, A. K. (2002). *Ethics and issues in contemporary nursing* (2nd ed.). Albany, NY: Delmar.

Carper, B. A. (1978). Fundamental patterns of knowing in nursing. *ANS. Advances in Nursing Science, 1*(1), 13–23.

Catalano, J. T. (2000). *Nursing now: Today's issues, tomorrow's trends.* (2nd ed.). Philadelphia: FA Davis.

Condon, E. H. (1992). Nursing and the caring metaphor: Gender and political influences on an ethics of care. *Nursing Outlook, 40*(1), 14–19.

Cooper, M. C. (1991). Principle-oriented ethics and the ethic of care: A creative tension. *ANS. Advances in Nursing Science, 14*(2), 22–31.

Crowley, M. A. (1994). The relevance of Noddings' ethic of care to the moral education of nurses. *Journal of Nursing Education, 33*(2), 74–80.

Davis, A. J. (1997). *Ethical dilemmas and nursing practice.* Norwalk, CT: Appleton & Lange.

Ellis, J. R., & Hartley, C. L. (2004). *Nursing in today's world: Trends, issues and management* (8th ed.). Philadelphia: Lippincott Williams & Wilkins.

Frame, M. W., & Williams, C. B. (2005). A model of ethical decision making from a multicultural perspective. *Counseling and Values, 49*(2), 165–179.

Fry, S. T. (1989). Toward a theory of nursing ethics. *ANS. Advances in Nursing Science, 11*(4), 9–22.

Gilligan, C. (1982). *In a different voice: Psychological theory and women's development.* Boston: Harvard University Press.

Hall, J. K. (1999). *Nursing ethics and law.* Philadelphia: WB Saunders.

Health Insurance Portability and Accountability Act (HIPAA). (1996). Retrieved October 2006 from www.hhs.gov/ocr/hipaa/.

Hoagland, S. L. (1990). Some concerns about Nel Noddings' caring. *Hypatia, 5*(1), 109–114.

Houston, B. (1990). Caring and exploitation. *Hypatia, 5*(1), 115–119.

Johnstone, M. J. (1999). *Bioethics: A nursing perspective* (3rd ed.). Orlando, FL: Harcourt.

Kohlberg, L. (1976). Moral stages and moralization: The cognitive-developmental approach. In T. Lickona (Ed.), *Moral development and behavior: Theory, research, and social issues.* New York: Holt, Rinehart & Winston.

Levine, M. E. (1989). The ethics of nursing rhetoric. *Image—The Journal of Nursing Scholarship, 21*(1), 4–6.

Liaschenko, J. (1993). Feminist ethics and cultural ethos: Revisiting a nursing debate. *ANS. Advances in Nursing Science, 15*(4), 71–81.

Liaschenko, J., & Peter, E. (2004). Nursing ethics and conceptualizations of nursing: Profession, practice and work. *Journal of Advanced Nursing, 46*(5), 488–495.

Mappes, T. A., & DeGrazia, D. (2006). *Biomedical ethics.* New York: McGraw-Hill.

Noddings, N. (1984). *Caring: A feminine approach to ethics & moral education.* Berkeley: University of California Press.

Overshok, T. (2002). The ethical decision making process: A demonstration. *Ohio Nurses Review, 77*(7), 14–15.

Patients' Bill of Rights in Medicare and Medicaid. (1999). Retrieved October 2006 from www.hhs.gov/news/press/1999pres/990412.html.

Reverby, S. M. (1987). *Ordered to care: The dilemma of American nursing, 1850–1945.* Cambridge, UK: Cambridge University Press.

Simon, S., Howe, L., & Kirschenbaum, H. (1992). *Values clarification: A handbook of practical strategies for teachers and students.* New York: Hart.

Steele, S. M. (1983). *Values clarification in nursing,* (2nd ed.). Norwalk, CT: Appleton-Century-Crofts.

Stewart, I. M. (1922). Some fundamental principles in the teaching of ethics. *American Journal of Nursing, 21,* 906.

Storl, H., DuBois, B., & Seline, J. (1999). Ethical decision-making made easier. The use of decision trees in case management. *Care Management Journals: Journal of Case Management, 1*(3), 163–169.

Sweeting, R. L. (1990). *A values approach to health behavior.* Champaign, IL: Human Kinetics.

Tong, R. (1998). The ethics of care: A feminist virtue ethics of care for healthcare practitioners. *Journal of Medicine and Philosophy, 23*(2), 131–152.

Tong, R. (1999). Moral understandings: A feminist study in ethics. *Hypatia, 14*(2), 121–124.

Walker, M. U. (1993). Keeping moral space open. *Hastings Center Report, 23*(2), 33–40.

Wilderding, J. (1992). Values clarification. In G. Gulecheck & J. McCloskey (Eds.), *Nursing interventions: Essential nursing treatment.* Philadelphia: WB Saunders.

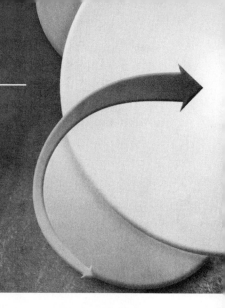

CHAPTER 5

Personal Knowledge Development

Self is a dynamic concept, ever deepening as we expand and broaden our relationships with others. The self is created in relation to others.

Beverly Hall and Janet Allan (1994, p. 112)

Personal knowing is the dynamic process of becoming a whole, aware self and of knowing the other as valued and whole. The other often is an individual, but small and large groups also can be known authentically and as a whole. Personal knowing is the basis for expression of authenticity, the genuine self, which in turn is essential in a healing relationship. Personal knowing expands that which is accessible to the self in the experience of the other. Personal knowing enables one to experience deeper levels of meaning in all of life's experiences, including those that are shared in interaction with others.

Figure 5-1 shows the personal knowing component of our model for knowledge development in nursing. In our model, personal knowing arises from the following critical questions: "Do I know what I do?" and "Do I do what I know?" The processes of opening and centering are the creative processes from which the authenticity of the self emerges. The processes of response and reflection hold the key to authenticating one's self—a lifelong process of becoming. The genuine self expresses directly, without words, who one is to others. Autobiographic stories are a written form of

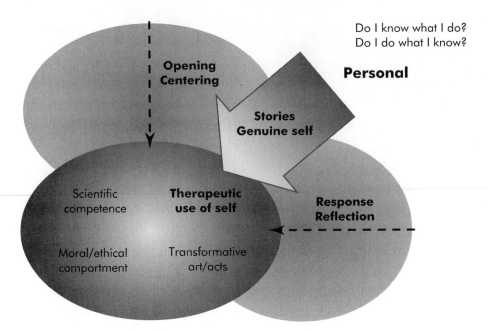

FIGURE 5-1 Processes for developing personal knowing and knowledge.

expression of personal knowledge. These expressions of knowledge provide opportunities for response and reflection within the discipline. In practice, personal knowing is expressed as the therapeutic use of self.

In this chapter we explore conceptual meanings of personal knowing on which the processes are founded for developing personal knowing as a component of nursing practice. We then provide descriptions of personal knowing processes that we have identified and used and that other nurse scholars also have identified and used. Within the descriptions of the processes we also explain the communicable forms of personal knowing that contribute to the development of personal knowledge within the discipline.

PERSONAL KNOWING IN NURSING

Personal knowing is fundamental to nursing by virtue of the nature of the interpersonal processes that are inherent to nursing practice. Meaningful interpersonal connections do not occur in a vacuum, and they are not happenstance occurrences. Well-developed personal knowing opens the way for being fully present with another. Interactions with others provide the experiential ground from which personal knowing emerges. As Hall and Allan (1994) state: "The self is created in relation to others" (p. 112). Personal knowing is the cornerstone on which wholistic practice is based, making possible wholeness of self and other in a context of relational experience.

The label *personal knowing* can be misleading in that it can imply a solitary and individual process, involving only the unique perceptions of the individual. Personal knowing involves deep inner reflection that is sometimes solitary, and it is an aspect of the whole of knowing that arises from within the individual. However, personal knowing also involves openness to experience in the world and with others and mutual, meaningful interactions with others. Contemporary popular notions of self-actualization and individuation reinforce images of the individual on a lone, often self-indulging journey of discovery. Moreover, contemporary cultures that primarily value empiric knowing reinforce the limited and mistaken notion that people essentially are rational egos seeking individual autonomy, rights, and freedoms (Hart, 1997). Despite these dominant cultural contexts, personal knowing does not emerge from processes of rational theory. The processes involved in personal knowing compel experience of the self as more than rational and as intimately connected to others.

Personal knowing is expressed as mind-body-spirit congruence, authenticity, and genuineness. Others experience and know the person as unique by virtue of those deeply personal qualities that are conveyed through being in the world within the context of the culture. Personal knowing also can be conveyed through autobiographic stories, written or told, which provide a glimpse of who the person is in a form that is not confined to the time and space of the moment. Personal stories are limited in their capacity to convey the fullness of the person, but they provide a means of communication with a wide audience. Personal stories convey essences of experience that are not communicated in theories or clinical histories. Personal stories are not trivial pastimes or entertainment; they are vital within a discipline that depends on meaningful interpersonal connections. Further, personal stories are important to the discipline to create a shared understanding of what it means to know and develop the self. Written expression of personal knowing opens opportunities for response from others and possibilities for deeper reflection.

CONCEPTUAL MEANINGS OF PERSONAL KNOWING

Carper's (1978) early description of personal knowing points directly to interpersonal interactions, relationships, and transactions as central defining qualities of nursing. Carper clearly identified the fundamental necessity of personal knowing for nursing as embedded in the concept of "therapeutic use of self."

One does not know about the self; one simply strives to know the self. This knowing is a process of symbolically standing in relation to another human being and confronting that human being as a person. This "I-Thou" encounter is unmediated by conceptual categories or particulars abstracted from complex organic wholes. The relation is one of reciprocity, a state of being that cannot be described or even experienced—it only can be actualized. (Carper, 1978, p. 18)

For Carper, an authentic person values others in their freedom to create themselves and make choices on their own behalf. This means setting aside generalizations, categories, and assumptions taken from empiric forms of knowing, as well as manipulative, controlling, and impersonal forms of treatment. Instead, personal knowing embraces and values the wholeness and integrity in each encounter and seeks to know and affirm the uniqueness of each person and that person's unique experience.

Spirituality and Personal Knowing

Personal knowing is intimately related to spirit and to what is sometimes referred to as spiritual (Bishop & Scudder, 1990; Hall, 1997; Hart, 1997; Huebner, 1985). The meanings of *spirit* and *spirituality* refer to the life journey of discovering personal meaning and purpose. *Spirit* is a term derived from the Latin word for "breath" and "breathing"; it conveys a sense of sustaining life, of an animating and vital principle inherent in "being" (Huebner, 1985). The "human spirit" is not something outside the person or a separate substance temporally residing within the body. It is the entirety of existence. It is as spirits that people become most authentically themselves.

Spiritual is a term that often is linked with religion, a tradition that Hall (1997) identified as deriving from the fact that Western culture limits expression of what is known either to science or to religion. Many people do connect their spirituality with religious beliefs; however, that which is spiritual does not of necessity link with religiosity (Campesino & Schwartz, 2006; Pesut, 2006). The spiritual is a complex of values, attitudes, and hopes linked to the transcendent that guides and directs a person's life. It is particularly connected to life experiences that bring one to the brink of uncertainty, the "existential boundary issues" of life and death, good and evil, hopes and dreams, despair and suffering. Personal knowing, linked with spirituality, means self-conscious awareness and nurturing of the interconnectedness of these life-challenging issues (Hall, 2004). Personal knowing as a spiritual dimension of life provides inspiration from which people give shape to their lives as they confront difficult challenges. Spirituality leads people to face the vulnerable realities of life that cannot be overcome and nurtures embodied spiritual agency for relating to these vulnerabilities (Hart, 1997).

Hall (1997) presented a conception of human spirit and spirituality as reaching within to learn to accept, love, and value what you find there, and learning to be yourself authentically and with confidence. What you find within the spirit may not be what you want to find. Personal knowing is the process of coming to know what is within and coming to live with, accept, and love what is within. This is not a process of self-centered exploration, nor is it linear. Rather, it is an unfolding process that is grounded in the context of everyday experience, in relationship with others.

Self-in-Relation

Hall and Allan (1994) explained the vital link between personal knowing and relationships with others in their concept of self-in-relation. Their ideas are grounded in traditional Chinese medicine, which philosophically views mind, body, spirit, and environment as an integrated whole. The embodied self is seen as an open system that belongs to a social world. Self-in-relation is the core of caring and healing, of wholistic nursing practice. The caring relationships that nurses enter into can reflect four dynamics that nurture self-in-relation, as follows:

Caring by giving, which requires being present and involved in relation with others. In this process, mutual sharing develops the self and the other by giving to one another, affirming the value and purpose of each life.

Empowerment develops a sense of the self as responsible for one's own health and the context within which health thrives for everyone. Empowerment in relationship gives rise to the ability to influence one's own health outcomes. When the self is fully in relation with the other, both are empowered, and true unconditional love occurs. Both learn the joy of reciprocity, wherein what each brings to the interaction is deeply valued.

Knowing the value of a human life comes from a mutual quest to find meaning in life. In a healing relationship, questions of life and death, of living and dying, come to the surface, inviting an openness to explore what is possible in this particular time and space. Openness while fully engaging with another person in this quest develops the self in each.

Sense of community is the most important and most elusive concept in wholistic healing practice. A caring community that supports giving in interrelationships provides the context for developing self-in-relation.

Discovery of Self and Other

Moch (1990) defined *personal knowing* as the discovery of self-and-other arrived at through reflection, synthesis of perceptions, and connecting with what is known. She identified the following three overlapping components of personal knowing: experiential knowing, interpersonal knowing, and intuitive knowing. Experiential knowing is the understanding and knowledge that comes from participating in the events of daily living; it is deepened by attending to the experience, studying the process of the experience, and connecting the experience to previous understandings. Attending to the experience involves being aware of what one is feeling and sensing and observing self and others.

For Moch, both cognitive and spiritual processes contribute to deriving meaning from experience. Interpersonal knowing is increased awareness through intense interaction or being with another. It emerges from intense attending, opening self to other, and conveying feelings to one another. Intuitive knowing is the immediate knowing of something without conscious use of reason.

Moch (1990) identified the following attributes of personal knowing:

- Personal knowing can be viewed only in the context of wholeness. There is no knowing apart from the knower.
- Personal knowing includes a process of encountering. The ideal encounter is one of mutual respect, which affirms those involved in the encounter and their existence.
- Personal knowing involves passion, commitment, and integrity. Passion is what affirms something as valuable, commitment motivates the search for personal meaning, and integrity brings thought and action together as an authentic whole.
- Personal knowing involves a shift in connectedness or transcendence. This is the instantaneous "aha" experience in which one's perspective shifts, either consciously or unconsciously.

Unknowing

Munhall (1993) reflected Carper's point that knowing the other requires setting aside personal assumptions and generalizations. She stressed the nature of a genuinely authentic encounter by conceptualizing a pattern of "unknowing" to signify the existential openness to the other that must occur in such an encounter. Unknowing creates a stance that is completely open to the experiences and perceptions of others as they experience them, not filtered by the nurse's own structures of understanding. Unknowing means setting aside all that is assumed to be known about the other, as well as setting aside previously held organizing structures that make sense of the world—or "decentering" from the stance of the self to move into the life of the other. The nurse takes a deliberate stance of complete openness and receptivity to the unique subjectivity of the other and remains open to a deep knowledge of the other being, to different meanings and interpretations, and to varying perceptions of the world. Unknowing is similar to the phenomenologic process of bracketing, but specifically refers to a kind of personal openness that is more than intellectual; it is a full mind-body-spirit openness that creates existential availability to know another deeply.

Despite certain distinctions in each of these conceptualizations of the meaning of personal knowing, there are important threads that are common to all of them. These threads include the primary importance of relationships and interactions in developing personal knowledge, an aspect of knowing that is beyond cognitive reasoning; the primacy of personal knowing in giving life its meaning and direction; and the imperatives of wholeness and integrity that embrace the entirety of existence and experience. These common threads form the conceptual understandings on which our approaches to developing personal knowing are based.

PROCESSES FOR DEVELOPING PERSONAL KNOWLEDGE: OPENING AND CENTERING

In our model of knowledge development in nursing, the pattern of personal knowing stems from the following questions: "Do I know what I do?" and "Do I do what I know?" Silva, Sorrell, and Sorrell (1995) posed the ontologic question of "Who am I?" and the epistemologic question of "How do I come to know who I am?" Each of these questions points to important aspects of the experience and processes involved in developing personal knowing. In this section we focus on the epistemologic aspects of how we come to know and express the whole, genuine self and the authentic being of the other.

Processes involved in developing personal knowing evolve in unique and individual patterns throughout a person's life, but there are dimensions of the experience of personal knowing that can be described. Personal knowledge in the discipline of nursing depends on nurses' dedicated involvement in processes that contribute to their own personal knowing—sharing their insights with other nurses, engaging in mutual response and reflection to deepen their understanding of personal dimensions of knowing in practice, and developing abilities in the therapeutic use of self.

The ability to engage in a genuine authentic presence requires deliberate preparation and intent. Figure 5-2 depicts the interrelationships of preparation processes. Preparation involves private opening and centering practices over time that ground the individual in the center of the self (represented by the heart in the figure) so that the self is known, valued, affirmed, and loved by the self. Among the practices that can be used are journaling, meditation, and various types of body-mind-spirit meditative practices such as yoga, tai chi, labyrinth walking, drumming, chanting, and other similar meditative practices. These practices bring mind-body-spirit into wholeness, create a time-space of inner calm and peace, and bring personal intentions and meanings to realization at a deep level that transcends consciousness.

From time to time, realizations that come from private centering practices enter into shared experiences with others, providing the opportunity to exchange responses and to integrate new perceptions and reflections. As you return to your private time-space of centering, responses from others deepen and enrich your experience of self. In the figure, the dotted loops represent reflection as it moves through the private centering practices, back and forth between the heart center and the interactive responses of others, to depict the circular movement among the aspects of preparation. Preparation provides the core strength and character that enter into

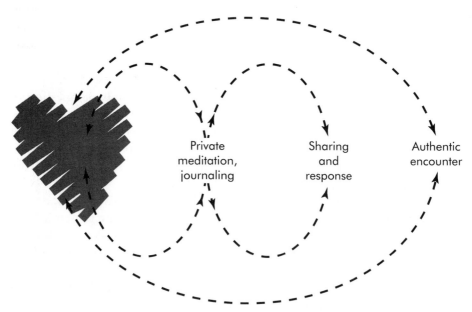

FIGURE 5-2 Preparation processes.

the authentic encounter, where the heart center of the person opens to be fully present with and for the other.

The opening and centering practices of personal knowing are different from "therapy." Therapy can assist a person in a quest for personal knowing, but therapy involves other purposes that focus on healing or restoring one's self from a troubled or disturbed situation to one that is less troubled and more able to cope with life's difficulties. Therapy involves an (often) unequal relationship in which one person provides therapeutic guidance and the other receives. Many practices used for opening and centering, such as meditation, journaling, labyrinth walking, or tai chi, can also be used for therapeutic purposes. But opening and centering are vital processes required to fully know one's self, to constantly deepen inner knowing and self-wisdom irrespective of therapeutic or healing needs. Opening and centering practices can be closely linked for some with prayer. However, prayer is generally a process of communing with a higher power, with a divine being, or with the universe, whereas meditative centering practices are ways of listening to your own heart, your own inner wisdom (Hall, 2004).

Preparation practices of personal knowing are integrated into daily life and focus on self-knowing as a whole, authentic being. They are practices that are self-healing and require the energy of the self without being dependent on outside sources. These practices can be facilitated by others or enhanced by joining with others who share a particular self-healing practice. However, they remain practices that require one's own deepest intentions and attention. In daily practices to nurture self-knowing, the individual reaches into an attentive mind-body-spirit center to come to know and love what resides within.

Opening and centering are interrelated processes that occur in many different ways and in as many different contexts. Opening and centering focus on the lived experience and the meaning of that experience. They are processes that can emerge spontaneously and can be felt within experience, defying description or analysis. Opening and centering occasions also can be deliberately sought as individual, solitary processes that contribute to self-knowing (Beckerman, 1994). In the following section we discuss the practice of journaling and related meditative practices as examples of the elements of personal practice that nurture self-knowing and prepare the self for authentic encounters. Although we focus here on journaling and meditative practices, other forms of practice can be used in similar ways.

Journaling and Meditation

Journaling, a practice that nurtures self-knowing, is a private encounter with the inner self. These practices require solitude away from other people and things. Meditation is a practice of clearing the mind and inviting deep inner awareness to emerge. Both journaling and meditation require consistent, regular practice and time devoted to the practice. There are multiple reasons for journaling, but in the context of developing personal knowing when you journal, what you write is never to be shared with others unless you yourself choose to do so. If you do decide to share something from your journal but are not comfortable sharing it in the form it appears in your journal, you can extract and revise segments from your journal with the intent of sharing with others. In order to be a useful practice for full discovery and knowing of your Self, your journal should be something that you write with the intention of keeping it private, maintaining your sense of safety for the expression of whatever feelings and perceptions emerge from deep within. In your journaling, you can let fears, anxieties, anger, and fantasies surface without even your own censoring. There are no critics peering into the inner self; even your own critical judgment is withheld as you seek to know and value your deepest self.*

Meditative practices can be used without journaling, but meditative practices also are a valuable part of journaling. As you settle into a time for journaling, begin by simply sitting still and quietly, turning your focus to your breath, then taking several deep breaths. Let the sense of your being settle into a centered space. You can move into the meditative practice of repeating a sound (mantra) or an affirmation that brings your focus closer to your center, to your deepest intentions, hopes, and desires. For example, you can repeat an affirmation such as "I trust my inner being" or "I am at peace with the path of my life."

When you feel ready, move to your journal to begin to bring your inner perceptions to the page. Journaling can include recounting facts and events but moves beyond the facts and events to explore how you feel and what is going on inside you. As other people enter your reflections, move back to your own center and explore your sense of being in the situation and the relationship. Journaling is a process of working from both the conscious and the unconscious and of engaging in an inner experience with the self. The inner experience sensitizes your perceptions of events, people, and situations and brings you to a place of harmony and wholeness with who you are in relation to your world (Beckerman, 1994).

---

*We stress this point for educators. We commend the use of journals for student learning and self-reflection, but when student journals are required to be shared with the teacher, the experience loses its fundamental value as a private, safe place where personal knowing can flourish. Personal reflective writings to be shared can be called "logs," "diaries," or "reflective essays" to distinguish their purpose from that of journaling. See Nelson (1994) for further insights regarding the use of reflective writing in teaching.

Abandon rules about written expression to fully express what you feel and your perceptions. You can doodle, draw, and let nonverbal images find expression on the page. Let the unexpected emerge without censorship or judgment. Imagine what you hope and dream for, what your deepest desires are. If you feel drawn to analyze and judge what is coming forth, move back to nonverbal meditation, focus on your breath, and turn your attention once again to being open and feeling unconditional love and value for who you are. The time to analyze and rationally think through problems will come from your journaling process, so you can let go of anything that is drawing your attention toward the rational processes of problem solving while you are journaling. Use the journaling process to deepen your own inner sense of worth and self-love, which will grant you greater clarity and strength to address problems. While you are meditating and journaling, always treat yourself as if you totally love yourself (Nelson, 1994).

You can enter into journaling with a specific intent, or you can enter the time-space with no particular intent other than to let your perceptions of your inner being come to the surface. If you are new to journaling or if you have had an experience or are involved in a situation that is saturating your consciousness, you can use a specific intent that focuses your journaling and meditation. The intent is not a problem-solving intent; rather, it is an intent to explore a particular aspect of your inner self. Box 5-1 gives an example of an intention that can be used to guide journaling.

Almost any image can be used as a focus for journaling as a means of using the process in ways that draw you into your inner self. Beckerman (1994) used works of art and focused her journaling on her perceptions of caring within the works of art. You can create an intention around your hopes and dreams, around memories, or around experiences. For example, you could write a prayer to express your deepest hopes and dreams. You could spend time journaling about different "selves" you have been throughout your life—your child self, your afraid self, your confident self. Typically, starting with a focus simply opens doors and begins the journey to deep reflection, and the path of the reflection then moves in directions that transcend conscious intent.

PROCESSES FOR AUTHENTICATING PERSONAL KNOWING: RESPONSE AND REFLECTION

Response and reflection come from being in the world of experience with others. The self is perceived as unique by others; it brings to each situation and interaction a dynamic that is recognized and known. As people respond

---

Box 5-1
Intentional Journaling

Centering: Set your journal and your pen at your side. Find a comfortable position for your body. Let your breath flow in and out in a natural rhythm. As you breathe, let go of all tension in your muscles. Focus your attention on your inner experience—your feelings, hopes and desires, fears, or worries. Notice what aspect of your inner experience comes most fully to the surface.

Opening: For a few minutes, give this inner experience your full attention and let it come completely into your consciousness. Remain open to whatever comes to you, without judging or censoring your experience. Do not try to find solutions or attempt to analyze the experience. Simply let the experience be, washing thoroughly through your mental awareness, your emotional feeling, and your physical sensations. You may need to laugh, cry, make sounds that match your experience, or move around to express what you are experiencing.

Journaling: Pick up your journal and your pen and put your experience in your journal. You may want to write words, or draw, or let the pen move in free form over the paper. Whatever you put in your journal, let it represent and describe your experience, just as it is.

Integrating: When you have finished journaling, set your journal and pen aside again and notice what your experience is like now. Notice your breath, any tensions in your muscles, your emotional and physical sensations. Notice what sounds or movements now seem to come to the surface.

Affirming: Find a word or phrase that now describes your inner experience and any shift that has happened in your experience. Place this word or phrase into an affirmation. For example, if you now feel released and free, you can use the affirmation "I am free to be." Write this affirmation in your journal, repeating it as many times as you are inspired to write it.

Returning: Take several deep breaths as you leave your journal and return to your usual activities. You can return again to your journal to explore other aspects of your inner experience or to more fully explore this same experience. Notice how your experience shifts in both your usual activities and in your journaling. From time to time, journal about the cycles and phases of your experiences.

---

to one another, they give messages that affirm, disappoint, celebrate, or negate aspects of the expressed self. Responses are taken in, felt, and perceived. In processes of reflection, returning to meditative practices, the person reflects and takes in meanings that arise anew from the interactive experiences.

In addition to responses and interactions that happen in the course of daily experience, insights from meditation, journaling, and other self-knowing practices can be shared with trusted friends and colleagues who are willing to listen and respond to what is offered. Drew (1997), in exploring nurses' meaningful experiences and expanding self-awareness, found that sharing the story of an experience with another person enlarged, solidified, and deepened the meaning of the experience and gave the experience meanings that provided a guide for future interactions.

Autobiographic stories and short essays that are developed from your journal are a way of sharing insights that come to you from journaling while keeping your journal as a protected private document. What you share from your journal should be only what you are sure you want to share. You may have journaled about feelings and emotions around a situation without writing the story of the situation. As you identify what you want to share, you might not include anything from your very personal journaling but use your journal to bring you back to the experience as you develop the story of the situation for sharing. Your journal also will draw you into deeper reflection as to the meaning of the situation, which you can weave into your story in language, metaphors, analogies, or symbols. In some instances you may find excerpts that you do wish to extract and share or integrate into a written or verbal story (Nelson, 1994).

As formally developed autobiographic stories are created and shared within the discipline, insights conveyed in the stories give others in the discipline an opportunity for reflection and response, which in turn enriches and deepens the personal knowing potential of others in the discipline. Although written stories are in one sense limited in their capacity to convey the essence of a person, they are rich in conveying inner processes and meanings that are not easily perceived in the interpersonal experience. Written stories provide opportunities for response and reflection that are different from those provided by the self alone.

FORMS OF EXPRESSION OF PERSONAL KNOWING

The genuine self, as Carper (1978) initially proposed, is the active, acted-in-the world form of expression of personal knowing. The authenticity of the self is appreciated by the self and others, and it grows over time in interactions with others. Autobiographic stories provide a written form of expression of personal knowledge.

The authentic, genuine self is conveyed most explicitly in nursing practice when the nurse engages in the "therapeutic use of self." Therapeutic use of self is the component of practice that arises from personal knowing. Therapeutic use of self can be discerned as a discrete aspect of a nurse's practice, but therapeutic use of self cannot be actualized without scientific competence, moral/ethical comportment, and transformative art/acts.

Formally developed autobiographic stories, written in the first-person voice of the nurse, provide a means of conveying personal knowing in a form that can be widely communicated within the discipline. This type of well-developed story also reflects a dimension of aesthetics, but because it is written as a nurse's first-person account, it reveals deep personal insights and experiences of personal knowing. Autobiographic stories also provide glimpses of ethical/moral comportment and scientific competence, but the main frame of the story remains within the realm of personal knowing.

The story in Box 5-2 was developed by Kathy Maeve (1994) from her personal reflections over weeks of caring for a woman named Dora. It speaks powerfully to her personal struggle to find meaning in the

---

Box 5-2

Regrets

To know Dora is to know regret. I regret the torture inflicted on her in the attempt to rid her body of this leukemia. I regret that we knew we couldn't. I regret the suffering she still has to go through as we finally allow the leukemia to take her life.

I regret that last night when I helped her to the bathroom, she very shyly covered herself, and wonder where such dignity comes from. I regret that because she cannot speak English, she has been treated like a little girl who cannot possibly know what is good for herself. I regret that the one time she acted for herself and boldly sneaked out of the hospital, everyone panicked and schemed about how to get her back. I regret that we did not honor her role as a mother and wife in a way that would have allowed her to realistically plan for these three small children she is leaving with a very young husband. I regret that he doesn't have a clue as to how to live without her.

For myself, I deeply regret that I could not speak directly to Dora, but always had to rely on others. I deeply envied Carmen and Gunda's ability to easily talk with Dora, and Dora with them. But I was her advocate with the system—I ran interference for her. And I was very careful. I knew there was no room for mistakes or misjudgments. I was careful and deliberate. If I had not been so, Dora would have stayed in the hospital the entire last few weeks of her life. As it was, she was in and out on a regular basis but had some time alone with her husband and children. And Dora loved me for this. Still, Dora and Carmen and Gunda got to be women together, and I envied this most of all. Last night Dora told Carmen to tell me that she wishes she could have known me longer so she could have taught me to speak Spanish so the two of us could have "talked as friends."

From Maeve, M. K. (1994). The carrier bag theory of nursing practice. *ANS: Advances in Nursing Science, 16*(4), 9–22. Copyright 1994, Aspen Publishers.

Box 5-2

Regrets—cont'd

The word "regret" hardly describes my sense of loss. So I have to make do with what I imagine about Dora. By my standards, she has had the worst of lives—20 years old, three children, an alcoholic husband who does not speak English and who has no real skills. Yet she had everything. For Dora was happy with who she was—so at home with her deep love for her children and for her husband too. And she had that beauty that young women have when they are full of love and passion and have their whole lives in front of them.

But we spoiled that beauty. We poked her body with needles at every opportunity. She lost her beautiful hair. She vomited so hard, and fried with fevers so high, we feared for her life continually. And then the leukemia finished off Dora's body. Her gums became infiltrated and grew over her teeth, giving her a somewhat gruesome smile. Her skin showed the signs of continual seeping of her precious blood into places where it could no longer sustain her life. And finally, she bled into her brain, shook before us, and never spoke or smiled again.

I look at her this night and see only her ashen body suffused with black and blue bruises and regret that such a beautiful young woman could ever look like this.

I regret that all I can hear now is her bubbling breaths—her voice will never sound again. I regret that because of the loss of her silky black hair, her 2-year-old son calls her a "cuckooee." This is explained to me as a kind of monster, and I regret that any child of this Mexican Madonna could ever see her in this way.

So, finally, I pump morphine into her at increasingly high rates, for I cannot bear to feel that Dora is feeling anything. Her moans are stabbing at me. I want to run away instead of seeing her like this, yet I love her and I must be here—it must be me. So I go in and out of the room and cry with Carmen and Gunda over this sweet child that we cannot save but willingly nurse through this ugly death.

And it is ugly. I don't think I can bear it, yet I can't take my eyes away from Dora, or her year-old baby in the bed next to her, as he plays with his feet, blows bubbles, and smiles at everyone. He looks at Dora with certainty—he has seen Mommy sleep before.

experience of being with Dora, of knowing Dora, and of caring for Dora. The story depicts caring for Dora, but the focus of the story is who Kathy is as a nurse caring for Dora—her own human experience as a nurse in relation to the caring experience. It is a story that speaks to other nurses and illustrates personal knowing.

REFLECTION AND DISCUSSION

In this chapter we explored various conceptual meanings of personal knowing, the processes for developing personal knowledge, how personal knowing is expressed in practice, and how personal knowledge is communicated within the discipline of nursing. The central message of this chapter is: Personal knowing is expressed through the authentic, genuine self and is the basis for the therapeutic use of self in practice. It involves deep inner reflection that is sometimes solitary, as well as openness to mutual, meaningful interactions with others.

To deepen your appreciation of personal knowing, consider the following questions related to the content of this chapter:

1. Bring to mind a patient or family with whom you had a particularly memorable relationship. Write about this person or family, and what you remember about your interactions with them. What did you learn about yourself in this situation?
2. When did you first begin to realize that you were a competent nurse? What experiences led you to this realization?
3. Begin using a meditative practice for 10 minutes each day for 1 week. At the end of the week, reflect on your experience of engaging in this practice. Has it had an influence on your experience? What have you learned about yourself?
4. Review the guidelines for intentional journaling in Box 5-1. Set aside about 20 minutes to journal using these guidelines. Set your journal aside for 2 or 3 days, then return to your journal and reflect on what you wrote. What new insights about yourself came to you as you journaled, and what new insights come to you as you reflect on your journal?
5. Consider a time when you left a nursing care situation feeling a great deal of regret and sadness. What were your regrets, and what brought about your feelings of sadness? What in your own personal past experience connected with this experience in practice?
6. Ask a trusted friend or colleague to share with you his or her impressions of who you are as a nurse. Let the person know that you are not seeking compliments or praise, but that you want an honest reflection of how you come across to others in your practice. Reflect on the perceptions this person shares with you. Are there aspects of his or her perceptions that you feel are not fully consistent with who you are? Did he or she describe traits that you would like to develop in different ways?
7. Consider a nurse you have known who you feel was fully authentic and genuine as a person. What is it about this person that you particularly appreciate? What have you learned from this person about what it means to be a nurse?

Reference List

Beckerman, A. (1994). A personal journal of caring through esthetic knowing. *ANS. Advances in Nursing Science, 17*(1), 71–79.

Bishop, A., & Scudder, J. (1990). *The practice, moral and personal sense of nursing.* New York: National League for Nursing.

Campesino, M., & Schwartz, G. E. (2006). Spirituality among Latinas/os: Implications of culture in conceptualization and measurement. *ANS. Advances in Nursing Science, 29*(1), 69–81.

Carper, B. A. (1978). Fundamental patterns of knowing in nursing. *ANS. Advances in Nursing Science, 1*(1), 13–23.

Drew, N. (1997). Expanding self-awareness through exploration of meaningful experience. *Journal of Holistic Nursing, 15*(4), 406–424.

Hall, B. A. (1997). Spirituality in terminal illness: An alternative view of theory. *Journal of Holistic Nursing, 15*(1), 82–96.

Hall, B. A. (2004). *Surviving and thriving after a life-threatening diagnosis.* Bloomington, IN: 1st Books.

Hall, B. A., & Allan, J. D. (1994). Self in relation: A prolegomenon for holistic nursing. *Nursing Outlook, 42*(3), 110–166.

Hart, H. (1997). Conceptual understanding and knowing other-wise: Reflections on rationality and spirituality in philosophy. In J. H. Olthuis (Ed.), *Knowing other-wise.* New York: Fordham University Press.

Huebner, D. (1985). Spirituality and knowing. In E. Eisner (Ed.), *Learning and teaching the ways of knowing.* Chicago: University of Chicago Press.

Maeve, M. K. (1994). The carrier bag theory of nursing practice. *ANS. Advances in Nursing Science, 16*(4), 9–22.

Moch, S. D. (1990). Personal knowing: Evolving research and practice. *Scholarly Inquiry for Nursing Practice, 4*(2), 155–165.

Munhall, P. L. (1993). "Unknowing": Toward another pattern of knowing in nursing. *Nursing Outlook, 41*(3), 125–128.

Nelson, G. L. (1994). *Writing and being: Taking back our lives through the power of language.* San Diego, CA: LuraMedia.

Pesut, B. K. (2006). Fundamental or foundational obligation? Problematizing the ethical call to spiritual care in nursing. *ANS. Advances in Nursing Science, 29*(2), 125–133.

Silva, M. C., Sorrell, J. M., & Sorrell, C. D. (1995). From Carper's patterns of knowing to ways of being: An ontological philosophical shift in nursing. *ANS. Advances in Nursing Science, 18*(1), 1–13.

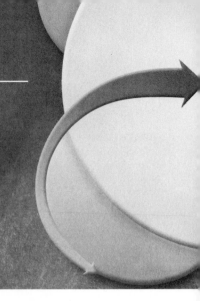

CHAPTER 6

Aesthetic Knowledge Development

The first requisite [of nursing] is the practical belief that the greatest
likeness among humans is their difference. The unspoken lesson of
anatomy, the autopsy room, chemistry lab builds up the insidious
biological impression of the body as a predictable entity—no wonder
normal and alike become confused!

Katherine Brownell Oettinger (1939, pp. 1224–1225)

A esthetic knowing in nursing is that aspect of knowing that connects
with deep meanings of a situation and calls forth inner creative
resources that transform experience into what is not yet real, but possible.
It is the dimension of knowing that connects with human experiences that
are common but expressed and experienced uniquely in each instance. In
practice the art of nursing is expressed in transformative art/acts. Expressions of aesthetic knowledge take the forms of aesthetic criticism and works
of art.

Figure 6-1 shows the aesthetic knowing component of our model for
knowledge development in nursing. In our model the aesthetic pattern of
knowing in nursing requires asking the questions "What does this mean?"
and "How is it significant?" From these questions the processes of envisioning and rehearsing nurture artistic expression of aesthetic knowing. Aesthetic knowing can be shared as aesthetic criticism; works of art such as

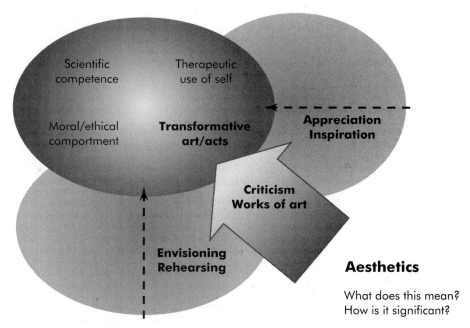

FIGURE 6-1 The aesthetic component of knowledge development in nursing.

poetry, stories, and photographs are also forms of expression of aesthetic knowing that provide for the discipline a source of appreciation and inspiration. In practice, aesthetic knowing is expressed in transformative art/acts, in which the nurse moves experience from what is to a new realm that would not otherwise be possible.

In this chapter, we begin with a discussion of the meaning of art and aesthetics as background for the conceptualization of art and aesthetics in nursing. Next we present a conceptual definition of the art of nursing and discuss our definition in light of other conceptualizations of the art of nursing that have appeared in nursing literature. Finally we focus on the epistemologic dimensions that address ways to develop aesthetic knowing and knowledge. These methods also incorporate important dimensions that address the ontologic processes of experiential perceptual sensibility, that is, cultivating ways of being that sensitize the self to the dimensions of aesthetic practice.

ART AND AESTHETICS

Aesthetics is a noun that derives from the Latin and Greek words referring to perception. It has evolved to refer specifically to the perceptual ability to appreciate artistically valid form. The adjective *aesthetic* identifies an object or experience as artistically valid. That which is artistically valid is coherent in form and substance, conveys meaning of a whole beyond the formative and substantive elements, and evokes a response.

Aesthetics does not necessarily equate to that which is viewed as beautiful or lovely. The standards by which something is taken to be appealing or beautiful vary widely in different disciplines and in different contexts and cultures. Individuals, given their unique perceptions and tastes, respond differently to an art object or experience. Within a given community or discipline, the cultural-disciplinary heritage and explicit or implicit collectively derived criteria of worth mediate the perception of artistic appeal.

However, there are general traits that distinguish that which is artistic or aesthetically valid, and that which is not. That which is artistically valid places various elements into a pattern to form a whole that symbolizes meaning beyond the elements themselves and evokes a feeling response. The meanings conveyed and the feelings that are evoked are connected to the cultural heritage from which the art form arises. But those outside the culture who may not fully recognize the culturally derived meanings still can discern the wholeness of the form, sense meaning inherent in the form, and recognize feeling that might be evoked from the form.

Ordinarily aesthetics is associated with what typically is seen as art. However, things that ordinarily may not be labeled as art have aesthetic characteristics (Sandelowski, 1995). A scientific theory, for example, is a creation that is formed from the elements of conceptual ideas into a pattern that conveys a meaning that the concepts taken alone could not convey. The appeal (a subtle feeling response) of a theory often derives from the aesthetic shape of the theory, its coherence. Without this quality the theory lacks a certain attractiveness or appeal to the community of scientists.

Art is the process of creating an aesthetic object or experience; it also is the term used to refer to the product that is created. Art as a process involves acquired skill in technical and mechanical aspects of working with the elements from which the product is formed, as well as inner capacities to imagine the whole before it becomes an expression and to intuitively bring into being the elements as an integral whole. This process can be readily illustrated in the fine arts, where, for example, the musician acquires technical and mechanical skills with an instrument and learns to bring the elements of sound into expression as a whole musical rendition that generates particular responses for the listener. Art as a product is a form that gives rise to feeling and transforms experience. Art draws the person (whether observer or participant) into a realm that would not otherwise be accessible to experience. Art expands perceptual capacities and possibilities.

Art is not limited to the fine arts. Art is present in all human activity that involves forming elements into a whole. The extent to which the process is satisfying and the extent to which the product assumes coherence as a whole that elicits a feeling response define the extent to which the experience can be called "art" (Eisner, 1985). Value judgments of the worth of any artistic expression do not define something as "art." Art is not limited to that which is called "good art" by some external standard. In many contemporary cultures, what can be called art has come to mean that which will sell or bring a profit. To the contrary, art is found in everyday experience and has multiple forms of expression (Gaydos, 2004; LeVasseur, 1999; Schlenker, 2004).

Likewise, aesthetic qualities (elements placed into a pattern to form a whole, symbolizing meaning beyond the elements themselves) can be reflected in all aspects of nursing practice—from notes written in a chart to theoretic formulations, from a single brief interaction with an individual to sustained interactions with groups and communities, and from an unexpected encounter to a thoughtfully planned design for a system of care. In all of these ranges of nursing experience, nurses draw on and use science, ethics, and personal knowing, as well as aesthetic knowing. It is the dimension of aesthetic knowing that endows the experience with its aesthetic qualities and differentiates it from the impersonal performance of technical acts and routinized procedures.

In philosophy, aesthetics addresses the nature and expression of beauty. Beauty is not taken to mean strictly that which, as a matter of taste, is perceived to be beautiful. Rather, it is that which takes a form that satisfies, or appeals. The substance of that which is addressed as "beauty" in philosophy may, in fact, represent something like sorrow, pain, or despair, but the form of expression conveys a sense of wholeness, a goodness of fit, congruity, integrity, rhythm, harmony, or flow. Further, the form of expression draws the observer into the experience so as to feel or resonate with the experience that is represented. Regardless of substance, the form reflects characteristics of congruence or fit to form a whole. As Carper (1978) stated in her early explanation of the aesthetic pattern of knowing in nursing, "The design, if it is to be esthetic, must be controlled by the perception of the balance, rhythm, proportion and unity of what is done in relation to the dynamic integration and articulation of the whole" (p. 18).

Aesthetic knowing has the following two components: knowledge of the experience toward which the art form is directed and knowledge of the art form itself. For example, the poet requires knowledge of a life experience that is reflected in the poem as well as knowledge of the techniques and methods used to create something that can be called poetry. The visual artist requires knowledge of the experience or situation that will be visually presented as a painting or a sculpture as well as knowledge of the technical aspects of painting or sculpting to achieve the desired visual symbols and representations.

In nursing, knowledge of experience encompasses knowledge of:

- The experience of nursing
- The experiences of health and illness

It is the lived experience of nursing and of health and illness toward which our aesthetics are directed, and it is the experience itself that our art is intended to transform. Background knowledge of experience is acquired through education, through hearing or reading stories about experience, from creating aesthetic knowledge forms such as poetry or paintings that represent nursing experiences, and from experience itself. Nurses learn, for example, about the experience of dying by studying theories of death and dying, by reading or hearing stories about dying, and by caring for people who are dying and their loved ones. Immediate knowledge of experience comes from experiencing another's feelings (Carper, 1978). It involves empathy but includes intuitive knowing and all other possible modes of perceiving another's reality, some of which may not yet be named.

In order to bring an aesthetic quality into the experience of caring for someone who is dying, you also need knowledge of nursing's art form itself, which is the focus of this chapter. We will explore a definition of the art of nursing; the elements that form the whole of the art as a product; the technical skills involved in creating the art/act; and the processes by which those elements can be shaped to form a satisfying, artistically valid whole. The conceptualization of the art of nursing and of the processes that bring the art of nursing into being forms the foundation for developing knowledge of the art form. From this foundation, we describe the processes involved in developing aesthetic knowledge in nursing.

CONCEPTUAL DEFINITIONS OF THE ART OF NURSING

As Johnson (1994, 1996) demonstrated, the idea of the art of nursing has had several different meanings reflected in the nursing literature since the time of Nightingale. Although no single clear definition of the art of nursing prevails, nurse scholars consistently have recognized a phenomenon that they call "the art of nursing" and believe that this aspect of nursing is vital to who nurses are and what they do. A large part of the difficulty in specifying "the art of nursing" is related to the fact that it resides in an ontologic plane; it is expressed in the being-knowing of the nurse. In this realm it does not seem reasonable or possible to fully separate that which can be viewed as aesthetic from that which can be viewed as other patterns of knowing. You can recognize aspects of being that clearly reflect aesthetic form and structure, but these are closely intertwined with scientific competence, therapeutic use of self, and moral/ethical comportment.

Another ontologic dimension that contributes to the difficulty in specifying "the art of nursing" is the embodied nature of art. *Embodied* refers to the whole body-mind-spirit experience; it is knowing-by-feeling. Art is directed toward experience. Human experience is a body-mind-spirit phenomenon in which the dichotomies that prevail in the conventional construction of knowledge cannot be sustained. In our dominant empirically derived approaches to developing knowledge, the rational mind is privileged. Knowledge of the art of nursing is aesthetically derived, calling on the whole mind-body-spirit where embodied perception of experience is one with the mind.

Recognizing the challenges derived from the ontologic dimensions of the aesthetic, of the whole, for this discussion we shift the focus to the following epistemologic question posed by Silva, Sorrell, and Sorrell (1995): How do I come to know the artistry? To address this question, it is necessary to conceptually define the phenomenon of the art of nursing as precisely as possible, integrating understanding of the ontologic dimensions of art. The definition of the art of nursing that we offer here was derived from discussions with practicing nurses who, without exception, recognized meaning in the phrase "the art of nursing" and provided rich discussion of their practices associated with this idea (Chinn, 1994, 2001; Chinn, Maeve, & Bostick, 1997). The inquiry drew on observations of nurses as they practiced nursing, photographs of the nurses as they practiced, journaling to explore deeper symbolic and personal meanings of the practices observed, discussions and storytelling among nurses concerning their experiences of the art of nursing, discussions of possible story lines elicited by viewing the photographs, and rehearsals of aesthetic elements (movement and narrative) of nursing practice as these components took shape. The definition that emerged from this inquiry, and that we are using in this text, is as follows:

> The nurse's synchronous arrangement of narrative and movement into a form that transforms experiences into a realm that would not otherwise be possible. The arrangement is spontaneous, in-the-moment, and intuitive. The ability to make the moves that are transformative is grounded in a deep understanding of nursing, including relevant theory, facts, technical skill, personal knowing, and ethical understanding; and this ability requires rehearsal in deliberative application of these understandings. (Chinn et al., 1997, p. 90)

This definition identifies synchronous narrative and movement as the elements that nurses use in forming the aesthetic experience—which is what, in this textbook, we call the *transformative art/act*. Synchrony is taken to mean the sense of coordination and rhythm of the engaged experience. It also is taken to mean the symbolic synchrony of intention and action coming together as an integral whole.

Synchronous narrative and movement as the elements that form the aesthetic in nursing are critical features of the Chinn, Maeve, and Bostick (1997) definition that have not appeared elsewhere in the nursing literature. As we show later in this chapter, conceptualizing the elements from which nursing art is formed provides substance to understanding and developing knowledge of the art form itself. Other aspects of this definition are connected to the meanings of the art of nursing that Johnson (1994) identified in the nursing literature, but our definition also conveys important distinctions. The following sections present the distinct conceptualizations of the art of nursing that Johnson identified in the nursing literature and discussion of the Chinn, Maeve, and Bostick (1997) definition in light of Johnson's conceptualizations.

The first distinct meaning for nursing art that Johnson identified in the literature is *the ability to grasp meaning in patient encounters*. In our definition of the art of nursing, the ability to grasp meaning in a complex nursing situation toward which our art form is directed is implied, in that a grasp of meaning in a situation is required if the nurse is to transform an experience from what is to what might be possible. In Johnson's (1994, 1996) interpretation of prior conceptualizations of the ability to grasp meaning, it is the meaning of the situation that is perceived intuitively and in the moment; that is, the intuitive aspect is engaged to perceive the health-illness experience of those for whom nurses care (the experience toward which nursing's art is directed).

In our definition, explicit reference to the intuitive, in-the-moment dimension refers to the intuitive element of the art form itself and not necessarily of the experience toward which nursing art is directed. In other words, as a nurse you may not have a grasp of what the moment means to a person or family but you sense something that the situation calls forth, and you act spontaneously on this sense of what is required in terms in caring for the person or family in the moment. This does not mean that you do not immediately grasp the meaning of the situation and the experience of the person or family. Rather, the focus from which your art form emerges is the intuitive use of your creative resources to form experience. You are open to making moves within an experience that you have not anticipated and planned, nor have you necessarily confirmed the patient or family's perceptions of the situation. Rather, your moves come from a perceptual grasp of the formative possibilities that reside within the experience and that are energized by the creative wellspring within your own nursing art-as-process. As a way to better understand what is meant by aesthetics, think about how you cannot really know how to be in a situation until you are actually in it. As an experienced practitioner, as you move into clinically complex care situations, you comprehend—all at once—what a situation is calling forth and you respond wholly. As you respond, your being, or behavior, calls forth in the other or others a response that, in turn, you intuitively read, wholly understand, and respond to. These sorts of all-at-once, instantaneous, and simultaneous response patterns, which transform the experience in the moment, constitute the art/act.

The intuitive aspect of creating form is what is referred to as creativity. It is a knowing-in-the-moment-of-creating that enables the artist to express unique possibilities that fit, that fall into the whole in right relationship. It then follows that intuitive perception of right relationship within the form depends, in a nursing encounter, on a deep grasp of meaning embedded in the situation.

Prior conceptualizations that concern the ability to grasp meaning either explicitly or implicitly refer to meaning as it relates to patient encounters. Our definition is clearly applicable to patient encounters but also can be found in nursing actions that do not involve a direct patient encounter. The ability to design a system of care is grounded in a grasp of meaning in the experience of people for whom the system is designed. Here, the spontaneous and intuitive aspects of the process of creating the design occur in the formation process, in which the nurse-designer is immersed in the experience of creating the design and is open to the flow of possibilities that emerge as the design takes shape.

The second conceptual meaning that Johnson (1994) identified in the nursing literature is *the ability to establish a meaningful connection with the person being cared for.* This aspect of the art of nursing is implied in our definition rather than being explicit, in that "transformative moves" require a connection of a certain type. This is closely related to the ability to grasp meaning in a situation; without a grasp of meaning, a meaningful connection is not possible. Transformative moves require presence with the other, literally or symbolically. In the context of relationship, synchronicity or rhythmicity can be perceived. The "synchronous arrangement of narrative and movement" elicits a synchronous interaction, with a timing and flow among all elements, including those present in the situation. The observable synchronicity symbolizes the deeper level of connection between the nurse and the person and is symbolic of the meaning in the connection.

The third conceptual meaning for the art of nursing that Johnson (1994) identified is *the ability to skillfully perform nursing activities,* which is one of the earliest conceptualizations of nursing art and a meaning that often was expressed by nurses who participated in Chinn's aesthetic inquiry (Chinn, 1994; Chinn et al., 1997). Nurses first pointed to tasks and procedures that are required in the "doing" of nursing, noting that it is how they do what they do that characterizes their art. The skills themselves do not constitute the art of nursing. Rather, the ability to "skillfully perform" is a characteristic of aesthetic form expressed in the nature of the nurse's movement and narrative, which may or may not involve tasks and procedures.

Skillful performance derives from a background of rehearsal that makes possible what Benner and Wrubel (1989) identify as "ready-to-hand" knowing. In our definition, skillful performance is explicit with respect to technical skill. However, the definition implies an integration of technical skill with relevant theory, facts, personal knowing, and ethical understanding, and the rehearsal that is required to develop the art of nursing is an integrated form of rehearsal in which all dimensions of being and acting are brought together to form a whole.

The fourth conceptual meaning that Johnson (1994, 1996) identified is *the ability to rationally determine an appropriate course of nursing action.* Research concerning clinical judgment and reasoning reveals the intuitive and aesthetic components that are necessary for sound practice (Benner, Tanner, & Chesla, 1996; Mattingly, 1994). However, in our conception, rational judgment is not a defining element of the art of nursing. In our definition, rational ability, like technical skill, is background necessary for aesthetic capability. It constitutes an important component of knowledge of that toward which nursing art is directed, but it does not point to knowledge of the art form itself. The artist must draw on rational understanding in the process of artistic creation, but rational understanding is not the key element of aesthetic sensibility.

A composer, for example, uses accepted theories of rhythm in constructing a musical score but in the process has spontaneous, intuitive inspiration to integrate rhythmic variations that may defy common conventions. In so doing the composer places a unique signature on the work that gives it artistic value and character. Likewise, as a nurse you apply theoretic understanding of a particular type of illness experience in developing a rational plan of care to point toward appropriate nursing action but remain open to spontaneous and intuitive inspiration to integrate variations as the caring process unfolds. It is the variations integrated with rational understanding that signify artistic form, and the particular ways in which the nurse shifts or moves through the experience convey an artistic signature, a particular and unique quality to the experience.

Finally, Johnson (1994) identified *the ability to morally conduct one's nursing practice* as a distinct conceptual meaning of the art of nursing that has appeared in the nursing literature. Like technical skill and rationality, our definition of the art of nursing points to ethical understanding as background essential for aesthetic practice. There is a value component in the idea of "transformative moves" that implies a significant ethical dimension inherent in the art of nursing, in that transforming creates a change in what would otherwise be. Nurses who participated in the aesthetic inquiry from which our definition was derived told many stories of their practice that involved ethical dilemmas and that elicited actions that they associated with the art of nursing. Although it can be said that an experience could not be recognized as artistically valid if it violates ethical sensibilities, aesthetic knowledge in itself does not convey ethical understanding (Vezeau, 1994b). Rather, aesthetic representation can reveal the significance of ethical and moral dilemmas and contribute to developing ethical sensibilities (Maeve, 1994). The ethical component that can be identified within the art of nursing comes from the integration of ethical comportment and transformative art/acts.

PROCESSES FOR DEVELOPING AESTHETIC KNOWLEDGE: ENVISIONING AND REHEARSING

The processes for developing aesthetic knowledge are envisioning possibilities, rehearsing, and forming the elements of the art into perceivable reality by creating representations of the possibilities. From these creative processes, aesthetic criticism can be constructed as a form of knowledge of the artistry of nursing that can be shared with others. Works of art also emerge as representations of what is known, and also are a form of aesthetic knowledge that can be made available to the broader audience within and outside of the discipline. Art forms that have been created in nursing to represent the meaning and significance of nursing and health experiences include poetry, photography and other visual art forms, story, drama, and dance (Chinn & Watson, 1994).

As nurses share and communicate insights derived from the processes of envisioning, rehearsing, and representing the artistry of nursing, the responses of others in the discipline place the work and the meanings represented within the context of the discipline. The connoisseur processes of appreciation and inspiration reflect back on the experience that is represented, the representations, and the symbolized meanings that are conveyed through the representations. Connoisseur processes, or expert judgment of aesthetic validity, deepen shared knowledge of the art of nursing.

Transformative art/acts are the in-the-moment, ontologic expression of the art of nursing in nursing contexts. These art/acts are characterized by synchronous forms of movement and narrative that transform the health-illness experience from what is into a realm that would not otherwise be possible. These art/acts usher the experience of those involved from one moment to the next, expanding the realm of possibilities into the future (Benner & Wrubel, 1989). In these instances everything comes together in synchrony, like a dance. It "works" for everyone involved in the situation. This experience has an element of mystery; it is perceived in the moment but not consciously or analytically understood. It involves feeling moved to a realm of possibility that had not been planned or anticipated but that is sensed as right for the moment.

Our conceptualization of transformative art/acts are consistent with descriptions of expert practice that Benner and her colleagues have identified (Benner, 1984; Benner et al., 1996). However, even though expert nursing practice involves artistic expertise, expertise is not a prerequisite for transformative art/acts and artistic practice. Novice and beginner nurses draw on aesthetic sensibilities as they practice. In fact, well-tuned artistic abilities at any level of expertise enrich the experience of caring for both nurses and patients.

Envisioning and Rehearsing

Envisioning and rehearsing are two interrelated processes from which creative possibilities emerge and within which aesthetic knowing is grounded. They are processes that can be perceived when nurses describe their art because nurses who have acquired artistic capacity intuitively have engaged in these processes in the course of their nursing practices. They have not been deliberately taught, nor have they conceptualized what they do in this way. In fact, many of the practices that Chinn, Maeve, and Bostick (1997) came to view as envisioning and rehearsing involve activities that the nurses hid from view, engaged in during their time away from job responsibilities, and previously assumed to be insignificant and trivial yet sometimes necessary to cope with difficult situations. For example, as nurses described situations that represented their art, they also consistently related how they told one another stories about the situation in phone conversations after work, over a meal, or in a secluded area during a down time. Their storytelling episodes always included an account of the response of the listener and the way their interactive talk formed and re-formed how they came to see similar situations and how they came to trust their own intuitive senses. When the nurses associated these and similar activities as necessary and important aspects of developing aesthetic knowing of their art form, they immediately grasped the connection.

A useful analogy for understanding the processes of envisioning and rehearsing is that of improvisation. In an improvisational art, which characterizes the art of nursing, the display (or performance) is possible because of carefully developed skills in the various moves and sequences that can be called forth in any unique situation. This requires intense rehearsal and development of finely tuned skills that are fully embodied. The artist develops skills covering a wide range of possible effects or feelings that the improvisation might call for and rehearses imagined passages before a coach or critic to receive direction concerning the symbolic meanings conveyed in each passage.

For example, in improvisational drama the actor practices sequences of movements, postural and facial expressions, and voice intonations that convey wide ranges of emotion, and narrative lines that give verbal expression to possible experience. The director (critic, coach, teacher) gives the artist feedback and guidance that lead the actor into new territory at times or guide the actor through repeated trials of an emerging sequence to perfect the sequence and bring the moves to a refined, embodied level. When, in the improvised interaction on stage, a particular attitude emerges, the actor has the skills so finely tuned that in the improvised moment, the actor's focus remains in the moment of the interaction and on the process that is emerging in the improvised situation. The actor does not convey authenticity if the moves are not fully embodied; the actor cannot pretend (a notion often associated with "acting"). Rather, authenticity can come only from moves that have become so fully embodied that the actor thoroughly feels and experiences the situation.

In the following sections we describe the processes for envisioning and rehearsing narrative and movement as elements of nursing practice. The processes we describe are not linear or sequential. Any one process can be the particular focus for a time, but they most often come together and interweave. They are presented separately here to describe in some detail what they are and how they function to contribute to aesthetic knowing. The processes include (1) creating and re-creating story lines, (2) creating and developing embodied synchronous movement abilities, and (3) rehearsing a situation and engaging a critic.

Creating and Re-creating Story Lines. When nurses tell stories to one another, they move into a realm that is created from the imagination and is not bound by the constraints of the workaday world. Even when the story begins with the intention of conveying an accurate account of a real experience, in the telling of the story the narrator creates emotion, stresses points of emphasis, exaggerates or downplays selected elements of the story, and selects certain features to include or exclude. Often the desires of the storyteller peek through in ways that surprise even the storyteller. Unexpectedly the storyteller gives, for example, an account of what she or he wishes had been done in the situation as if it actually happened, rather than accounting for what did happen. If the story were viewed through the lens of empirics, the story would have little or no worth. Viewed through the lens of aesthetics, the story has exquisite value as a frame from which to explore possible avenues of understanding and meaning, to shift experiential ground and expand perceptual capabilities called forth by the new ground, and to create visions and possibilities for the future (Maeve, 1994).

A story that is grounded in aesthetic knowing is told in the voice of the person who receives nursing care. Stories told in the voice of the nurse are more often reflective of personal knowing and explore inner personal meanings. Stories told in the voice of the person receiving nursing care reflect a deepening understanding, empathy, and embodied knowing of the experience of the other. The story illuminates the health and illness experience toward which nursing's art form is directed. The story can come from actual experience, but aesthetic storytelling does not require adhering to the factual "truth" of a situation, as an empiric case study or anecdotal account requires. The storyteller purposely exaggerates, fictionalizes, emphasizes, and reshapes the actual experience to enhance listeners' perceptions of certain meanings that are intended to be conveyed in the story. The story comes from the imagination more than from the actual experience, although the imagination is inspired by actual experience. The well-developed story will reveal a deeper truth of insight, understanding, and wisdom—the deepest meanings and possibilities in human experience that often are not manifested in empiric reality or perceived cognitively.

In the process of creating a story line, the essential characters are placed in a situation that presents a tension that moves toward an uncertain ending. The story line might be based on an actual situation, the ending of which is known, but for the purposes of aesthetic development the ending is left open and variable. The tensions that move toward the ending are central to the process of creating different story lines. Characters other than the essential characters can shift and move in and out of the story; each character can take on different roles as the story lines shift.

Creating and re-creating story lines serve several purposes related to aesthetic knowing. Most important from the perspective of aesthetics, each story line brings forth new perceptions of meaning that could be possible in the situation. The varying story lines bring to awareness how various meanings are symbolized in human experience and open new possibilities for creative engagement with each emerging meaning. Stories elicit profound reflection on meaning, both personal meaning and the meanings that others represent in the story. In this way the story brings to awareness knowledge of that toward which our art is directed—the experiences of those whom nurses care for and the meanings that can be embedded in those experiences.

Creating and re-creating story lines also provide narrative experience and rehearsal, which in turn develop knowledge of and skill with the art of nursing itself. Creating story lines provides a way to experience a situation vicariously and to place one's intention into action as an integral whole. It also becomes a rehearsal in which the present is integrated with insights from the past and possibilities for the future. The exact words that emerge in the process of creating and re-creating story lines are not those used in the actual practice situation, but the facility to form narrative lines develops an ability to use narrative effectively in practice. The narrative that is used to tell a story places the plot within a context; conveys the "feel," the attitude, and the mood of the story; and integrates the various elements of the story line to form a whole vicarious experience placed in narrative time and space. Narrative that is used in practice serves the same functions, in that it places the isolated real experiences of the person into a larger plot; contributes to creating an atmosphere within which the experience unfolds; and integrates the various elements of experience into the whole of the past, present, and imagined future. In the rehearsal of creating and re-creating story lines, you work with complete or nearly complete narratives. In practice the complete story line may never unfold, but the narrative moves of the nurse serve to shift experience into and through an emerging life plot.

In creating a story line you can develop your ideas in writing (Sorrell, 1994) or conversation. The creation of a story line can begin with an anecdotal account of a real experience. The experience can be your own, or it can be an experience that you observed or have heard about. The first account of the experience is likely to seem relatively simple and inadequate to represent the significance of the experience itself, and it may sound "clinical" because of the culturally acquired propensity to focus on anecdotal accounts of a sequence of events, or clinical case studies.

To create a story line, first explore what about this experience compels your attention; identify the key characters involved in the experience; and imagine each character's perspective, motives, and intentions. Explore the context within which the experience is set and key elements of the situation that seem important to the unfolding of the story. Imagine various endings

toward which your experience could have moved or might move. Ultimately you will select a preferred ending, but various endings provide possibilities for building tensions within the middle of the story around what is
possible and toward uncertain endings.

Next, sketch out the essential characters that you wish to place within your
story line. You can shift the characters as your story line unfolds and changes,
but the characters will remain central to the story line. As you sketch the
characters, the elements of the story line will begin to emerge because
characters change over the time line that is portrayed in the story line. Imagine several different possibilities for the movement of the story line, and let
one of the possibilities emerge into the story. This will be your first narrative,
material with which you can work in re-creating the story line with other
possible endings.

The principles associated with creating and re-creating story lines
(Mattingly, 1994) are as follows:

- The interactions between the characters of the story and their motives
  provide key structuring devices. Unlike clinical accounts of illness, a
  story line shifts attention away from the contingencies of the illness,
  disability, or health challenge to the way the characters in the story
  structure their experiences. Actions, interactions, and motives move
  the story line along toward the end of the story without revealing the
  end (Mattingly, 1994). In Toni Vezeau's story titled "Hair, Smells,
  Spaces" (Vezeau, 1994a, pp. 181–186), Elena is giving birth. She uses
  vivid descriptions of the smells of Elena, her mother, and the nurse
  who are present in the room and fully experiencing the hopes, joys,
  pain, and fear of the experience. Xavier, the father, stands outside the
  room but his smell also enters the room, emanating in part from his
  fear that the baby might not be his, in part from the hope that it is. An
  unnumbered group of disinterested observers are present, but do not
  give off any smells.
- The story line is organized within a time-space of desire for a good
  ending. What is happening as the story unfolds is a time-space that
  cannot remain static because it is a place of tension where readers/
  listeners do not want to be, where the ending might be one that is
  dreaded. The story line compels movement toward an ending and
  elicits a desire for an ending in the listener or reader of the story. The
  valence of desire toward a valued end elicits an account of what the
  nurse wishes she had done, rather than what actually was done
  (Mattingly, 1994). In "Hair, Smells, Spaces" there are two good

endings that drive the story line—the successful birth of Elena's child, and how the mystery of fatherhood might be resolved (Vezeau, 1994a).

- Change is central to a story line. People and things change over time. Time moves toward an end, but within the line of the story, time can play tricks of reversal and circularity, boomerang around, and cross time lines situated before the story begins. The ending of the story represents a transformation from the state of affairs at the beginning of the story, and the agency that is the most important in creating the transformation is human motive and action (Mattingly, 1994). Vezeau provided a masterful portrayal of change, using metaphors of smell and hair and space throughout her story. The time of the story is only the short time of a difficult labor and birth, but the metaphors of smell and hair place the story in the larger context of each of the character's lives (Vezeau, 1994a).
- Conflict, struggle, and tension are ever present. The beginning of a story line sets up the focus of the tension, and as the story line proceeds, the obstacles to be overcome in dealing with the tension unfold. The story line simultaneously builds the desire to resolve the tension. As the story line moves forward, the voices of the key players express different perspectives on the tension and the desired ending and leave the ending uncertain (Mattingly, 1994). The beginning story line of "Hair, Smells, and Spaces" builds conflict, struggle and tension into the rich symbolic descriptions of the hair, smells, and spaces so central to birthing (Vezeau, 1994a).
- Endings remain uncertain throughout the story line, sometimes even through the ending of the story. Several different anticipated endings never happen. As the story line unfolds, what is positioned between the past (the beginning) and the future (the end) is a landscape of what is possible. The ending of the story need not be logically necessary, but rather it illustrates what is possible. The ending of the story line must be plausible, but it is only one of several plausible endings (Mattingly, 1994). In Vezeau's story, the reader is drawn into the unfolding story line, hoping for the desired endings but never sure until the very end. The anticipated birth provides a surprise that the disinterested observers view with alarm and dread—the baby has six toes on his left foot. Xavier immediately recognizes the extra toe as the resolution of his conflict—he himself has a sixth toe on his left foot (Vezeau, 1994a)!

These same principles used in creating a story line characterize the real-life story that unfolds for a person experiencing illness, disability, or other health challenges (Mattingly, 1994). The difference is that the story unfolds in small increments placed in experienced time. The interactions, motives, and intentions of the people involved in the situation are the key structuring device that develops the plot of the story and moves the real-life story (experience) forward. What is happening usually is not a situation the key players desire to be in, or they know they cannot stay in the situation (like the moments after the joyful birth of a child). The desire to move forward and to move into a different place is strong. Change is central; every day—sometimes every moment—brings with it a new challenge. Conflict, struggle, and challenge are ever present, and there are obstacles to be overcome. The ending of the story remains uncertain, with the unfolding life story positioned between the past and the future, where the landscape is what is possible.

Creating and re-creating story lines provide aesthetic narrative skills that the nurse uses as a participant in the emerging real-life stories of those for whom care is provided. The experienced unfolding story is shaped and transformed by the emerging possibilities of the present time situated between past and future. Mattingly (1994) described this process as "therapeutic emplotment." The story that unfolds is not constructed in the same way a story line is constructed and usually is not told as an explicit story. Instead, the plot of the story is lived. The aesthetic challenge is to gradually structure isolated episodes into a plot that moves toward a possible end and bring to the experience actions and narrative lines that emplot the experience and that move the experience toward a possible ending.

The synchrony among all the participants of the real-life story signifies their mutual participation in the creation of the plot, the selection of a possible ending, and the creation of the shifts of action that bring about changes and transformations as the real-life story unfolds. The plot unfolds in moment-by-moment interaction; it cannot happen as a plan or a design. The possible desired end toward which the participants wish to move provides a force toward which movement is directed. The nurses' ability to participate in this essentially aesthetic process is nurtured by skills they develop through rehearsal in creating and re-creating story lines.

For example, consider your experience of working with someone who had a life-altering experience such as a major trauma or disabling illness. You enter the person's life story at a time when the imagined future that the person had anticipated is inalterably changed. The person and the family face a period of tension and uncertainty in which the new imagined future is a dreaded future, one that was never imagined before. As their nurse, you begin with small, everyday acts of nursing care. With each nursing interaction, you begin to create with the patient and family a new plot that cannot be fully anticipated in advance. Based on your experience and background as a nurse, you are able to help the patient and family imagine a new future, perhaps not a desired future, but one that they can begin to embrace. Some elements of the new future are small, everyday things like learning to function with only one arm. Other elements of a new future are more complicated, like imagining new options for making a living.

Creating story lines that move the situation toward a desired future provides a vision of what might be and a rehearsal of ways in which nursing care can be enacted to energize movement in a new direction. As the actual experience unfolds, that which is envisioned by the nurse and by the client and family is shaped by everyday experiences. As the nurse assists the person to take a few first steps after a traumatic injury, for example, the possibility for mobility begins to take form, and along with this possibility comes the potential for returning to a job or re-engaging in a desired activity. The imagined scenarios of one's new life story gradually begin to take shape, formed by the mutual interactions of nurses, family members, and others involved in caring for the person.

The purpose for creating stories is twofold. First, your stories develop a deep sense of connection with human experience that only aesthetic expressions can convey. This sense of connection begins for you as you develop the story. It also then becomes a possible reality for all who read or hear the stories you create. Second, your stories can provide an avenue for you to explore, and in a sense rehearse, new possibilities for practice. If you place a dynamic in your story that reflects a situation in practice that you had hoped for but never happened, or that you imagine might be possible, then this imagined situation is akin to having actually experienced it in practice. Your story provides a vicarious experience that brings your nursing practice closer to becoming real.

Creating Embodied Synchronous Movement. Movement is inherent to the practice of nursing, and yet very little attention is given to systematic development of movement skills, other than body mechanics. Movement is taken for granted; people enter nursing with a lifetime of experience in moving through space and with a cultural understanding of the symbolic significance of various moves, gestures, and postures. Within the frame of the art of nursing, movement takes on a very different level of significance. Movement is a mind-body-spirit integrity, in which what is expressed in a body move represents a complex flow of intention, concerns, hopes, desires, and fears.

As an element of the art of nursing, movement becomes the medium for expression of meaning that parallels visual representation in the fine arts. Like the picture that conveys a thousand words, your movements as a nurse express a multitude of meanings on many levels. The communicative power of movement includes what is popularly known as body language, sending messages grounded in the culture that require no language and, in fact, at times defy language. In addition, movement communicates who you are as a nurse, the nature of your intentions, how you regard your self, your genuineness as a nurse and as a human being, your capacity for being in a relationship, and your level of technical and scientific competence.

Movement, including posturing, engages synchronous interaction. How you move in and around a situation sets a rhythm, a style, a dynamic, a pace, and an attitude that invites engagement. It is a fundamental symbolic marker of your synchronous abilities as a nurse artist.

Important dimensions of your artistic ability can be perceived only when others' responses in the environment are viewed as an integral whole with the nurse's movement. If the way in which you move into a room, for example, conveys to people who are in the room that you are in a rush, or impatient, their reactions to your entry will reflect their personal response to the message conveyed by your movement. Some people who perceive your impatience might be apologetic for bothering you; others might feel angry that you seem inconvenienced by what they legitimately need and feel entitled to. If you do not intend to show your sense of impatience or being rushed, then your challenge is to acquire ways of moving into a situation that do not convey this message to others.

Movement brings physical and symbolic touch into being. The meaning of touch, considered vitally important in nursing practice, is conveyed through the movement that brings the touch into being and that moves away from the touch. As an example, consider a scene in the movie *Silence Like Glass*, in which Eva, a rising star ballerina, faces a devastating malignancy and can no longer dance. Her dance partner, with whom she had dreamed of touring the world, comes to visit. As he is leaving, she reaches out to touch his hand in a loving gesture that also conveys the regret and sorrow of the moment. He quickly withdraws his hand from her touch, with a subtle upper body shift backward and a facial expression of repulsion. Here, if you observe just the moment of touch in a snapshot of her hand touching his, you might conclude that it was a gesture of caring and love, and the fuller meaning of the episode—his movement of withdrawal from her touch—would be lost.

Movement provides a means for a nurse to define the time-space within which care and concern will be expressed (Chinn et al., 1997). As the nurse enters an encounter, body moves, gestures that sometimes include touch, and visual scanning define the space within which the nurse turns attention throughout the encounter. The nurse's moves remain primarily within this space until near the end of the encounter, at which time there occurs a gesture or move, often along with words, that signifies retreat from the encounter.

Movement brings about actions of protection, assistance, comfort, and healing. The intentions that bring these types of moves into being are inherent within the moves and serve to define the moves. The actual body movement and posturing can be done without conscious intention, but without intention, movement is mechanical and void of meaning. With conscious intention, your movement can be deliberately shaped so that subtleties of posture and sequence of movement carry meanings that help to shape the interaction. Your intention that energizes the movement can be sensed by others, because your intention is embedded in the style of the move, and in the physical form and shape of your movement.

Movement is the medium that conveys aesthetic performance of technical abilities. Like movement that provides comfort and healing, technical performance can be empty and mechanical. What creates an aesthetic performance of a technical ability is the nurse's intention to bring the various elements of the experience and the situation into a coherent, integrated whole, in which all movements fall into right relationship. Being able to do this requires practice (rehearsal) and well-developed skill, but unless the caring/healing intention is inherent in the performance, the act of doing the technical task remains mechanical. Intention saturates the movements of technical ability with meaning; finely tuned style, timing, finesse, and coordination convey artistic as well as scientific competence.

The aspects of mind-body-spirit movement that contribute to its artistic quality are as follows:

- *Coordinated balance* is the concurrent movement of all parts of the body within a whole, smooth, integral pattern. Coordinated balance includes breath patterns as a foundation for the more visible coordination of muscle movement. Breath forms the rhythm of the movement and undergirds the movement with strength, both physical and symbolic. Coordinated balance among parts within a sequence of movements requires embodied knowing of the intended flow of the sequence. You may have cognitive awareness of the flow of sequence of movement, but the more your moves arise from embodied intelligence and are not cognitively processed, the finer and more balanced your coordination.
- *Finesse* is the refinement and versatility with which moves are made. Finesse depends on embodied familiarity with the environment, the objects, and the processes with which you work. It reflects integrated knowing of the material world and the capabilities of the body. Finesse

comes with practice and experience and can be nurtured with rehearsal, but each individual has different aptitudes for developing finesse with different moves.

- *Style* is the unique character that each individual brings to movement—the heart of the movement. It is the particular way that you use movement in the process of bringing intention and action together, and your unique artistic expression that emerges in the creation of an integrated whole. Style cannot be taught because it arises from who you are as a unique person. Style can be encouraged; as others respond to your unique ways of acting and being in the world, you begin to appreciate your own personal style and refine your abilities to use your own style to express your intentions. Style can be described and characterized by the observer, but it cannot be duplicated because it resides as an integral element within the self. There can be no value judgments with respect to style itself, but style is an important aspect that contributes to artistic value. Artistic value resides not in the style per se but in the form of the whole, the meaning that is conveyed, and the responses that are evoked.

- *Timing* involves rhythm, pace, and the placement of various moves with a time sequence of an unfolding experience. The saying that timing is everything certainly applies to the artistic validity of nursing art. Timing is an important factor in narrative interactions as well as movement; *when* you say something is vitally important. Timing is a key marker of intuitive ability because timing cannot be planned in advance, and it is not cognitively processed. Rather, timing emerges from apprehension in the moment as an experience unfolds.

- *Synchrony* is the ability to bring together elements of the environment, the responses of others, and the situation into an integrated whole. Synchrony depends on coordination, finesse, style, and timing. It brings all elements of movement together in interaction with the situation.

Movement is a medium that creates the shape of the emerging story of a lived experience. It is an avenue of communication that shows, demonstrates, opens, assists, and inspires the shift from one moment to the next. When movement is considered as a foundational element of the art of nursing, it acquires symbolic meaning that shapes the form of the whole and the intended feeling response.

The aspects of coordination, finesse, and style can be rehearsed in isolated practice sequences and deliberately planned exercises. Timing and synchrony need to be rehearsed within a situational context because they are guided by the situation. Timing and synchrony can be refined by placing various situations in a story line to rehearse alternative timing and elements of synchrony. Reflecting on practice situations provides material from which new story lines can be imagined and rehearsed.

Movement exercises, particularly those that are meditative (such as tai chi or yoga), can be used to develop embodied movement skills of coordination, finesse, and style. These forms of movement provide rehearsal in bringing intention and imagery into expression through physical movement. The posturing and movements of these body meditations are consistent with good body mechanics, developing an embodied sense of balance, rhythm, and coordination.

Rehearsal and Engaging a Connoisseur-Critic. Rehearsal can focus on specific aspects of narrative or movement, or it can involve a real-life situation in all of its complexity. It most often brings several elements together into a situation that is performed either in a protected studio where you might role-play various situations, or in a relatively safe actual nursing situation. A connoisseur-critic is an experienced nurse who is well versed in the art of nursing and who is able to envision the best forms of artistic nursing practice. A connoisseur-critic is also committed to teaching and coaching others as they develop artistic abilities.

Engaging a connoisseur-critic to observe your rehearsal is a vital aspect of developing aesthetic ability. Developing your art form depends on being able to convey a sense of the whole and a sense of feeling. As the one who is "performing" you cannot be situated in the role of the observer. Only from the observer's perspective can artistic validity be fully perceived. It is in interaction with the responses of the critic that you gain insight into the integrity of your expression, deepen your knowledge of your art form, and discover avenues for moving your art to a new realm of possibility (Reed, 1995).

Connoisseur-critics have deep familiarity with and appreciation of the art form. They have developed sufficient skill in the art form to understand the technical expertise that is required. They have studied the theories that pertain to the art form so that they have knowledge of that toward which the art is directed, as well as knowledge of the art form itself. They know the history of the art form and understand how it has changed over time. They are familiar with the cultural context within which the art form currently is placed and the possibilities for new directions that are emerging within the art. Given their expertise, they have developed a keenly trained "eye" and "ear" and "feel" for the art (Chinn et al., 1997). The intention of the connoisseur-critic is to nurture the artist's ability to a new dimension of expression. It is this intention, and its translation into action, that creates a safe environment that nurtures the artist's skill. A skilled teacher is a connoisseur-critic, and a skilled connoisseur-critic is a skilled teacher.

Connoisseurship is integral to the process of developing the art. Skilled critics nurture critical abilities in the novice artist and build the reflective capacities necessary for refining aesthetic ability. Knowledge of the art expands beyond knowing how to place elements into a form. The novice also acquires aesthetic sensitivity to meanings in the art as it is being performed, an educated appreciation of the work of expert practitioners, and openness to inspiration from the work of others.

The primary function of the connoisseur-critic in a rehearsal context is to provide guidance that moves the art form to a new level of development. The critic provides substantive information about aspects of the performance that are well developed, elements of the performance that show promise for development, and specific guidance for taking the performance to a new level of skill. Ideally the critic works with the artist over time so that the critic becomes familiar with the unique abilities and style of the performer and can place each rehearsal in the context of evolving ability. The critic becomes sensitive to signals of emerging ability and moves with the artist to encourage the next move toward artistic competence.

The critic does not give generalized value judgments of "good" or "bad." Value judgments are empty of substantive insight about the performance. The critic does give authentic indicators of the feeling response that the performance elicited, as well as substantive information as to what about the performance elicited response. For example, in response to a nurse's unexpected move that clearly turns an evolving situation in a new direction, the critic might say, "When you did ... [summarizing the move], at first I said to myself 'Oh no!' because it was so unexpected and seemed so daring, so out of place. Then, as soon as I saw what happened next, I was overjoyed because clearly you made a breakthrough when you did that." Here, the value-laden responses of fear and joy are grounded in the particular perspective of the critic and explicitly linked with the nurse's actions.

When the critic observes something that could change or that needs to change, rather than render a value judgment of "bad," the critic gives specific guidance for the next step and, if possible, places the element within the context of the performer's history. For example, in response to a move that is awkward and poorly timed, the critic's response might be the following: "I sensed that you were distracted and tense today when you ... [summarizing the move]. One thing that you might try next time is to pause and breathe for a moment before you jump into this kind of challenge. Spend a moment getting clear about your intentions as you gather your equipment, and breathe!" Or the critic might respond, "You lacked finesse when you were ... [summarizing the incident]. Here is a small sequence of moves that you can practice over the next week that I think will help. Start out slowly, and practice breathing and establishing a rhythm, a flow."

Connoisseurship implies a creativity of its own in that the critic engages in observing the rehearsal with a sense of openness to insights that previously have not been conceived. It also implies a discipline in that the critic offers a trained perspective and expectation concerning artistic validity. The elements that the critic observes in light of expectations for artistic validity include the following:

- *Voice intonation and expression in narrative.* The way that narrative is delivered carries the feeling of the narrative. The critic notices the feeling that is elicited from the narrative and notes specific elements of expression that appear associated with the response.
- *Substance of the narrative interactions.* The critic notices words, phrases, and narrative sequences and how they are framed within the whole.
- *Synchrony of movement.* The critic observes how movement is situated within the context and provides guidance for developing skill in areas that interfere with integrity and synchrony.
- *Synchrony between movement and narrative.* The critic observes the ways in which movement and words come together to form a whole within the interaction and ways in which movement and narrative fall into place in right relationship.
- *Perceived intention and emotion.* The critic senses the intention that is communicated by the nurse, which may not coincide with the nurse's felt intention. When the perceived (received) intention and the nurse's felt intention do not coincide, elements of artistic form might need to shift to adequately convey the felt intention.
- *Synchrony of interaction.* The critic notices the responses of others in the situation and the rhythm and flow in the interactions, which reveal possible avenues for developing the art.

AESTHETIC KNOWLEDGE FORMS: CRITICISM AND WORKS OF ART

Works of art that are developed to show and symbolize artistic qualities that are expressed in nursing practice are an unwritten form of aesthetic knowledge. Works of art can take the form of visuals such as paintings, drawings, or photographs; literary works such as poetry and fiction; dance; music; or any other art form. Works of art embody meanings in the nursing experience as the artist perceives them; they are expressed in the unique creation of the artist. Those who see or hear or read what is expressed in a work of art also engage in an aesthetic experience of perceiving meaning in a situation, often a meaning that would not otherwise be perceived, except for the experience of engaging in the art form as an observer.

Aesthetic criticism is the formalized written expression of aesthetic knowledge. Aesthetic criticism can focus on the art/act as enacted in nursing practice or on a tangible work of art inspired from nursing experience. Aesthetic criticism gives insight into the art form, interprets the work of selected artists, and deepens appreciation of the art. It is constructed from the work of the connoisseur-critic, who selects the work of one or more artists as a point of focus. The critic engages in deep reflection into the meanings of the art and the technical adequacy of the art, systematically explores the significance of one or more interpretations of the art, and places the art in a historical and cultural context.

Aesthetic criticism includes the following essential elements (Chinn et al., 1997):

- *Historical integration.* Historical integration occurs on two levels: the history of the art as an art form and the personal artistic history of the artist. The significance of an artist's work can be interpreted only in light of that which has come before. The critic examines evidence of change and continuity in the artist's own history and interprets the meanings of each of these threads. The critic also presents threads of change and continuity in the art form and places this artist's work within the context of those threads. Johnson's (1994) philosophic analysis of literature concerning the art of nursing, although explicitly not a historical study, provides evidence of past conceptualizations of the art of nursing and identifies certain consistencies that have appeared within the literature over time. The aesthetic critic would draw on this and other sources to use as a mirror from which to reflect the meaning of the work that is the focus of the criticism.
- *Comparative description of the art form.* The critic examines the form that this artist takes in the artistic process and compares this artist's work with that of known forms of the art. By drawing comparisons, the critic substantiates the unique aspects of this artist's work and the significance of this artist's work for the discipline.
- *Consideration of plausible interpretations of meaning.* The critic transfers perspectives among a number of plausible interpretive meanings of the art and explores what the various meanings contribute

to aesthetic understanding in the discipline. The critic may develop a preferred interpretation, but the stance remains open and fluid.

- *Translation of future possibility.* The critic explores the directions that this artist might take and what the work of this artist contributes to the future development of the discipline. This aspect of criticism sets the stage for inspiration—for the artist and for others in the discipline.

PROCESSES FOR AFFIRMING AESTHETIC KNOWLEDGE: APPRECIATION AND INSPIRATION

As with the other patterns of knowing, for knowledge to become meaningful within the discipline, members of the discipline engage in collective processes to affirm what is valuable for the discipline. In the sphere of aesthetics, collective affirmation of aesthetic knowledge involves appreciation and inspiration. There are three guiding principles on which appreciation and inspiration are founded: (1) unique, creative expression grounded in the immediacy and enduring wholeness of human experience; (2) expanded dimensions of plausible meanings; and (3) illuminated possibilities for the future.

Shared works of art provide the discipline representations that are unique in temporal time and space but that are grounded in the wholeness of human experience. Aesthetic criticism reveals the particular uniqueness by highlighting and bringing to conscious awareness aspects of creativity that may not be readily perceptible to the casual observer. Unique features serve to distinguish this work from any other and reveal possibilities in human experience and expression that have not existed before and will not be replicated. At the same time, valued works of art touch chords of immediacy and call forth human responses in the moment. The capacity to call forth human response in the moment reflects the art's power to reflect enduring wholeness—that which is shared and common in the human experience.

Valued works of art, because of their uniqueness and their ability to call forth human response, offer expanded dimensions of meaning to the discipline of nursing. Aesthetic criticism explores various dimensions of meaning that are conveyed through the art and offers plausible interpretations of the meanings. The response that is elicited by the art deepens the observer-participant's appreciation of experience and meaning to an extent that would not otherwise be possible.

Valued works of art inspire new and different directions for the future. Aesthetic criticism articulates possible directions, but any observer-participant also can find inspiration within the aesthetic experience. Other artists gain inspiration for their own work by deepening their appreciation of the valued art. The observer-participant gains inspiration relative to life experience; new possibilities, new directions, and different paths to travel enter the imagination and become seeds of possibility.

REFLECTION AND DISCUSSION

In this chapter we have reviewed meanings of art and aesthetics in nursing and presented methods for developing aesthetic knowing and knowledge in nursing. The central message of this chapter is: aesthetic knowing in nursing brings together all of the elements of a nursing care situation to create a meaningful whole, to place everything in the situation in right relationship with all other elements. It is expressed in practice as transformative art/acts that shift the situation from what is, to what is envisioned as possible. Aesthetic knowledge in nursing is communicated to the discipline through works of art representing nursing practice, and through aesthetic criticism that deepens understanding of creative aspects of nursing practice.

To deepen your appreciation of aesthetic knowing, consider the following questions related to the content of this chapter:

1. What comes to mind when you hear the phrase "the art of nursing"?
2. Consider a situation in which you felt that you practiced artfully—a situation in which you felt deeply satisfied that you made a real difference in the turn of events. Write or tell a story based on the situation from the patient's or family's perspective. Rewrite or tell the story again, with a story line that reflects what might have been if you had not been the nurse in the situation. Rewrite or tell the story a third time with a story line that reflects what might have happened if you had taken entirely different approaches in your role as a nurse. What do you learn from each of these three versions of your story?
3. Find a photograph or a painting that depicts a nurse caring for a patient. Using the four elements of aesthetic criticism, develop your own interpretation of the meanings embedded in the picture. What new insights come to you as you study the picture as a critic?
4. Ask two or three nursing colleagues to rehearse or role-play a situation in your practice that left you feeling dissatisfied, or one in which you felt at a loss. Discuss the situation as you experienced it, and ask your colleagues to come up with ideas about how it could have been different. Develop at least two scenarios to role-play, each with a different script and a different kind of outcome. What insights do you gain about this situation? What might you now do differently in another similar situation in the future?

5. Observe a colleague whose practice you admire. Using the elements of artistic validity, describe what you observe. What characterizes the nurse's movements? The nurse's verbal expressions and interactions? What emotions and intentions are conveyed in the nurse's movements? The nurse's words? The nurse's tone of voice and verbal style? Were the nurse's movements and verbal expressions in synchrony with one another, and with the patient?

6. Invite one or two colleagues to discuss a poem, short story, or novel depicting an experience of health or illness for the purpose of gaining deeper understanding of the experience. What do you learn about this experience that might change how you practice in a similar real-life situation?

Reference List

Benner, P. A. (1984). *From novice to expert: Excellence and power in clinical nursing practice.* Menlo Park, CA: Addison-Wesley.

Benner, P. A., Tanner, C. A., & Chesla, C. A. (1996). *Expertise in nursing practice: Caring, clinical judgment, and ethics.* New York: Springer Publishing.

Benner, P. A., & Wrubel, J. (1989). *The primacy of caring: Stress and coping in health and illness.* Menlo Park, CA: Addison-Wesley.

Carper, B. A. (1978). Fundamental patterns of knowing in nursing. *ANS. Advances in Nursing Science, 1*(1), 13–23.

Chinn, P. L. (1994). Developing a method for aesthetic knowing in nursing. In P. L. Chinn & J. Watson (Eds.), *Art and aesthetics in nursing* (pp. 19–40). New York: National League for Nursing.

Chinn, P. L. (2001). Toward a theory of nursing art. In N. L. Chaska (Ed.), *The nursing profession: Tomorrow and beyond* (pp. 287–297). Thousand Oaks, CA: Sage.

Chinn, P. L., Maeve, M. K., & Bostick, C. (1997). Aesthetic inquiry and the art of nursing. *Scholarly Inquiry for Nursing Practice, 11*(2), 83–96.

Chinn, P.L. & Watson, J. (Eds.), *Art and aesthetics in nursing.* New York: National League for Nursing.

Eisner, E. (1985). Aesthetic modes of knowing. In E. Eisner (Ed.), *Learning and teaching the ways of knowing: Part II.* Chicago: University of Chicago Press.

Gaydos, H. L. B. (2004). "Making Special": A framework for understanding the art of holistic nursing. *Journal of Holistic Nursing, 22*(2), 152–163.

Johnson, J. L. (1994). A dialectical examination of nursing art. *ANS. Advances in Nursing Science, 17*(1), 1–14.

Johnson, J. L. (1996). Dialectical analysis concerning the rational aspect of the art of nursing. *Image—The Journal of Nursing Scholarship, 28*(2), 169–175.

LeVasseur, J. J. (1999). Toward an understanding of art in nursing. *ANS. Advances in Nursing Science, 21*(4), 48–63.

Maeve, M. K. (1994). Coming to moral consciousness through the art of nursing narratives. In P. L. Chinn & J. Watson (Eds.), *Art and aesthetics in nursing* (pp. 67–89). New York: National League for Nursing.

Mattingly, C. (1994). The narrative nature of clinical reasoning. In C. Mattingly & M. Fleming (Eds.), *Clinical reasoning: Forms of inquiry in a therapeutic practice.* Philadelphia: FA Davis.

Oettinger, K. B. (1939). Toward inner freedom. *American Journal of Nursing, 39*(11), 1224–1229.

Reed, P. G. (1995). A treatise on nursing knowledge development for the 21st century: Beyond postmodernism. *ANS. Advances in Nursing Science, 17*(3), 70–84.

Sandelowski, M. (1995). On the aesthetics of qualitative research. *Image—The Journal of Nursing Scholarship, 27*(3), 205–209.

Schlenker, E. C. (2004). A place for aesthetics: Aesthetics' place is in life—and in nursing! *Journal of Holistic Nursing, 22*(4), 374–378.

Silva, M. C., Sorrell, J. M., & Sorrell, C. D. (1995). From Carper's patterns of knowing to ways of being: An ontological philosophical shift in nursing. *ANS. Advances in Nursing Science, 18*(1), 1–13.

Sorrell, J. M. (1994). Remembrance of things past through writing: Esthetic patterns of knowing in nursing. *ANS. Advances in Nursing Science, 17*(1), 60–70.

Vezeau, T. M. (1994a). Narrative in nursing practice and education. In P. L. Chinn & J. Watson (Eds.), *Art and aesthetics in nursing* (pp. 163–188). New York: National League for Nursing.

Vezeau, T. M. (1994b). Narrative inquiry in nursing. In P. L. Chinn & J. Watson (Eds.), *Art and aesthetics in nursing*. New York: National League for Nursing.

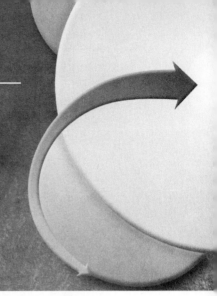

CHAPTER 7

Empiric Knowledge Development: Conceptualizing and Structuring

Looking at human behavior is like running into a cloud whose origins and direction is unknown. You can see the cloud, dynamic and three dimensional, but when you reach out to grab a handful to test you come away with nothing visible but a clenched fist. You may be buffeted by the forces within the cloud that moves on, still visible and dynamic and still three dimensional and you think "I can see the cloud, I can feel the forces it contains, but how do I study it when it refuses to lend itself to anything more than a fleeting encounter?"

Marjorie R. Wright (1966, p. 244)

In this chapter we focus on methods for conceptualizing and structuring empiric phenomena. Figure 7-1 shows the empiric quadrant of our model for nursing knowledge development, highlighting the role of conceptualizing and structuring ideas into knowledge expressions such as theories and formal descriptions. Theories and formal descriptions, in turn, become shared as empiric knowledge in the discipline and serve to enable scientific competence in practice.

The following two processes are involved in structuring and conceptualizing empiric phenomena: (1) creating conceptual meaning and (2) structuring and contextualizing theory. In the discipline of nursing, theory is

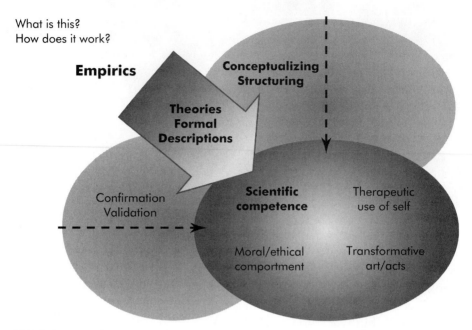

What is this?
How does it work?

FIGURE 7-1 The empiric pattern of knowing: Conceptualizing and structuring empiric phenomena to create formal expressions of empiric knowledge and to develop scientific competence.

generally considered the most formal, most highly structured of the empiric knowledge forms, and it is this type of theory that we focus on in this chapter. However, there are many varieties of empiric knowledge to which these processes can also apply.

WHAT IS EMPIRIC THEORY?

The idea of theory carries varying conceptualizations within and outside the discipline of nursing. There are many definitions of theory. This can be confusing, but each definition can be useful depending on how you are using the term. It is a challenge to select the best definition when you are developing theory because your definition will guide your methods of theory development. Your definition also will reflect your underlying beliefs and values related to science, knowledge, and what constitutes an adequate scientific method. You will see our values and beliefs reflected in our explanation of how we came to the definition used in this text.

Theory has common, everyday connotations apparent in phrases such as "I have a theory about that" or "My theory is. ..." These usages imply that theory is an idea or feeling or that it explains something. In this text, we use a definition that is consistent with the more everyday meanings of theory as a collection of ideas or explanatory hunches. But our definition goes beyond this to a characterization of theory as something deliberately designed for a specific purpose.

Beliefs about the nature of theory arise in part from the various fields of inquiry from which nursing knowledge is developed. Some nursing theorists come from traditions in which the ideal of theory is logically linked sets of confirmed hypotheses. Others view theory as loosely connected ideas that are conjectured but not confirmed. Still others think of theory as philosophically based sets of beliefs and values about human nature and action. As a result, the nursing literature contains varying definitions of theory, but this diversity serves to stimulate further understanding and development of theory. The following four definitions in the nursing literature emphasize different perspectives and different underlying values concerning theory. These definitions each highlight important aspects of theory that we draw on in our own definition:

- A logically interconnected set of confirmed hypotheses (McKay, 1969). This definition implies a specific form of expression based on rules of logic. It also requires that the hypotheses are tested and confirmed by using methods of research to qualify as a theory.
- A conceptual system or framework invented to some purpose (Dickoff & James, 1968). In this definition, the purpose for which a theory is created is emphasized. The term *invented* implies a creative process, not necessarily the type of testing and confirmation that McKay suggests. This definition emphasizes the importance of the theory having a purpose.
- An imaginative grouping of knowledge, ideas, and experiences that are represented symbolically and seek to illuminate a given phenomenon (Watson, 1985). Watson also emphasizes creativity. For Watson, the purpose for which a theory is created is to enhance understanding of a given phenomenon. As Dickoff and James explain in their work, from their point of view a theory's purpose should be a specific practice-oriented application. For Watson, a theory fulfills the purpose of understanding what a phenomenon is, which may or may not have direct application in practice.
- Conceptual and pragmatic principles forming a general frame of reference for a field of inquiry (Ellis, 1968). This definition does not address a specific kind of purpose for theory, and it does not suggest any particular method for developing theory. For Ellis, theory provides a philosophic view that guides inquiry in a discipline. Theory contains

abstract (conceptual) and pragmatic principles that provide a general frame of reference.

From our perspective, theory is a creative and rigorous structuring of ideas. The ideas are expressed by word symbols that form a conceptual structure. The structure is created using some method that draws on the creativity of the theorist. The theorist can describe the method used to develop the theory and can explain how the method was applied. The concepts contained within the theory must be defined, and they must have a logical relationship with one another to form a coherent structure or pattern. Theory is purposive; theorists create theory for some reason. Theoretic purposes may take many different forms, but the purpose needs to be clearly evident. Theory is not a finalized prescription or a formula for practice; it cannot describe exactly what can be objectively observed. Instead, theory projects tentative ideas that open new perceptions and possibilities concerning what might be beyond our surface understanding of the world. Theory is grounded in assumptions, value choices, and the creative and imaginative judgment of the theorist. You may or may not share these values, but your exposure to another way of viewing what might be can expand your own thinking about your experience, your profession, and the direction of your own work. Our definition of theory is as follows:

Theory A creative and rigorous structuring of ideas that projects a tentative, purposeful, and systematic view of phenomena.

The word "creative" underscores the role of human imagination and vision in the development and expression of theory. It does not mean that "anything goes" or that theory is improvised. Creative processes required to develop theory also are rigorous, systematic, and disciplined, yielding a well-developed conception that bears the mark of the creator. In our view, theoretic statements are tentative and open to revision as new evidence and insights emerge. The statements are developed toward some purpose or within a specific context. Our definition does not require that a hypothesis be tested before the statements can be considered as theory. Ideas that the creator systematically develops based on experience and observation can be considered as theory before formal testing.

Given our definition, it is possible to contrast how theory differs from related terms such as *science, philosophy, paradigm, theoretic framework,* and *model.* Like the word "theory," these terms are highly abstract and have many different meanings for different people. Sometimes the meanings overlap, and sometimes the meanings seem very different. When there are confusing overlaps and differences, you can resolve the confusion by clarifying and creating your own definitions. Your definitions cannot be arbitrary or simply based on your personal beliefs. Like our definition of *theory*, your definitions of any terms will reflect your beliefs. In addition, your definitions must be consistent with common threads of meaning that generally are accepted within the discipline and grounded in a logical rationale that is coherent to other members of the discipline. Definitions also must be suitable for the context in which they are created and the purpose they serve. If you are defining the word "self-esteem" for a research study, for example, your definition might include the foundational meanings that are consistent with a tool you are using to measure self-esteem. If you are defining "self-esteem" for a clinical project that is designed to assist women make prenatal health choices, your definition may or may not reflect the underlying meanings of a measurement tool.

We have defined theory for the purpose of explaining to you, the reader, our view of what theory is, how to develop it, and how to evaluate it. Definitions of related terms help to make clearer the meaning of the central term—in this case theory. Our definitions of several related terms for the context of this text are shown in Table 7-1. The definitions of related terms—like our definition of *theory*—may not be universally accepted, but we believe that they are reasonable and reflect common meanings. Also, no matter how rigorous the attempt to differentiate like terms by providing definitions, there will be elements of shared meaning among them.

EMPIRIC THEORY AND METHODOLOGY

Methodology refers to the general framework of assumptions, philosophy, and approach used in the process of developing knowledge. In our experience, approaches to empiric knowledge development carry with them assumptions of more traditional objectivist science. Empirical methodologies are often equated with nontheoretical, objective observation: that is, a "standing apart" from what you are observing in order to know its meaning. This further assumes that meaning is located in what you are observing, and that you are able to stand apart objectively to observe and report what that meaning is. Because meaning is assumed to be located within what is observed and not the observer, once described, meaning can be reliably shared with and understood similarly by others.

A second meaning for *empiric* is located in the context of illness care. In this context an "empiric treatment" is one that is based on knowledge that the treatment works. Experience, rather than theoretical knowledge, forms the basis for establishing and confirming knowledge.

A third meaning of *empiric* is one grounded in the philosophy of knowledge development. This meaning defines empiric knowledge as knowledge

TABLE 7-1 Conceptual Definitions of Terms Related to the Concept of Theory

Term	Definition
Science	An approach to the generation of empiric knowledge that relies on accessible sensory experience to create knowledge and to form understanding. The term also refers to the results of using systematic methods of empirics. The process involves critical and logical thought; the results yield the facts, theories, and descriptions. Natural science assumes that the scientist and the object of study are separate and that what is being studied is governed by laws and rules that do not vary. Human science approaches take into account the thinking, feeling, and intentional characteristics of human nature and assume that the scientist influences what is studied.
Philosophy	A form of disciplined inquiry that discerns the nature of reality and of knowledge and knowing, ways of discerning reality, and principles of value. Philosophy relies on logic and reasoning, rather than empiric evidence, to create knowledge.
Research	An application of formalized methods of obtaining reliable and valid knowledge about empiric experience.
Fact	That which generally is held to be an empirically verifiable object, property, or event, meaning that the phenomenon is experienced and named consistently and similarly by others in a given similar context.
Model	A symbolic representation of an empiric experience in the form of words, pictorial or graphic diagrams, mathematic notations, or physical material (such as a model airplane).
Theoretic or Conceptual Framework	A logical grouping of related concepts or theories, usually created to draw several different aspects together that are relevant to a complex situation, such as a practice setting or an educational program.
Paradigm	A worldview or ideology. A paradigm implies standards or criteria for assigning value or worth to both the processes and the products of a discipline, as well as for the methods of knowledge development within a discipline.

derived from perceptual experiences—our sensory perceptions and observations. This meaning of *empiric* is broader, and perceptual experiences can include subjective accounts, indirect observations, and interpretations of that which is observed. However, that which is perceived or observed is subject to some form of confirmation. It is this third meaning of *empirics* from philosophy—sensory, perceptual experience as the source of knowledge—that most closely fits our usage.

Thus, anytime knowledge developers use sensory perceptions as a basis for knowledge development, they are using empirical methods. Not all empirical methods are scientific according to some meanings of the term *scientific*. This is the case especially when *scientific* is defined as a process that can only be applied to the physical world. In our view, empirical methods for knowledge development are scientific to the extent that they are methodical and precise.

This means that we would admit a variety of approaches to inquiry within the quadrant of our model defined as "Empirics." One core requirement is that empirical knowledge be grounded in perceptual experience. This would include knowledge developed using controlled experimental studies as well as a variety of naturalistic methods that rely on interacting with and understanding the nature of others' experiences. These knowledge forms are empirical because they are grounded in perceptual experience. They are also scientific because they are developed using rigorous methodologies and are expressed in language that is understood similarly within the discipline. The requirement for rigor and their expression in language means they have a structure that can be communicated to other members of the discipline and subjected to procedures of confirmation and validation.

For some methodologies, the structure of knowledge is more formalized, as in phenomenological themes that impart understanding, or groupings of like concepts that create a core variable in grounded theory. For other methodologies, the structure is less formal, but still is formalized in language as in thick ethnographic descriptions. The degree of formalization may affect the degree to which the knowledge structure can be confirmed or validated. However, even the thickest of descriptions, if carefully done, have a degree of confirmation within the context of their development.

In short, it is our position that noncritical naturalistic inquiry methods— methods that gather and utilize qualitative data—are justifiably empiric as well as scientific. They are empiric in that they rely on perceptual experience to gather and understand data, and they are scientific in that they are methodical and precise. These methods generate formal descriptions that can be considered theory as we have defined it.

In the following sections important processes for conceptualizing and structuring empiric theory are addressed. Formalized methods for creating conceptual meaning are proposed; however, conceptual meaning is created and communicated apart from utilization of these formal processes. These processes can be used to deliberately address conceptual meaning embedded in theory developed by any other means. Likewise, the structuring processes outlined are representative of formalized approaches to structuring theory. These processes are also embedded to different degrees within a variety of methodologies used to develop empiric theory. The structuring processes that we describe in the next sections constitute one common approach to structuring theory.

CREATING CONCEPTUAL MEANING

Creating conceptual meaning is a theory-building approach that depends on mental thought processes. The process of creating conceptual meaning carefully examines the ideas and thoughts generated when word symbols are encountered. In similar cultures, the meaning behind word symbols is both common and unique. For example, in nursing similar meanings for the concept of hypothermia are shared among those who belong to a professional discipline. At the same time, a person's own subjective meaning may be unique, and more "real" to the individual than any other possible interpretation of the world. For example, if I am in a room with a comfortable ambient air temperature and feel cold, when everyone else in the room is comfortable, my own perception and experience of being cold is most real to me even though I recognize that I am the only one who feels cold. When you are creating conceptual meaning for a theory, you use your mental capacity to recognize when your own perceptions are unique and to assess the extent to which your unique experience represents an oddity and the possibility that it opens a new prospect for others to consider.

Conceptual meaning does not exist as an "out there" reality to be objectively discovered; it is created. It is deliberately formed from experience. The process of creating conceptual meaning brings dimensions of meaning to a conscious, communicable awareness. Any language is limited when it comes to expressing the fullness of experience, and the process of creating conceptual meaning makes it possible to expand what we understand about a phenomenon that is beyond the definitions and meanings of single words. At the same time, language systems shape perceptions and meaning (Crowe, 2005; Muller and Dzurec, 1993; White, 2004). If someone is called clever, that person begins to form an awareness of self that may be helpful and affirming, or the word "clever" may not adequately express the person's rich inner experiences and instead may trivialize how the person experiences the world. If the word represents a desired value, the description given contributes positively to self-awareness.

Although the process of creating conceptual meaning provides a foundation for developing theory and is a logical starting point for theory development, it does not necessarily have to be accomplished first. It is a process that can be done by the beginning or advanced scholar and by the novice or expert practitioner. Although this process is critical to all theory development, it is often overlooked (Norris, 1982). Most theorists provide definitions of terms used within theory, but forming word definitions is not the same as creating meaning. Conceptual meaning conveys thoughts, feelings, and ideas that reflect the human experience to the fullest extent possible, which is not possible with a definition. A word definition provides an anchor from which to situate common mental associations with a term. Conceptual meaning displays a mental picture of what the phenomenon is like and how it is perceived in human experience.

What Is a Concept?

We define the term *concept* as a complex mental formulation of experience. By "experience," we mean perceptions of the world, including objects, other people, visual images, color, movement, sounds, behavior, interactions—the totality of what is perceived. Experience is considered empiric when it can be symbolically shared and verified by others with sensory evidence. The following three sources of experience interact to form the meaning of the concept: (1) the word or other symbolic label; (2) the thing itself (object, property, or event); and (3) feelings, values, and attitudes associated with the word and with the perception of the thing.

Conceptual meaning is created by considering all three sources of experiences related to the concept: the word, the thing itself, and the associated feelings. The same word may be used to represent more than one phenomenon. For example, the word "cup" may be used to represent several different kinds of objects or ideas. Each use of the word carries with it different perceptions. If the object is a fancy teacup, a very different mental image forms than if the object is the cup into which a golf ball falls on a putting green. The word "love," a more abstract concept, can be used to describe a feeling toward a parent, child, pet, car, job, friend, or intimate partner, with each use implying an essentially different but related feeling. In creating conceptual meaning, you examine a range of applications for a word symbol, find what is common among all of the uses and what is different, and decide what elements of meaning are important for your purpose.

All concepts can be located on a continuum from the empiric (more directly experienced) to the abstract (more mentally constructed) (Jacox, 1974; Kaplan, 1964). In one sense, all concepts are both empiric and abstract. They are empiric because they are formed from perceptual encounters with the world as experienced. They are abstract because they are mental images of that experience.

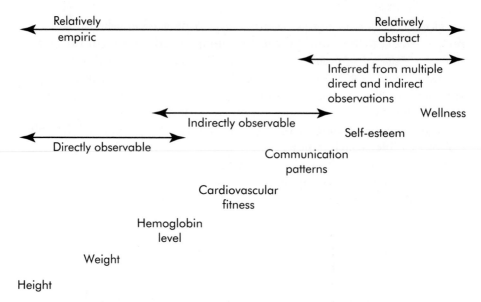

FIGURE 7-2 Example of continuum and empiric abstraction.

Some concepts are formed from very direct experiences that can be more readily verified by others. Others are formed from experiences that are commonly recognized but inferred indirectly. Figure 7-2 illustrates this continuum. Relatively empiric concepts are ideas that are formed from direct observations of objects, properties, or events. As concepts become more abstract, they are inferred indirectly. The most abstract concepts are mental constructions that encompass a complex network of subconcepts.

The most concrete empiric concepts have direct forms of measurement. Concepts formed about objects such as a cup or properties such as temperature are examples of highly empiric concepts because the object or property that represents the idea (empiric indicator) can be directly experienced through the senses and confirmed by many different people. A relatively empiric property such as biologic sex also can be observed directly by noting the primary and secondary sexual characteristics that identify a person as male or female or, more precisely and especially if sex is ambiguous, by identifying chromosomal patterns. Properties such as height and weight can be measured with standardized instruments.

As concepts become more abstract, their observational qualities, or their empiric indicators, become less concrete and less directly measurable. Assessment of an abstract concept depends increasingly on indirect means. Although an indirect assessment or observation is different from direct measurement, it is considered a reasonable indicator of the concept.

Hemoglobin level is representative of a concept that cannot be directly observed but can be indirectly measured with the aid of laboratory instruments. This type of measurement depends on more complex and less direct forms of instrumentation.

Cardiovascular fitness is an example of a concept that is middle-range on the empiric–abstract continuum. Concepts increase in complexity in this range, and several empiric indicators must be assessed. Because no object such as cardiovascular fitness exists, a definition is required if we are to know what it is. Even though definitions for less empirically based concepts are thoughtfully formulated, they are arbitrary because many different definitions could be chosen. As concepts become increasingly abstract, definitions become more dependent on the theoretic meaning of the concept and the purpose for defining it.

Self-esteem is an example of a highly abstract concept for which there is no direct measure. The instruments or tools that are developed to assess self-esteem depend on theoretic definitions serving a specific purpose and are built on many behaviors and personality characteristics that experts agree are associated with that concept. Ideas about these characteristics may be derived from a theory or from concept clarification. Each behavioral trait contained in the tool can be considered as a partial indicator of self-esteem. When the composite behaviors and personal characteristics are built into an assessment tool, it usually is a more adequate indicator for the abstract concept than any one behavior taken alone. The composite score obtained from the tool is then considered to be a measurement constructed as an empiric indicator.

Highly abstract concepts are sometimes called constructs. Constructs are the most complex type of concept on the empiric–abstract continuum. These concepts include ideas with a reality base so abstract that it is constructed from multiple sources of direct and indirect evidence. An example of a construct is wellness. Although the idea of wellness exists, it cannot be directly observed. Figure 7-2 illustrates the idea that highly abstract concepts are constructed from other concepts. All concepts shown on the continuum (as well as others) can be included in the concept of wellness.

Some abstract concepts have little meaning outside the context of a theory. For example, Levine (1967) coined the word *trophicogenic* to mean "nurse-induced illness." Rogers (1970) discussed three "principles of homeodynamics." Rogers' term *homeodynamics* is a combination of the Latin root word *homeo*, meaning "similar to" or "like," and the common English term *dynamics*, meaning "pattern of change or growth." The reader can infer the meaning "change processes" for the term *homeodynamics*, which is consistent with Rogers' intent.

Abstract concepts also may acquire additional meaning through gradual transfer into common language usage. Freud's concept of ego is an example. The word "ego" once had no common meaning outside Freud's theory, but today, with gradual changes in its meaning and broad usage outside the theory, most everyone who speaks American English and many other English speakers around the world know the meaning of "a big ego."

A single phenomenon also can be represented by several different words. Each word conveys a slightly different meaning, often nuances that relate to socially derived value meanings. For example, the words "car," "Model T," and "hot wheels" can all refer to one thing—an automobile. Using any of these words to describe the object conveys more about the perspective or value of the person using the word than it does about the object itself. As the words acquire contextual and value meanings, they shift further toward the abstract.

Feelings, values, and attitudes are inner processes that are associated with experiences and words. For example, the word "mother" carries feelings, values, and attitudes that form in human experience with an actual person. Varying experiences with mother (the person) account for a range of feelings that different people associate with the word "mother." At the same time, human meaning of the concept *mother* is formed from shared cultural and societal heritages. A concept such as *mother*, which can carry specific or highly complex meanings, changes in level of abstraction, depending on the context of usage.

Many nursing concepts are highly abstract. Although theory and other common forms of empiric knowledge such as models, frameworks, and descriptions incorporate and depend on highly empiric facts, nursing theory does not generally reflect factually based concepts. Box 7-1 contains an exercise that may be useful in understanding the challenges involved in exploring and creating conceptual meaning.

Although it usually is not possible, nor necessary, to identify precisely where concepts fit on an empiric–abstract continuum, it is important to understand that concepts vary in the degree to which they are connected to what is perceived as experience and the extent to which their meaning is mentally constructed. When you begin to study an abstract concept, it is natural to wonder why it is difficult to grasp the meaning of the term and understand all that is conveyed by the concept.

Methods for Creating Conceptual Meaning

Creating conceptual meaning produces a tentative definition of the concept and a set of tentative criteria for determining whether the concept is useful in a particular situation. We use the word "tentative" because both the

---

Box 7-1

An Exercise in Creating a Concept and Exploring Various Complex Dimensions of Concepts

Close your eyes and imagine a "cup." Take a few minutes to notice what the cup is like. Notice what feelings are associated with it. Notice where it is and any other features of context. You might want to make a mental or written note when you open your eyes.

Congratulations! Well, maybe this wasn't such an unusual feat, but you did create a concept.

If you haven't already done so, write a definition of *cup* based on what you saw.

Now, examine the definition. Did your cup have a handle? Did it have a hard surface that you described? Was it decorated? Was there anything in it? Did you smell anything?

Did you describe a cup that is used for drinking something? If you did (which we are betting on!), think about as many other images of "cup" as you can.

What did you come up with?

Did you think of the cup on a golfing green? A cup of a woman's brassiere? Did you think of anything like a "cup of cheer?" There is an image associated with that sort of cup, but can you see it and touch it? No, but you could recognize it.

Place your cup images on an empiric–abstract continuum.

A coffee type of cup is more empirically based (we can see and touch that!), but a cup of cheer is much more abstract. Remember Aunt Gracie who dutifully offered that wedding toast to a nephew she really didn't like much? She went through the motions, but did she mean it? Would her intention influence your use of the phrase "cup of cheer" to describe her action?

What did you notice about context when you described your initial cup image? When you take your original cup image and insert it into another context, what do you notice?

Would you imagine a group of groggy campers around a morning campfire sipping coffee from bone china cups on dainty saucers? Probably not, but these still are cups. Different sorts of cups are associated with different social contexts.

Now make a list of all features common to your cups.

Ours all held something—even the cup of cheer. If we omitted the cup of cheer image, all our cups were made out of material to hold something solid. If we omitted the woman's brassiere and the golf-green cups, then we could say they also had handles.

Let's assume the type of cup you are interested in is a cup for drinking liquid. You now have (1) an object that is made out of solid material that (2) holds something, which means it has an open end and a closed end with (3) a handle.

How do you know this is not a drinking glass that also is used for drinking liquid?

If you said, "It's the handle," you agree with us. We drink liquid from glasses, and they must be made from solid material to hold what we drink. Cups, it seems, need that handle because they usually hold something hot.

Continued

Box 7-1
An Exercise in Creating a Concept and Exploring Various Complex Dimensions of Concepts—cont'd

Are you getting tired about now? Well, you are in luck, because your best friend just came by with some take-out coffee. Out of the bag it comes. Here is a coffee cup without a handle! How can that be?

The technologic development of new materials has omitted the necessity for a handle on cups that hold hot liquids. This tells us that the images associated with cups may change in our lifetime.

Think about the implications of this short mental gymnastic. *Cup* is a very empiric concept that should be fairly easy to define, yet it isn't. Nursing practice concepts are highly abstract. If *cup* can get complicated, what challenges will abstract concepts pose when we try to create conceptual meaning?

The point: Conceptual meaning is complex to determine, context determines meaning, and it is critical to know the level of precision needed!

---

definition and the criteria can be revised. The term *tentative* does not mean that anything goes or that any definition that suits the author will do. It does mean that the definition is open and can be changed as new insights and understandings come to light. This process is a deliberative, disciplined activity. The person who is creating meaning draws on many information sources, examines many possible dimensions of meaning, and presents ideas so that they can be tested and challenged in the light of the purposes for which the conceptual meaning is intended.

There are various methods for creating conceptual meaning. Norris (1982) described several methods for concept clarification. Walker and Avant (2004) described a method of concept analysis based on the work of Wilson (1963). Morse (1995) described methods of concept development and analysis that draw on qualitative and quantitative research approaches to validate meanings that are projected by analytic processes. Rodgers and Knafl (2000) propose an "evolutionary" method of concept analysis which recognizes that conceptual meaning is dependent on context. Our approaches to creating conceptual meaning draw on these sources and our experiences of creating conceptual meaning for various purposes.

Selecting a Concept. Selecting a concept is a process that involves a great deal of ambiguity. Concept selection is guided by your purpose and expresses values related to your purpose. If you are a student in a nursing class, your concept selection may be guided by expediency as well as interest. If you are a postdoctoral student, you may create conceptual meaning to resolve a dilemma you encounter in moving through the research process.

Values that influence your selection of a concept include your beliefs and attitudes about the nature of nursing. We believe concepts selected should justifiably relate to the practice of nursing. An example would be a concept that represents a human response to health or illness, such as fatigue. Characteristics of clients, such as hardiness, also may be selected, particularly if they are important determinants of health. Characteristics of nurses, care systems, or nurse-client-family interaction also might be chosen if they are important determinants of health.

Often, multiple disciplines share interest in the same concept and to claim a concept is justifiably related to nursing does not mean it is only a "nursing" concept. Fatigue, for example, is a concept that is of interest to nurses, but also to physicians as well as clinical pharmacists. Fatigue becomes more of a nursing concept when a conceptual meaning is created for *fatigue* that is useful and important within a nursing context—for example, when the meaning reflects what nurses have control over and what they do. Locating the concept of fatigue within a theory that conceptualizes fatigue as a human response to chemotherapy and developing criteria for fatigue that can be assessed and alleviated by oncology nurses makes it a nursing concept. Physicians might develop criteria for fatigue that index it in relation to the safety of continuing a regimen of treatment (their role) whereas clinical pharmacists might create criteria that would assist drug manufacturers to formulate pharmaceuticals that are more effective in alleviating fatigue.

In choosing concepts, then, the role and context of nursing is important to the choice. More important, as you create conceptual meaning, is making choices that help ensure the meaning created is useful to nurses as they manage human responses and help persons toward health. The important question is not "Is this a nursing concept?" but rather "Is this concept of interest to nursing and is the meaning created useful for nursing's purposes?"

Sociopolitical considerations also will influence your choice of a concept, often in ways that are subtle and difficult to perceive. For example, if you choose to examine the concept of transition for daughters who must place their mothers in nursing homes, you eventually will come to examine the consequences of women's caretaking within a society that devalues the elderly and that disregards women's work in caring for aging parents as real work.

Some concepts are not appropriate as a focus for the process of creating conceptual meaning. Some are too empirically grounded, and others are too expansive to yield a useful outcome. Concepts that represent empirically knowable objects (such as antiembolic stockings) usually are not good choices because they are highly empirically grounded and can be demonstrated by a display of the thing itself. You do not need to examine the concepts to understand their meanings, and having criteria for recognizing them will not help you clinically in any significant way. Broad concepts such as *caring* and *stress* pose another set of problems. Because these types of concepts are so vast, creating meaning can result only in a broad understanding that omits detail and may be misleading. This is not to say that creating conceptual meaning for very narrow or broad concepts is never useful, and for some purposes it may be justifiable. In our experience, the concepts that are most often amenable to creating conceptual meaning are those in the middle range. It often is helpful when choosing a concept to place it within the context of use to narrow its scope in relation to your purpose.

It often makes sense to choose a concept that is poorly understood or that tends to have competing or confusing meanings. However, most concepts carry a certain degree of ambiguity, and your meanings will alter as contexts for use change. Moreover, much of what is in the literature about concepts will be found to be inadequate or erroneous when you examine the concept in a new light. For example, much of the early information on fatigue was generated from research on airplane pilots and proved inadequate to understand cancer fatigue. As a result, nurses began to generate knowledge about this particular type of fatigue. Remember that other disciplines do not have the same perspectives and motives for generating conceptual information as do nurses. Although knowledge of nursing concepts within other disciplines may be useful, these other circumstances need to be carefully examined. Other disciplines have a different perspective, and scholars in those disciplines are not likely to take into account perspectives common to nursing. Their work can inform our perspectives, but usually the conceptual meanings derived from other disciplines will not be adequate for nursing purposes.

With these guidelines in mind, you can select a word or phrase that communicates the idea you wish to convey. Despite your best efforts to make the perfect initial choice, it probably will change as you explore various meanings. Trying out alternative words becomes part of the process itself. For example, there is no adequate single term for the idea expressed in the phrase "the use of humans as objects." The term *objectification* is close, but it implies some experiences that do not involve the use of humans. The process of working with various terms related to this idea will help you to explore various meanings that are possible. Because experience is not adequately expressed in common language, words may seem quite inadequate at first. You may select a common word for a concept and eventually assign a specific definition to the word to suit your particular purposes, or you may borrow a word from another language, combine two or more common words to specify a particular meaning, or make up a phrase or a word. Many significant concepts for nursing have not been adequately named. As nurses engage in processes for creating conceptual meaning, a more adequate language for nursing phenomena will be created.

Clarifying Your Purpose.   To provide a sense of direction, you must know why you are creating conceptual meaning. One purpose is to set boundaries or limits so you do not become hopelessly lost in the process. For example, your purpose might be to work with the concept *dependence* for a research project. Eventually you will need a clear conceptualization of dependence, as well as ideas about how to measure or assess dependence. Another purpose might be to differentiate between two closely related concepts such as *sympathy* and *empathy*. In this case, your concern is to create definitions that differentiate, based on thorough familiarity with meanings that are possible.

Another reason for creating conceptual meaning is to examine the ways in which concepts are used in existing writings. The concept of *intuition,* for example, commonly appears in nursing literature with many different but related meanings. The meanings conveyed reflect different assumptions about the phenomenon. As you become aware of these meanings, you can explore the extent to which the meanings are consistent with your own purpose.

Other purposes for creating conceptual meaning include generating research hypotheses, formulating nursing diagnoses, and developing computerized databases for clinical decision making. Creating conceptual meaning also is a valuable process for learning critical thinking (Kramer, 1993). When you keep your purpose as clear as possible, you have an anchor that provides a sense of direction when you seem to be hopelessly lost.

Sources of Evidence.   Once a concept has been selected, the process of creating conceptual meaning proceeds by using several different sources from which you generate and refine criteria for the concept. The sources you choose and the extent to which you use various sources depend on your purposes. Early in the process of gathering evidence for the concept, tentative criteria are proposed, and those criteria are refined in light of additional information provided by continued gathering of evidence. We recommend beginning the process of criteria formulation early so that useful information is not lost. Criteria are succinct statements that give essential characteristics and features that distinguish the concept as a recognizable entity and that differentiate this entity from other related ideas.

Exemplar Case. An exemplar case is a description or depiction of a situation, experience, or event that satisfies the following statement: "If this is not X, then nothing is." The case can be drawn from nursing practice, literature, art, film, or any other source in which the concept is represented or symbolized. If the case is depicted as an object or in some form of media, many rich aspects of the phenomenon can be conveyed by displaying the media for others to experience. Regardless of format for presentation, the case is selected because it represents the concept to the best of your present understanding. For concrete concepts such as *cup*, an exemplar case is relatively easy. An ordinary teacup, for example, can be presented for everyone to see and hold. The people who examine the object can then verify, "If this is not a cup, then nothing is." To demonstrate the concept *red* (a property), a model case is more difficult. You can physically present to the group something that you perceive as red in color and find out whether they agree that this is what they also would perceive as red. However, a more precise and consistent identification of red would result from measurement using a spectrophotometer.

When you deal with highly abstract concepts, the task of constructing and selecting exemplar cases is even more difficult, and often these concepts can only be measured indirectly. Many such measurements depend on scales that rely on self-report. For example, the concepts of *anxiety* or *pain* are typically measured by self-report rating scales. Usually, exemplar cases of abstract concepts involve experiences and circumstances that are described in words. Exemplar cases may be created from your own experience, or you may find cases in the literature that have been constructed or described by others. For example, to demonstrate an abstract concept such as *sorrow*, a scenario from a novel or film or a rich description of an experience from your practice can be shared with others who respond to the scenario as a representation of the phenomenon of sorrow.

If you create your own exemplar case, work with your ideas and revise your description until you are satisfied that the case fully represents your concept. For a concept such as *mothering*, your exemplar case might describe the following event: an infant cries, and an adult picks up the infant. The event is a start, but your observers might object, saying that this description represents only the physical act of picking up a crying child and is not necessarily mothering. Your exemplar case develops until there is enough substance that people respond to the case by forming a mental image of mothering. As you build on the scenario of an adult picking up an infant to represent mothering, you could include various circumstances, behaviors, motives, attitudes, and feelings that surround the act of picking up the infant. You paint a picture or tell a story so that people can confirm that this is indeed mothering. As this and other exemplar cases are created, you can compare various meanings in the experience and define what is common and what is different about the various cases that you consider.

It often is useful to alternatively include and exclude various features of exemplar cases to reflect on how central each feature is to the meaning you are creating. In the exemplar case of mothering, the adult initially might be portrayed as female. Later you might portray a male in the same case. In the absence of any evidence one way or the other, you might tentatively decide that the idea of mothering you are creating will be deliberately limited to instances involving women. Because your decision is tentative, you can change your construction for another purpose or circumstance. You can acknowledge the fact that some men mother, but for your purpose, your idea deliberately includes the experience of women.

While you are working with exemplar cases, pose the following question: What makes this an instance of this concept? The responses to this question form the basis for a tentative list of criteria. In early stages, the criteria may be quite detailed and may be the essential characteristics associated with the concept, given the meanings you deliberately decide to include. The criteria are designed to make it possible to recognize the concept when it occurs and to differentiate this concept from related concepts. For example, in the case of mothering, you would want to be able to recognize mothering when it happens and distinguish mothering from related phenomena such as caring, nurturing, or helping.

Impressions about the criteria begin to form as you work with your exemplar case. You begin to form ideas about which features are essential for your purposes and why, as well as their qualitative characteristics. These ideas become the criteria for the concept. Sometimes exemplar cases are presented after clarification is complete. In these instances the exemplar case is similar to a definitional form for the concept. Here we use exemplar cases as a way to create meaning, not to represent it.

Definitions. One source that provides information about conceptual meaning is definitions and word usages of the concept you are exploring. Existing definitions often are circular and do not give a complete sense of meaning for the concept, but they do help to clarify common usages and ideas associated with the concept. Existing definitions often help to identify core elements about objects, perceptions, or feelings that can be represented by the word. They also are useful to trace the origin of words, giving clues to core meaning.

Dictionary definitions provide synonyms and antonyms and convey commonly accepted ways in which words are used. They are not designed to explain the full range of perceptions associated with a word, particularly a word that has a unique use within a discipline or represents a relatively abstract concept.

Existing theories provide a source of definitions that sometimes extend beyond the limits of common linguistic usage. Theoretic definitions and ways concepts are used in the context of the theory convey meanings that pertain to the domain of the discipline from which the theory comes.

The term *mother* as defined in the dictionary, for example, refers to the social and biologic role of parenting and includes a few characteristics of the role, such as authority and affection. In the context of psychological theories, the meanings conveyed with respect to the values, roles, functions, and characteristics of people who are mothers are almost endless and include parenting, physical care, guilt, responsibility, power, and powerlessness.

Visual Images. Visual images that already exist, such as photographs, cartoons, calendars, paintings, and drawings, are useful sources for creating conceptual meaning. If you are choosing existing images, they may be explicitly labeled or named as the concept of interest, or you may judge them to reasonably represent it. If you can find images that others have explicitly labeled as an instance of the concept, such as a picture that the artist labels "Sorrow," the artist's linking of the visual image to the concept provides further validation of the meaning of the concept, enriches the range of meaning, and helps to minimize any bias inherent in your own views of meaning for the concept. In some instances you might deliberately create images that represent the concept being clarified rather than use existing sources. Whether you personally create and examine an image or ask others to create images, the idea is to compare them for similarities and differences. Advertisements and photographs documenting the concept *depression,* for example, provide information about conceptual meaning. Often, visual imagery will highlight some aspect of the concept that is significant. On other occasions, visual imagery may raise questions about the essential nature of the phenomena that are important to refining criteria. Visual images that represent concepts very well also highlight difficulties in expressing meaning linguistically. A photograph may express rich dimensions of the concept of *dignity,* yet the essence of dignity expressed by the photo is impossible to describe. This is an example of how aesthetic expressions of concepts contribute to empirical knowledge.

Popular and Classical Literature. A variety of literature resources can provide information about conceptual meaning. Literature reflects meanings arising from the culture and provides rich sources of exemplars for concepts. Classical prose and poetry often are good sources of meaning for concepts used in nursing. For example, images of love and longing may be found in the poetic works of Emily Dickinson. Louisa May Alcott's classic book, *Little Women,* provides information about the nature of intimacy and caring. The popular current literature also is a source of valuable data about conceptual meaning. Popular self-help books on topics such as overcoming negative thinking and co-dependency often can clarify commonly understood (or misunderstood) conceptual meanings. Fairy tales, myths, fables, and stories provide relevant insights, depending on the concept you are exploring. Usages for words that are expressed in popular jargon and cartoons may highlight borderline meanings. For example, when a 5-year-old jumps up and down and exclaims, "I'm so anxious for my birthday to be here!" the meaning of *anxious* is not the same meaning that concerns nurses. What the child's usage does convey is the physical agitation that accompanies the experience of anxiety within the context of nursing practice.

Music and Poetry. The imagery of music or poetry may be useful in creating conceptual meaning. Music or poetry can be chosen by seeking out lyrics or titles that name the concept under consideration. The music itself, or the metaphoric images in the title or lyrics, may reasonably suggest the concept. Music and poetry can effectively convey meanings through rhythm, tones, lyrical or linguistic forms and metaphors, or musical moods that reflect experiences in life events with which nurses deal. For example, the Shaker folk tune "Simple Gifts" suggests criteria for concepts of authenticity, genuineness, centeredness, and community. The tune itself conveys a sense of inner happiness and peace; the lyrics reflect relationships between inner peace and the ability to build strong relationships. The popular song "Don't Fence Me In" conveys through the musical mood, rhythm, and lyrics what it feels like to be confined emotionally and projects a yearning to be free.

Professional Literature. Meanings for concepts can be explored from within the context of professional literature. This literature often provides meanings that are pertinent to the practice of nursing. For example, philosophers, as well as nurses, have written about the concept of *presence* as a way of being with another. When the work of a scholar in another discipline coincides with your experience as a nurse, the work of other scholars can augment your conceptual meaning. When you find contradictions with your experience as a nurse, the contradictions prompt you to clarify your own insights about the phenomenon.

Anecdotal Accounts and Opinions. Peers, co-workers, hospitalized individuals, other professional workers, and people who are not connected to nursing can provide valuable information about the meaning of a concept. It may be useful to seek others' opinions about the meaning of a concept, particularly if your direct experience with the concept is limited. Nurses who work with the concept daily may be able to shed light on nuances of meaning that will markedly affect how meaning is integrated into theory. For example, a nurse who works with people whose lung function is severely compromised might observe that anxiety, although usually characterized by increased activity, evokes a different reaction. Rather than random activity, anxiety may be accompanied by a deliberate quieting of behavior to conserve energy. Asking others to share their ideas about a concept is an informal exploration different from standard research procedures that might investigate conceptual meaning. Rather, it is an exploration of opinions and understandings of others to ground your meaning in everyday perception or to test your professional meanings in light of everyday assumptions about a phenomenon.

Methods for Testing Tentative Criteria and the Exemplar Case. As you examine various sources of evidence, you will begin the process of testing the soundness of your conceptualization created in light of your purpose. You may find alternative meanings that are reasonable or plausible but not well suited for your purpose. For example, for someone who is interested in a cup used for the purpose of drinking liquids, a golf-green cup, although a plausible instance of the concept of *cup*, does not have the defining features required for drinking liquids. To stimulate your thinking about nuances of meaning, you can turn to a number of cases that challenge your conceptualization and consider alternative contexts.

Contrary Cases. Contrary cases are those that are certainly not an instance of the concept. They may be similar in some respects, but they represent something that most observers would easily recognize as significantly different from the concept you are considering. For more concrete concepts, contrary cases are relatively easy. A saucer or a spoon can be presented, and most observers in Western cultures would agree that these things are not cups. A spoon may hold liquids that people sip, but it is not a cup. A saucer that a cup sits on also is clearly not a cup. A contrary case for the color red might be the color green. For the concept of *restlessness,* calmness could be presented as a contrary case.

As you consider contrary cases, ask the following: What makes this instance different from the concept I have selected? By comparing the differences between exemplar and contrary cases, you will begin to revise, add to, or delete from the tentative criteria that are emerging. If your purpose includes designing an exemplar case for your concept, you also might use this information to refine the exemplar case. For example, one of the traits that distinguish a cup from a saucer or a spoon is the shape of the cup. You already might discern that this feature is essential by looking only at the cup. When you see the spoon and saucer, however, the shape stands out in sharp contrast, and your description of essential features of the shape of the cup can be more complete and precise. As you compare the objects, you also may decide that the volume of liquid that a cup holds is an important distinguishing characteristic. Later, when you consider miniature teacups as cases, you might decide that volume is not an essential quality, especially if your other criteria are sufficient to distinguish which objects can be called a cup and that is your purpose.

Sometimes in creating narrative contrary cases, the tendency is to simply reverse the situation depicted in the exemplar case. Usually this does not add new information of significance for creating conceptual meaning. If you are having difficulty with constructing a negative case, ask someone else to suggest a contrary case or something that is definitely not what you are trying to describe. Sometimes you can locate a contrary case in the literature. Contrary cases that contribute to meaning often reveal important aspects of the exemplar case that are hidden in assumptions that you may be making about the concept.

Related Cases. Related cases are instances that represent a different but similar concept. Related cases usually share several criteria with the concept of interest, but one or more criteria will be particularly associated with it. A different word generally is used to label the related instances. If you find that one word typically is used to refer to essentially different phenomena, you may need to select language for your concept that differentiates it from the related meanings. For example, if you were focusing on the concept of love between a parent and child, you may need to use the word label *parental love* to signify that you see essential differences between this experience of love and other related experiences of love.

In the case of a cup, you might consider a drinking glass. For the concept of *red*, you might consider a red-orange hue or magenta. For the concept of *mothering*, you could design a case of tending that would be similar to the exemplar case. You might make a child-care worker the adult or substitute an elderly person for the infant. Again, you consider differences and similarities between the exemplar and related cases and revise the tentative criteria to reflect your new insights.

Borderline Cases. A borderline case usually is an instance of metaphoric or pseudo applications of the word. A borderline case is found when the same word is used in a different context. For example, if you are examining fatigue in chronic illness, a useful borderline case of fatigue would be military fatigue clothing. Poetry and lyrics to music provide rich sources of metaphoric uses of words. In the evolution of language the metaphoric meanings of words carry powerful messages that often persist as new usages emerge and thus illuminate core meaning. The metaphoric meanings for the concept of red are excellent examples. *Red* as a word and as a color has become in Western culture a metaphoric symbol for communism, violence, passion, and anger. To give a "cup of cheer" is an exemplary borderline usage of the term *cup.* This highlights the feature of cups as capable of holding something.

Slang terms and terms to describe technologic operations or features are rich sources of borderline cases when they are first entering the language. After they become well accepted, they are no longer borderline, moving to more central conceptual meanings, sometimes even exemplary cases. Slang, which can develop from a quirky application of a word, provides rich sources of borderline cases. The language that emerges for new technology also is a rich source of borderline cases. In the early 1990s, the word "web" probably would have prompted a mental image of something that a spider creates and the Internet would have been considered a borderline case. By the end of the 1990s, the word "web" was so fully associated with the Internet that it might have become a model case of *web.*

For the concept of *mothering,* a borderline case might be a computer motherboard, because this term, and its related concept, is not part of the typical computer user's conceptual realm and remains primarily a technical term. You might choose this borderline usage to help clarify features of the concept of *mother* that can be seen as foundational to the concept of mothering. These features could include the central importance of mother in some cultures for defining the scope of relationships or structuring the energy of all relationships in the system. Ask what happens to your meaning if you perceive mothering as a process that structures and directs the nature of relationships in a system.

Paradoxic cases are variants of borderline cases that are useful to highlight central meanings of concepts. These cases, paradoxically, embody elements of both exemplar and contrary cases. For example, in exploring the meaning of *dignity,* you might create a case in which actions that violate dignity occur in order to preserve a central feature of dignity. Your case might be an emergency cardiopulmonary resuscitation of a person in a public space to preserve the life of the person. Such a case is paradoxic in that it violates some criteria for dignity but highlights the importance of a central criterion for discerning the concept.

You probably will invent other varieties of cases in the process of creating conceptual meaning. How cases are classified is not critical. Their important function is to assist you in discerning the full range of possible meaning so that you can design a meaning that is useful for your purpose. Even though creating conceptual meaning is a rigorous and thoughtful process, cases are somewhat arbitrary and are historically and culturally situated. What you call them is not essential to the process. What is important is the meaning that you derive from the conceptual exploration and investigation.

Exploring Contexts and Values. Social contexts within which experience and the values that grow out of experience occur provide important cultural meanings that influence mental representations of that experience. Consider, for example, the concept of *judgment* if you are a student taking an examination, a real estate agent assessing a home for sale, an official scoring a gymnastics meet, or a magistrate preparing to impose a sentence. When you explore the various meanings acquired by virtue of the context, you probably will become aware of meanings you previously had not considered.

One way to imagine various contexts is to place your exemplar cases in different contexts and ask the following: What next? You mentally imagine the practical outcomes of your conceptual meaning in its context. For example, if you place your exemplar case of the color red in the context of a magazine advertisement, what symbolic meaning is conveyed? What advertising results does the advertiser intend? If the color red is placed in the context of traffic signs and symbols, what meaning does the color now convey? What behavioral responses do you now expect? What about a woman wearing a red suit in a boardroom where everyone else is dressed in dark suits? As you consider various possible combinations of context, you will clarify how meanings are influenced by the context.

Values also are revealed by placing the concept in a subtly differing context. The concept of *mothering* has a relatively positive connotation for most people. Most people agree that humans need "good" mothering to grow and develop adequately. However, people differ widely in what they consider to be good mothering; these differences often have to do with the cultural context. For example, there probably would be considerable disagreement as to whether what happens in a schoolroom, in a hospital, or in counseling can be considered mothering. What is considered mothering reflects deeply embedded cultural values. When you consider your exemplar case placed in several different social contexts, you create an avenue for perceiving important values and make deliberate choices concerning them.

Formulating Criteria for Concepts. We focus on criteria as an expression of conceptual meaning because they are a sensitive and succinct form for conveying essential conceptual meaning. Criteria are particularly useful as tools to initiate other processes of empiric theory development. Your exemplar case is itself a full expression of conceptual meaning, but the criteria make explicit the features and characteristics of the exemplar case that represent your conceptual meaning. Other forms of narrative, diagrams, and symbols can express meanings that move beyond the limits of empirics alone.

Criteria for the concept emerge gradually and continuously as you consider definitions, various cases, other sources, and varying contexts and values. As you develop the criteria, you naturally will refine them so that they reflect the meaning you intend. Criteria often express both qualitative and quantitative aspects of meaning and should suggest a definition of the word. Because criteria are more complex than is a limited word definition, they amplify the meaning and suggest direction for the processes of developing theory.

To illustrate the function of criteria for a concept, consider how you might convey the idea of one U.S. dollar in coins to a person who is not familiar with American money. One way is to present all possible combinations of coins to the individual, who then memorizes the combinations to consistently collect the right coins together to yield an equivalent of a dollar. Another approach is to provide guidelines that enable the individual to recognize and compose the various combinations independently. An exemplar case might use three quarters, one dime, two nickels, and five pennies. Because many other combinations are possible, criteria are created from the exemplar case to cover all other possible combinations. The exemplar case is chosen deliberately to include all the types of coins available, so that in examining the case several characteristics of all possibilities emerge. One feature is that the units of the various coins add up to an equivalent of 100 pennies—the smallest possible coin value. However, this criterion alone may not be sufficient for someone who is not familiar with this monetary system, and other criteria are created to ensure that all other possible combinations are recognized. You might consider the weight of the possible coin combinations, the colors of the coins, their metallic makeup, or the exchange value of each coin. All of these features may be used, but criteria should convey, as simply as possible, the information needed by a novice to collect one U.S. dollar in coins. The fact is that any color combination or any number of coins up to 100 may be used as criteria. Metallic content of the coins might serve as an adequate criterion and may even be the most precise of all possible criteria. But if your purpose is to assist a person from another country to understand how to make a dollar's worth of change, you would not select the metallic content as a criterion because it is impractical for that purpose.

For concrete objects, criteria may be relatively simple. For the concept of a cup, examples of criteria may be as follows:

- The object is cylindrical or conic in shape.
- The object is capable of containing physical matter.
- The height normally is between 3 and 7 inches, and the widest diameter is 3 to 4 inches.
- When the object contains liquid, it is capable of safely holding hot liquids.

Notice that this set of criteria is phrased so that a disposable foam cup or golfing green cup can be included. This choice is guided by the purpose. If you needed to make sure that the golfing green cup was not included as a cup, you might revise the criteria to include "the object is capable of being held in the hand, regardless of what it contains." This criterion places a limit on the volume and weight of the cup and implies that it must be a portable object.

Developing criteria for more abstract concepts is a more complex process, and the criteria often are more abstract. Criteria for the concept of *mothering* might include the following:

- The mothering person must have visual contact with the person who receives mothering in a manner that can be observed.
- The person who receives mothering must be physically touched by the mothering person.
- Some positive feeling must be experienced by the mothering person and by the person who receives mothering.
- There must be a reciprocal interaction between the mothering person and the person who receives mothering.
- Vocalization by the mothering person must occur.

These criteria do not limit the mothering person by sex, age, or species. The mother could be an elderly, male person. The criteria also do not specify that the person who receives mothering is an infant. If the purpose of applying the criteria is to distinguish between instances of mothering and fathering, these criteria would need to be revised to specify at least sex. If the purpose is to differentiate between mothering and neglect, they might be adequate.

The following question arises in the course of creating conceptual meaning: How do I know that the meaning I have created is adequate? You can examine your conceptual meaning for adequacy in relation to the processes used for creating meaning, as well as the conceptual meaning itself that you have created. Fuller (1991) suggests examining the process and the product of conceptualization in terms of both validity and reliability. A conceptualization is valid if it is based on multiple examples that are fully representative of the range of meanings for the concept, if you used multiple interpretive stages during the clarification process, and if the essential structure (or pattern) of the concept can be understood from the criteria. The conceptualization is reliable if the concept can be consistently recognized on the basis of the criteria that you have created. The meaning you create also is adequate if it reflects a reasonable and communicable understanding that is useful for your purposes. If your aims reflect valued nursing goals, if you have been careful in choosing and using resources, and if you understand why you have made the choices you have, you will have created an adequate and useful meaning. Additional processes for theory development will provide a check on conceptual meaning and will contribute to further refinements in your conceptual meaning.

Conceptual Meaning and Problems of Theoretic Development. Problems associated with conceptual meaning often underlie other problems involved in developing theory. A major challenge with respect to structuring and confirming theoretic relationships is the selection of direct and indirect empiric indicators for a concept. When research reports give conflicting results, the differences are sometimes tied to the use of different definitions and empiric indicators for the concept. If you explore the conceptual meanings within research reports, you often can clarify the extent to which differing conceptual meanings account for the differing research findings. As you carry out the processes for creating conceptual meaning, you will be able to suggest a full range of possible empiric indicators for a concept that are pertinent to your specific purpose. You also will be able to identify the limits of empiric approaches in specifying indicators for a phenomenon.

Consider, for example, the concept of mothering and the sample criteria we gave in the previous section. These criteria include characteristics that can be observed empirically. They are reciprocal interaction, visualization, touch, and vocalization. The criterion that states that "some positive feeling must be experienced by the mothering person and by the person who receives mothering" might be one of the most important distinguishing features of your intended meaning for mothering, but it does not easily lend itself to objective observation. It can be assessed indirectly by asking mothers to describe their feelings.

Conceptual meaning is fundamental if you must distinguish one concept from a closely related one. This often is the case when you are forming theoretic relationships or structuring and contextualizing theoretic statements. The processes of creating conceptual meaning make it possible to propose differentiating features of similar concepts that are useful to guide theorizing and related research activities. Consider the concepts of *tending* and *mothering*. Individuals tend to the needs of others in many different contexts, and mothers tend children. A question to be resolved might be the following: Is there a particular kind of tending that occurs in mothering? You can examine a related case of a nanny who is tending children to determine whether any characteristic of tending is within your idea of mothering. As you explore various differentiating features of the central concept, your ideas will become clearer and the structure of your theory or research study will improve. Creating conceptual meaning helps you make decisions about the qualitative dimensions of criteria, such as whether they always need to be evident or whether they may be expressed with different intensities. For example, you may decide that for the concept of mothering, the expression of positive feeling must be present, but the degree to which it occurs may vary.

In creating conceptual meaning, the challenge is to evolve a useful and adequate meaning from a range of possibilities. The processes for creating conceptual meaning are in and of themselves useful. When you also create meanings that can be used in conjunction with other activities of theory development, you move toward refinements of meaning that are useful for research and ultimately practice validation that can further refine the theory.

Structuring and Contextualizing Theory

Structuring and contextualizing theory involves forming systematic linkages between and among concepts. Many approaches can be used (Dubin, 1978; Newman, 1979; Reynolds, 2006; Tomey & Alligood, 2006; Walker & Avant, 2004). The choice of a particular approach depends on your purposes for developing theory, what you already know or assume to be true, and your underlying philosophic ideas about the nature of nursing knowledge. If you begin with an entirely new idea about something and with very little reported about it in the existing literature, the form of the theory that you construct may be a categorization of the concepts into a relational taxonomy that essentially describes your ideas. If you begin with an idea that builds on other theorists' descriptions, you might develop a theoretic structure that provides explanations of complex interrelationships between concepts. If you are structuring theory as an outcome of grounded research, the interrelationships between data clusters guide the theoretical structure you create. Approaches to structuring and contextualizing theory are described in detail in the sections that follow and include the following:

- *Identifying and defining the concepts.* Concepts are important elements that convey the focus and meaning of the theory. Definitions of concepts can evolve from the processes of creating conceptual meaning, be thoughtfully borrowed from other theories, or be formulated from other sources. They should indicate as clearly and concisely as possible the theoretic meaning of important concepts within the theory.
- *Identifying assumptions.* Assumptions are the basic underlying premises from which and within which theoretic reasoning proceeds.
- *Clarifying the context within which the theory is placed.* Contextual placement describes the circumstances within which the theoretic relationships are expected to be empirically relevant. Clear statements regarding context are particularly important if the theory is to be used in practice.
- *Designing relationship statements.* Projected relationships between and among the concepts of the theory, taken as a whole, provide the substance and the form of the theory.

Identifying and Defining Concepts.   Structuring theory requires that you identify the concepts that will form the basic fabric of the theory. The concepts can come from life experiences, clinical practice, basic or applied research, knowledge of the literature, and the formal processes of creating conceptual meaning just described. Often theory emerges because of a conviction that existing knowledge and theories are not adequate to represent an experience.

Some concepts are better suited for theory development than are others. Concepts that are extremely abstract carry broad meanings and refer to a wide range of experience. They usually are not suitable as a beginning point for theory development. Concepts such as *social structure, politics,* or *love,* for example, refer to such a broad range of experience that defining them within the limits of empiric inquiry is extremely difficult; these concepts are better suited to philosophy than to empiric theory. Such concepts, however, can be useful in considering the context within which the theory is placed.

If concepts are extremely narrow and concrete, they refer to only a narrow range of experience, and the level of abstraction may not be sufficient for theoretic purposes. For example, concepts such as *toothache* or *postappendectomy surgical pain* apply to relatively few instances of pain. *Chronic or acute pain* may be a more suitable concept from which to develop theory. What is considered a suitable level of abstraction for theory varies in nursing. The recent trend toward middle-range, situation-specific theory and evidence-based practice provides a useful guideline for decisions about the level of abstraction for theoretic concepts.

As the concepts are specified or begin to form, early ideas about the structure of their relationships begin to emerge. There usually are one or two primary or central concepts around which the theoretic relationships build. Thinking about possible relationships helps to clarify what concepts the theory needs to include. Previous research, existing theories, philosophies, and personal experience provide a background for forming theoretic relationships. Initially, you might simply note concepts that you think are related on the basis of your experience, what you find in the literature, or ongoing research.

Assumptions stemming from cultural history also influence conceptual structure. For example, an assumption that is inherent in most empiric theory is the concept of linear time, which in turn determines the relationship linkages that various concepts have with one another.

Antecedent, coincident or intervening, and consequent concepts imply prediction within a linear time frame. Antecedent concepts are those experiences that you identify as coming before other concepts. Coincident concepts are those that coexist in time. Intervening concepts also are coincident and have a particular influence on relationships among concepts that are specified in the theory. Consequent concepts are those that follow another.

Some theories place antecedents in a causal relationship with those that follow. Other theories rest on a philosophic view that rejects the idea of causation. Instead, the ideas of influence or affect are used to explain relationships over time. If a primary concept within your developing theory is *anger,* you might propose that previous childhood experiences cause the anger experience, or you might consider childhood experience as an antecedent that influences the anger experience.

Consequents also can imply causation. For example, once a person experiences stress, consequents of that experience can be thought of as resulting from the stress. Changes in mental functioning, in sleep and rest patterns, and in relationships with other people might be theoretic concepts structured to reflect phenomena caused by the stress.

Intervening concepts can be used to shift from a view of causation to one of influence. Intervening concepts are those that influence the relationships between antecedent experiences, the event itself, and its consequents. For example, the central concept of fear might be viewed as being influenced by the antecedent experiences of childhood, and sleep patterns might be viewed as an intervening variable that influences the relationship between the childhood experience and present fear.

As initial ideas are formed concerning relationships between concepts, the concepts themselves become clearer, and processes of creating conceptual meaning can be used to make the meanings explicit. Some concepts might be grouped together and assigned more abstract terms to compose a new concept. This occurs especially when theory is structured and conceptualized with inductive theory development processes such as grounded theory. For example, you might begin to see that *time of day* and *season of year* could be grouped to become components of the more abstract concept of *biologic rhythms.*

As the concepts of the theory are identified and conceptualized, theoretic definitions emerge. Theoretic definitions form the basis for and reflect empiric indicators and operational definitions for concepts that are needed for research and convey the general meaning of the concept. Empiric indicators are different from theoretic definitions in that they specify as exactly as possible how the concept is to be assessed in a specific study. For example, a theoretic definition for the concept of *mothering* might read as follows:

Mothering An interaction between a human adult and a child that conveys reciprocal feelings of attachment. The interaction is behaviorally expressed by reciprocal visual contact, touching, and vocalization.

This theoretic definition gives a general idea of the concept's empiric indicators (sometimes referred to as operational definitions). The first part of the definition provides a general meaning for the term. The second part suggests behaviors associated with the concept that can be assessed. Empiric indicators would specify specific observational tools, or measurements, that would be used in a research study. Measurements of vocalizations, for example, clearly would be defined in terms of the characteristics consistent with the conceptual idea of vocalizations consistent with the concept of mothering, and the tools, or instruments, used to measure these vocalizations, and the range of outcomes, would be specified.

Notice that the theoretic definition is consistent with tentative criteria for the concept of *mothering,* but the definition serves a different purpose. The criteria are specific and useful as a foundation for construction of theory and for empiric study of the concept. The theoretic definition summarizes the insights that are formed in creating conceptual meaning and concisely conveys the essential meaning of the concept.

Identifying Assumptions as Part of Theory. Assumptions are underlying givens that are presumed to be true. In the context of empiric theory they can be challenged philosophically and may be assessed empirically. Philosophic assumptions form the grounding for a theory. If they are challenged, the substance of the entire theory also is challenged on philosophic grounds. Assumptions that could be empirically assessed but are not within the context of the theory also affect the value of the entire theory. For example, a theory about the best way to teach a diabetic person about foot care may assume that diabetics do want to learn such care. Although this assumption could be empirically assessed, for purposes of the theory it is assumed and reasonably so. If the guidelines inherent in the theory are used when diabetic individuals have no desire to learn foot care, it will not be helpful and another approach will be required.

Stated assumptions are easy to recognize, but many assumptions are implied or not stated and are difficult to recognize. An example of an underlying assumption that usually is not stated is that human beings are separate from, but interact with, their environment. For theories that involve human experience, this statement can be taken as reasonably true. However, many commonly accepted truths about human existence gain new significance within a theoretic context, and they need to be stated even if they seem self-evident. For example, if a theory includes the concept of death, certain underlying assumptions about the nature of life and death would influence the essential ideas of the theory, and these assumptions need to be stated. A theory of grief that is based on a view of death as a transition to another form of life will be very different from a theory of grief that views death as the end of life.

Rogers (1970) made her assumption explicit that human beings are unified wholes, possessing their own integrity and manifesting characteristics that are more than and different from the sum of their parts. On the surface, this statement seems perfectly reasonable and sensible, but it is significant because it is an assumption that is not common to all nursing theory. As an assumption, it does not require empiric evidence, but it is fundamental to the relationship statements Rogers proposed. In theory, it is the relationships, not assumptions, that are empirically validated and confirmed.

Assumptions influence all aspects of structuring and contextualizing theory. If the assumption of wholism is used as a basis for a theory of mothering, interrelated concepts must be consistent with a wholistic view of human experience. Patterns of behavior that reflect the whole would be reflected in the theoretic concepts. They might include patterns of movement and communication. In contrast, if human beings were assumed to be biologic and social organisms, the concepts of a mothering theory might include physical responses and cultural mores.

Clarifying the Context. Theoretic relationships must be placed within a context if the theory is to be useful for practice. If a theory of mothering is meant to apply only to the interactions of women and children in Western cultures, these limits on the applicability of the theory must be considered and stated. As the theory is extended, it might be useful for other cultures and for other kinds of intimate relationships such as adult–child, adult–adult, or adult–animal interactions.

Contexts that are very broad or very narrow reflect the range of applicability of theory. A theory that is structured for many cultures may not be useful for any culture. Conversely, a theory that is structured within the context of a single institution (for example, one hospital) may not be useful for other settings. Historically, as nursing incorporated an emphasis on middle-range theory the context for which theories were developed narrowed. Broad frameworks that addressed phenomena such as adaptation or conservation were still considered theory and were useful in many nursing situations. Middle-range theories tended to focus on phenomena that did not emerge in all nursing situations but were commonly recognized in nursing; phenomena such as uncertainty or hopelessness are examples for a fuller discussion. Situation-specific theory narrowed context even further to particular situations of uncertainty or hopelessness (Im & Meleis, 1999). Thus, a middle-range theory of hopelessness or uncertainty would need to be adapted and developed for use across different contexts. For example, a middle-range theory of uncertainty would be made situation specific if it addressed factors significant to the experience of uncertainty such as ethnicity or age of clients.

Designing Relationship Statements. Relationship statements structurally interrelate the concepts of the theory. The statements range from those that simply relate two concepts to relatively complex statements that account for interactions among multiple concepts. Theories usually contain several levels of relationship statements, which comprise a reasonably complete explanation of how the concepts of the theory interact. The relationships begin to take form as the concepts are identified and emerge, but the process of designing the relationship statements requires specific attention to the substance, direction, strength, and quality of interactions between concepts.

Consider a relationship statement that might be formulated about the concept of mothering. A theorist might propose that, as an adult's visual contact with an infant increases, the infant's visual contact with the adult also will increase. This relationship statement speculates that one event (increased adult visual contact) precedes a second event (increased infant visual contact). This relationship also describes a substantive interaction (visual contact) as a component of mothering. It implies direction (an increase) as part of the interaction.

A more complex relational statement addresses further dimensions of quality, contexts, and circumstances that are proposed. Such a statement might take the following form:

> *Under the conditions of C1 ... Cn, if X occurs, then Y will occur.*

The illustration involving the concept of mothering might take the following form:

> *When an adult mothering figure and*
> *an infant are in close proximity (C1),*
> *and*
> *when the adult has a negative feeling toward the infant (C2),*
> *and*
> *when the frequency of physical contact is limited (C3),*
> *then,*
> *if the adult's frequency of visual contact decreases,*
> *the infant's frequency of visual contact also will decrease.*

A relationship also may be designed to introduce new concepts to the potential theory. Initially, such a relationship might read as follows:

> If the infant's frequency of visual contact is not sufficient to satisfy the mother, the adult's frequency of visual contact will increase in a conscious effort to engage the infant in interaction.

This relationship introduces the concept of awareness as well as the subjective value of "sufficient to satisfy." The idea of awareness and a value of sufficiency are not objectively identifiable or empirically observable. As the theory is developed further, possible empiric indicators for satisfaction might be created, or this dimension of the theory might be viewed as something to be subjectively assessed. In this way the theory not only stimulates the creation of new empiric knowledge but also opens possibilities for exploring and integrating other ways of knowing. Although empiric theory primarily is designed to propose and create empiric relationships, it often contains concepts and relationships that integrate and require ethical, aesthetic, personal, and emancipatory knowing. Ethical considerations around inappropriately disturbing the mother–infant relationship and the aesthetics of creating measurement approaches that do not create distress for either party need to be considered. The possibility that researchers in assessing a subjective variable such as "sufficient to satisfy" might bring their own experience-based bias about mothering to the research project reflects the personal knowing dimension. Emancipatory knowing is used as researchers ponder whether social practices have created expectations for mothers that demand, or expect, maternal-infant bonding, creating the possibility that mothers will not exhibit authentic expressions of satisfaction.

A hypothesis is a type of propositional statement. It is a single statement of a proposed relationship between two or more variables. Hypotheses can take several forms and still provide a basis for developing theory. A neutral hypothesis asserts that one variable (X) is related to a second variable (Y) or that one variable (X) changes in relation to another (Y) without indicating the direction of change. A directional hypothesis indicates the direction of association between variables in which as one variable (X) increases or decreases, a second (Y) also increases or decreases.

A confirmed hypothesis is a relationship statement for which there is research support. It can be either directional or neutral. Hypothesis testing requires that certain controls and procedures be adhered to and that statistical exemplars be applied in the confirmation process.

The traditional form of expressing hypotheses requires statements that conform to rules of logic. The logic may be either deductive or inductive. The following sections provide an overview of each of these forms of logic. Boxes 7-2 and 7-3 explain deductive and inductive forms of logic that often are used or that provide a foundation for constructing formal hypotheses.

Comparison of Induction and Deduction. Deductive logic is reasoning from the general to the particular. Inductive logic is reasoning from the particular to the general. In inductive logic, particular instances are observed to be consistently part of a larger whole or set, and the set of particular instances is merged with that larger whole. This larger set can then be considered in relation to still another set of events or phenomena in another logical system.

In deductive logic, the premises as starting points embody two variables that can be categorized in relation to each other as broad or specific. In Box 7-2, humans (a broad concept) were said to use cups with handles (a specific feature). In the other premise, neonates were said to be a class of humans: that is, neonates were specifically members of a broader class (humans). The conclusion contains both specific variables: neonates use cups with handles. In deductive logic, the movement is from premises embodying broad and specific variables to a conclusion in which the variables are more specific.

Box 7-2
Understanding Deduction as a Formal System of Reasoning

FORMAT	EXAMPLE A	EXAMPLE B
A is B (premise).	The "fit" survive.	Humans use cups with handles.
C is A (premise).	The most numerous are the "fit."	Neonates are humans.
C is B (conclusion).	The most numerous survive.	Neonates use cups with handles.

WHAT TO KNOW

Sound conclusions can be empirically empty, as in example A, in which both premises are definitionally true but give no new information.

Conclusions are only as sound as premises, as in example B, in which the format is correct but the first premise is not true.

Premises go by several labels: hypotheses, suppositions, axioms, or propositions.

Conclusions go by different labels: laws or theorems.

Reasoning moves from general to particular: the conclusion is a specific instance of the first premise.

Deduction is associated with the hypotheticodeductive methodology of traditional science.

Challenge: to use premises that have enough empiric confirmation to yield useful theoretic constructions.

Like most other words, deduction and induction have common meanings related to, but different from, their meaning within systems of logic. People often state that they deduce hypotheses from theory or deductively develop theory. These deductions are not the result of applying rules of logic but arise out of careful thought without specifically using a system of logic. Used like this, deduction implies that a more general theory was a source of specific hypotheses or relational statements.

With induction, people induce hypotheses and relationships by observing or experiencing an empiric reality and reaching some conclusion. These related meanings of *induction* and *deduction* should be noted because sometimes the terms refer to systems of logic and to rules and conventions for the ordering of reasoning. At other times the terms refer to a general approach to thinking that is short of logical rules but similar in form.

Box 7-3
Understanding Induction as a Formal System of Reasoning

FORMAT	EXAMPLE A	EXAMPLE B
X1 is a member of set Y associated with Z.	A grackle is a black bird and can fly.	A bunionectomy is a painful surgical procedure.
X2 is a member of set Y associated with Z.	A starling is a black bird and can fly.	A laparotomy is a painful surgical procedure.
X3 is a member of set Y associated with Z.	A crow is a black bird and can fly.	A tooth extraction is a painful surgical procedure.
X4 is a member of set Y associated with Z.	A raven is a black bird and can fly.	A closed reduction is a painful surgical procedure.
X5 is a member of set Y associated with Z.	A vulture is a black bird and can fly.	A tendon repair is a painful surgical procedure.
Therefore, X6, X7, ... Xn are members of set Y and associated with Z.	Therefore, all black birds can fly.	Therefore, all surgical procedures are painful.

WHAT TO KNOW

The observation of multiple particular instances of the same phenomena that share a common characteristic is required to generalize that all subsequent cases also will share that characteristic.

Induction reasons from the particular to the general case.

Induction is associated with the inductive research methodologies.

Challenge: to observe enough episodes of individual instances to have confidence in the generalization.

REFLECTION AND DISCUSSION

This chapter provided an overview of methods for creating conceptual meaning and structuring and contextualizing theory. Specific techniques for evolving criteria for concepts and forming linkages among concepts to create theory were presented. A centrally important message of this chapter is that conceptual meaning is not given, but is created. The creation of meaning appropriate for the purpose of the theory determines how concepts are structured and assessed. This, in turn, determines the utility of the theory for practice goals.

To deepen your appreciation of theory development processes consider the following related to the content of this chapter:

1. Identify a situation or phenomenon in nursing (a concept) that you believe has not been named or clarified. Consider why. Is this an important concept to attend to?
2. Locate a research study that embodies a broad concept such as *stress* or *quality of life*. How was the concept measured or assessed? Did the assessment adequately represent the fullness of the concept?
3. Examine a standardized tool for assessment or measurement of a broad concept and consider groups and individuals for whom the measurement tool might not be appropriate and why.
4. Identify a middle-range concept of importance to nursing. Relate the concept to another concept and then to a nursing goal. As an example, relate *distress* and *hardiness* to the goal of *hope*. Consider the various ways the concepts could be structured. Do they need to be narrowed before a reasonable structure is possible?
5. Find a research study that "tested" a middle-range theory. How were the key concepts assessed? Were they assessed or measured in a way that is practical for nurses to use?
6. Choose a middle-range theory, or any research grounded in the theory, and think about how all knowing patterns were used (or should have been) in the design of the theory or the conduct of the research.

Reference List

Crowe, M. (2005). Discourse analysis: Toward an understanding of its place in nursing. *Journal of Advanced Nursing, 51*(1), 55–63.

Dickoff, J., & James, P. (1968). A theory of theories: A position paper. *Nursing Research, 17*(3), 197–203.

Dubin, R. (1978). *Theory building* (Rev. ed.). New York: Free Press.

Ellis, R. (1968). Characteristics of significant theories. *Nursing Research, 17*(3), 217–222.

Fuller, J. (1991). *A conceptualization of presence as a nursing phenomenon*. Salt Lake City: University of Utah.

Im, E.-O., & Meleis, A. I. (1999). Situation-specific theories: Philosophical roots, properties, and approach. *ANS. Advances in Nursing Science, 22*(2), 11–24.

Jacox, A. (1974). Theory construction in nursing: An overview. *Nursing Research, 23*(1), 4–13.

Kaplan, A. (1964). *The conduct of inquiry*. New York: Thomas Y. Crowell.

Kramer, M. (1993). Concept clarification and critical thinking: Integrated processes. *Journal of Nursing Education, 32*(9), 1–10.

Levine, M. E. (1967). The four conservation principles of nursing. *Nursing Forum, 6*(1), 93–98.

McKay, R. P. (1969). Theories, models and systems for nursing. *Nursing Research, 18*(5), 393–399.

Morse, J. M. (1995). Exploring the theoretical basis of nursing using advanced techniques of concept analysis. *ANS. Advances in Nursing Science, 17*(3), 31–46.

Muller, M. E., & Dzurec, L. C. (1993). The power of the name. *ANS. Advances in Nursing Science, 15*(3), 15–22.

Newman, M. A. (1979). *Theory development in nursing.* Philadelphia: FA Davis.

Norris, C. M. (1982). *Concept clarification in nursing.* Rockville, MD: Aspen Systems.

Reynolds, P. D. (2006). *A primer in theory construction.* Upper Saddle River, NJ: Allyn & Bacon.

Rodgers, B. L., & Knafl, K. A. (2000). *Concept development in nursing: Foundations, techniques and applications.* St. Louis: Saunders-Elsevier.

Rogers, M. E. (1970). *An introduction to the theoretical basis of nursing.* Philadelphia: FA Davis.

Tomey, A. M., & Alligood, M. R. (2006). *Nursing theorists and their work*, (6th ed.). St. Louis: Elsevier-Mosby.

Walker, L. O., & Avant, K. C. (2004). *Strategies for theory construction in nursing*, (4th ed.). Upper Saddle River, NJ: Prentice-Hall).

Watson, J. (1985). *Nursing: Human science and human care: A theory of nursing.* Norwalk, CT: Appleton-Century-Crofts.

White, R. (2004). Discourse analysis and social constructionism. *Nursing Research, 12*(2), 7–16.

Wilson, J. (1963). *Thinking with concepts.* London: Cambridge University Press.

Wright, M. (1966). Research and research. *Nursing Research, 15*, 244.

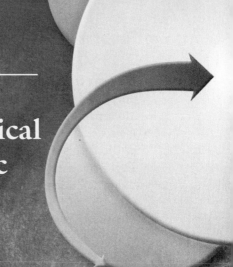

CHAPTER 8

Description and Critical Reflection of Empiric Theory

We converse with one another of knowledge, research, assumptions and so forth, overconfident that we understand.

Norma Koltoff (1967, p. 122)

Once theories are developed, the questions "What is this?" and "How does it work?" can be asked. These questions stimulate development of empiric theory and serve as an organizing framework for deliberately examining it. This chapter explains analytic and evaluative processes that are useful in understanding the nature and value of theory. These processes describe and critically reflect theory—that is, examine its value for various purposes. A clear understanding of the nature of any theory flows from description and critical reflection. This is important if you are going to use a theory in research processes or practice.

The definition of empiric theory we use in this text, as stated in the following, points to the elements of a theory that can form the basis for describing what the theory is all about.

> *Theory* A creative and rigorous structuring of ideas that projects a tentative, purposeful, and systematic view of phenomena.

The descriptive components that this definition suggest are as follows.

- *Purpose:* If a theory is purposeful, then a purpose can be found. The purpose of a theory may not be stated explicitly, but it should be identifiable.
- *Concepts:* If a theory represents a structuring of ideas, the ideas will be in the form of concepts that are expressed in language.
- *Definitions:* If the concepts of a theory are integrated systematically, their meanings will be conveyed in definitions. Definitions vary in precision and completeness, but conceptual meaning should be identifiable in a theory. The meanings for the concepts created by the theorist give the theory its particular character.
- *Relationships and structure:* If the concepts are related and structured into a systematic whole, then the overall whole of the theory is identifiable.
- *Assumptions:* If theory is tentative, assumptions form the underlying "taken for granted" truths on which the theory was developed, leaving open possible theoretic interpretations that would come from different sets of assumptions.

Theory, by definition, contains these identifiable components. Describing theory is a process of posing questions about these components and responding to the questions with your own reading or interpretation of the theory. Some elements will seem clear; some will depend on tentative interpretations; some will remain unclear. Despite ambiguities, the process of describing theory creates a description that can then form the basis for critical reflection.

WHAT IS THIS? THE DESCRIPTION OF THE THEORY

In this section we discuss the processes for describing theory. Once a theory is formalized it can be described, and the description can be used as a basis for critical reflection. Critical reflection processes follow this section on description of theory.

What Is the Purpose of This Theory?

The general purpose of the theory is important because it specifies the context and situations in which the theory is useful. Purpose can be approached initially by asking the following: "Why was this theory formulated?" The responses to this question provide information that pertains to theoretic purposes.

Some purposes are specific to the clinical practice of nursing. In these theories the concepts of the theory include nursing actions and behaviors that contribute to the purpose. Pain alleviation and restored self-care ability are examples of purpose that require clinical practice and suggest that nursing actions are part of the theory. Note that these purpose statements have a value orientation: alleviation and restoration. These ideas imply change toward a certain goal, not just change for the sake of change. Such value connotations are important to notice when describing the purpose of theory.

Some purposes may not require the direct clinical practice of nursing but are useful for understanding phenomena that occur in the context of nursing practice. These purposes can contribute to achieving practice purposes, or they may not be directly relevant to practice goals. Consider, for example, a theory with a central purpose of explaining variables affecting blood flow velocity in the skin. Clinical practice is not necessary to explain blood flow velocity, but a theory with this purpose might be linked to a theoretic explanation of how blood flow velocity influences the incidence of decubiti or the extent of peripheral neuropathy in people with diabetes. A theory that explains skin blood flow velocity and factors affecting it might have potential to help practitioners prevent skin breakdown and peripheral neuropathy.

Theoretic purposes that do not require direct clinical nursing actions but are of concern to nursing also may involve professional issues in nursing. For example, the purpose of an empiric theory might be to describe features of organizations that empower nurses. This valued and necessary purpose is not directly related to the specific nursing actions of giving care, but it is certainly useful for changing practice.

It is important to clarify whether purposes are embedded in the theoretic structure or are reasonable extensions of the theory. For example, consider a theory of mother–infant attachment that links together the following concepts: (1) birth or adoption experience, (2) maternal support systems, (3) degree of bonding, and (4) healthy infant development. The linkages are formed in a way that suggests that maternal attachment is influenced by the nature of birth or adoption experience, which determines the extent of maternal support and bonding, and that these, if positive, encourage healthy infant development. In this example healthy infant development is an example of a clinical outcome—or purpose—that is structured within the theory. Suppose the theorist stated that the purpose of the theory was quality of life for the family unit, but how the concepts within the theory interrelate to create quality of life was not structured by the theorist. Quality of life as a purpose would constitute an extension of the theory because the concept is not located within the structure of the theory. Purposes that are embedded within the structure of the theory usually are explicit. Purposes that are reasonable extensions of the theory are important for understanding the clinical usefulness of the theory, though not clearly linked to the central concepts within the theory. Often purposes that are extensions of theory are linked to the concepts and structure of the theory by implicit assumptions. Purposes outside the context of the theory also suggest directions for further development of the theory. In the example just cited, research or logical reasoning would be indicated that links healthy infant development with quality of life indicators.

Purposes within a theory may be found for different individuals or groups of individuals who might use or benefit from use of the theory. For example, if a theory is developed toward the clinical goal of pain alleviation, the theory can be examined for purposes appropriate for the individual nurse, the physician, and the person receiving care, as well as for the family. Consider theory developed with a clinical purpose of promoting high-level wellness. The theoretical purpose for the nurse might be distinctly different from that implied for the person receiving nursing care. The nurse's purpose might be to design a system that promotes recovery. The purpose for the person receiving care might be to recover and to provide responses that indicate how effective the system is in promoting recovery. Taken together, these two purposes might be viewed as an overall purpose of creating an interacting recovery process.

In addition to whether or not purposes can be found for various individuals using or affected by the theory, questions related to scope of purpose can be asked. For example, does the overall purpose focus on an individual, a family, groups, or society in general? An organized society or an expanded collective consciousness are examples of broad purposes that apply to relatively unbounded groups of people. Purposes such as environmental health or political activism may apply to communities or may be linked to definable groups within those communities. When there are multiple purposes within theory, the scope of those purposes may vary. You may find narrower scope purposes for individuals and families, and broader scope purposes for a community. When multiple purposes within theory are found, if clarity is not compromised, you should be able to order purposes in a hierarchy that flows toward one central purpose.

The following question often arises: "How are purposes to be separated from the concepts of the theory?" Purposes that are part of the matrix of the theory also are concepts of the theory. One approach to identifying which concept also is the central purpose is to describe or to designate the concept toward which theoretic reasoning flows. This is related to the structure of the theory. Ask the following questions: "What is the end point of this theory?" and "When is this theory no longer useful?" Responses to these questions provide clues to purpose and help to clarify the context in which the theory can be used. In Hall's (1966) theoretical framework, for example, the theory would cease to be valuable when the client has engaged in self-actualization, and self-actualization may be deemed the overall purpose. This purpose of self-actualization in the structure of Hall's theoretical framework represents the end point of theoretic reasoning. In the context of Hall's theory, self-actualization is a purpose that requires nursing practice. Outside the context of Hall's theory, self-actualization is a purpose that is shared with other professions.

What Are the Concepts of This Theory?

Concepts are identified by searching out words or groups of words that represent objects, properties, or events within the theory. You can begin to describe concepts by listing key ideas and tentatively identifying how they seem to interrelate. As you begin to discern relationships, your perception of the key concepts of the theory will become clearer. One initial difficulty in identifying concepts is determining which concepts are integral to the theory and which are part of some supporting narrative. There is no easy way to deal with this difficulty. By beginning to identify concepts and deriving interrelationships, decisions can be made about which concepts are central to the theory.

As you identify important theoretic concepts, ask questions about the nature of the concepts and their organization. Is there a major concept with subconcepts organized under it? Are there several major concepts with subconcepts organized under them? Are concepts singular entities? Are some concepts singular entities and others organized with subconcepts? What are the relationships and interrelationships between and among concepts? Are some concepts mentioned that do not seem to fit the emerging structure? What is the relative scope of the various concepts? Once concepts are identified and questions such as these are addressed, the relationships and structure will begin to emerge.

Other questions deal with the numbers of concepts. How many concepts are there? How many might be termed major concepts? How many are minor concepts? Do not get stuck trying to distinguish between major and minor. Rather, notice whether one concept or a few concepts really stand out as important whereas others seem less so, and why. As you consider the organization and number of concepts, address qualitative features of the concepts as well. Do the concepts represent abstractions of objects, properties, or events? Is it possible to identify what they represent? Are the concepts more empirically grounded, or are they more abstract? What proportion is empirically grounded? What proportion is highly abstract? Are the concepts fairly discrete in meaning, or do several have similar meanings? When similar meanings for concepts exist, do they all seem to express a single idea, or are they different? How? Concepts that are alike may represent one central idea that is fairly clear or several different images. For example, the concepts of *rehabilitation, restoration,* and *recovery,* which share common meanings, may appear in the same theory with similar meanings or with different meanings.

When you are addressing the question of a theory's concepts, the concepts within it must be examined carefully for quantity, character, emerging relationships, and structure. The description of concepts is crucial because their quantity and character form understanding of the purpose of the theory, the structure and nature of theoretic relationships, the definitions, and the assumptions.

Purposes, Concepts, and Scope of Theory. Categorizations of scope can be found in nursing's theoretical literature. The same or similar labels can be used differently, are relative to one another, and typically are used to classify the scope of theory in relation to purpose and concepts. To label theory as micro or atomistic, for example, suggests relatively narrow-range concepts and purpose, whereas *macro* implies that the theory has a broad purpose and covers a relatively broad range of concepts. These categorizations often differ according to the scope of practice within the discipline. What is micro for one discipline may be middle-range in others. A theory with a wholistic purpose likely would be broad in scope in almost any discipline and would deal with patterns reflecting the whole. Grand theory, like macro theory, refers to very broad-scope theory in most disciplines. The term *atomistic* implies a narrow-scope theory and carries the connotation that parts are a legitimate focus for study and understanding their interrelationships will yield credible understanding of the whole. Conversely, *wholism* often connotes that the sum of parts cannot reflect the whole.

Micro theory may reflect purposes that can be known only indirectly because evidence to validate their achievement requires perceptions keener than those provided by unaided senses. The purpose of altering action potential is representative of this category. Improving regional blood flow is an even broader purpose than is altering action potential because in some cases it is indirectly perceptible, whereas action potentials cannot be assessed without sensitive signal-processing equipment. Concepts contained in such theories are narrow and often specifically defined.

When purpose represents a portion of an accepted overall purpose for a profession or discipline, middle-range theory is being approached. We use the term *substantive* middle-range theory to reference concepts that reflect the clinical practice of nursing. A theory of pain alleviation is an example of substantive middle-range theory, as pain alleviation usually assumes the need for clinical practice. Micro theories might attempt to explain the physiology of pain phenomena, whereas substantive middle-range theories would deal with pain alleviation as a segment of nursing's total interest. Concepts contained in substantive middle-range theory, then, reflect a "part of the whole" orientation; they are broader than those contained in micro theories but still do not reflect the totality of nursing's purpose.

Macro theories have a broadly conceptualized purpose. Health, expanded consciousness, and high-level wellness, not just for individuals but for humanity in general, are examples of such purposes. Macro theories deal with the whole of nursing's concern. Concepts within these theories tend to be broad in scope and related to individuals as wholes rather than as portions of the person's structure or function.

An example may serve to illustrate how the purpose of a theory provides information that can be used in responding to questions about scope. Abdellah, Beland, Martin & Matheney (1960) proposed that nursing purposes can be described as the solution of problems in 21 different categories. Each problem is complex in itself, and taken together they represent the totality of nursing function. Problem 11 is "to facilitate maintenance of sensory function." Theory regarding the management and prevention of sensory function as a problem could be considered more middle-range than grand or macro theory in that it is only 1 of 21 problems of concern to nursing. Narrower theory is possible concerning the development or maintenance of sensory function in diverse groups, such as those with chronic illness, the young or aged, or any of numerous subdivisions. Theory of sensory neural transport would represent micro theory in relation to this problem area. Assume that the maintenance of function in all 21 problem areas constitutes health, whereas the solution of existing problems constitutes movement from illness toward health, with health a valued purpose for individuals. Macro theory would be theory that interrelates all 21 problem areas so that the general purpose of health restoration or maintenance could be approached.

In some ways, these multitudes of ways to categorize theories around scope is "much ado about nothing." Two things, however, are significant. First it is important to know that terminology for categorizing theory by scope has a variety of nuanced meanings in the literature and is therefore confusing to understand. Making a firm decision that a theory is or isn't macro or middle-range when there is legitimate disagreement is not important. However, understanding how degree of scope affects utilization and further development of a theory is critical.

What Are the Definitions in This Theory?

A definition is an explicit meaning that is conveyed for a concept. Definitions exist to clarify the nature of the abstraction that the theorist constructs in a way that others can comprehend. Definitions suggest how word representations of an idea (concept) are expressed in experience.

It often is difficult to determine from a listing of key words which concepts are basic to the theoretic structure and which comprise definitions and assumptions. Carefully reading the theory and relying on your own judgment should provide this information.

Concepts may be defined in a list of definitions, or they may be defined in narrative form in the text but not labeled as definitions. It is not always easy to recognize narratives as definitions because they are not labeled and may contain information that is not directly pertinent to the definition of the concept.

Concept definitions also can be implied by how the theorist uses the conceptual terms in the context. If, for example, a theorist uses the concept of *wholism,* but this term is not explicitly defined, you can examine the use of the term and infer the meaning or definition. If the theorist describes various dimensions of wholistic health, for example, then the definition of wholism is akin to "the sum of the parts." If the theorist does not use parts or dimensions in speaking of wholistic health, then the theorist may be using a definition more closely associated with wholism as being more than the sum of its parts.

Because concepts may be defined both explicitly and implicitly, ask the following questions: How are concepts defined? Explicitly? Implicitly? Both? Are implied definitions consistent with explicit definitions? Can common language meanings be taken as the meaning intended? Would a common language approach lead to differing interpretations of the meanings of the concepts?

Another way to describe definitions is to characterize the extent to which the definitions are general or specific. It is possible for both explicit and implicit meanings to be either general or specific. Assess how general or specific definitions are. How clearly does the definition suggest an associated empiric experience? Is the definition specific about what a phenomenon is, or does it suggest what its use is? Does it provide possibilities for empiric indicators that represent the phenomenon?

For abstract concepts found in many nursing theories, specific definitions are difficult to formulate. Attempting to create specific meanings of abstract concepts prematurely may interfere with exploring a wide range of possibilities that lead to discovery. Definitions that specify general features can conjure very specific mental images of the actual experience. An early definition that is broad and nonspecific encourages the exploration of many possible meanings. General meanings are preferred in broad-scope theory or theory that is not likely to be empirically tested. Most definitions have both specific and general features. Examine how definitions are both specific and general.

Once definitions are identified, ask the following questions: Are similar definitions used for different concepts? Are differing definitions used for the same concept? Are some concepts defined differently than common convention? Are definitions expanded as the narrative proceeds? Is it difficult to judge whether definitions are provided at all? Can definitions fit other terms within or outside the structure of the theory?

What Are the Relationships in This Theory?

Relationships are the linkages among and between concepts. The nature of relationships in theory may take several forms. Often relationship statements that are uncovered may be peripheral to the core of the theory.

As concepts are identified, ideas about relationships between them begin to form. Suppose you uncover the following relationship statement: "The individual is composed of three dimensions and is an integral part of the environment." This statement suggests that the individual is related to an environment and that there are three interrelated subcomponents of the individual.

Once a tentative identification of relationships is made, ask the following questions: Are there concepts that stand alone, unrelated to others? Are there concepts interrelated with other concepts in several ways and others related in only one or two ways? Are there concepts to which several other concepts relate but that, in turn, are not related to other concepts?

The ways in which the relationships emerge provide clues to the theoretic purposes and the assumptions on which the theory is based. Some concepts may be linked to the theory by assumptions, which may explain why the concept seems to fit within the matrix of the theory but a theoretic relationship containing the concept is not explicitly stated. The theoretic purpose may be represented by linear relationships of several concepts that converge on one specific concept that, in turn, is not linked to any other concepts—that is, the linkages end with a specific concept. As linkages between concepts are identified, you can address the nature or character of relationships. If a relationship is unclear, ask yourself what relationships might be possible and their character; your ideas can provide clues for further development of the theory.

Examine the nature of the relationships. Are the relationships basically descriptive, or do they explain something about the phenomenon of interest? Do they create meaning without explaining? Do they impart understanding? Is there evidence that some relationships are predictive? Relationships within theory that create meaning and impart understanding often link multiple concepts in a loose structure. In other forms of description, concepts are interrelated without elaboration on how and why conceptual relationships are arranged. Concepts that are interrelated often explain how empiric events occur and may provide some detail about how and why concepts interrelate. Prediction implies if-then statements about the occurrence of empiric phenomena. When empirically based predictions of human behavior are shown to be valid, they usually are based on explanation.

The statement "Individuals are composed of three dimensions" is mainly descriptive. It implies that one concept, the individual, is composed of three parts called dimensions. If expanded to "The individual is composed of three dimensions that overlap and share common core areas," the statement becomes more explanatory. It proposes that each dimension has a shared area with another dimension and that there is an area shared by all three. When "interrelated whole" is added, the "how" of the relationship becomes even clearer because the dimensions must overlap to interrelate the parts of the individual.

Predictions are fairly easy to detect. Sentences that translate into if-then statements are predictive. It is not possible to make an if-then statement out of "The individual is composed of three dimensions," unless it is the following that is implied: "If not three dimensions, then not the individual." The statement "The individual is an interrelated whole composed of three dimensions that overlap and share common areas" implies that disturbances in one sphere would be reflected in other spheres. This prediction, however, is implied and not explicit.

Suppose the statement read, "Because the individual is an interrelated whole composed of three dimensions that overlap and share common areas, a disturbance in one dimension is reflected in disturbances in other dimensions." This statement is clearly predictive. The distinctions among *description, explanation,* and *prediction* are not always clear. Generally description means that the statement projects what something is or the features of its character. Explanation suggests how or why it is. Prediction projects circumstances that create or alter a phenomenon. Our use of the terms *descriptive, explanatory,* and *predictive* in describing the nature of theoretic relationships refers only to the form of the theory. For the purposes of describing a theory, research findings are not required to confirm the nature of relationship statements as descriptive, explanatory, or predictive.

What Is the Structure of This Theory?

The structure of theory gives overall form to the conceptual relationships within it. The structure emerges from the relationships of the theory.

Consider the following two concepts within a theory: individual and environment. In one theory, individuals are part of the environment; in another theory, individuals are separate from the environment. In both theories there is an identifiable relationship between individuals and environment, but the structure of the relationship differs.

Although your responses to questions concerning the relationships of theory usually suggest the form, in some cases they do not. Many theories do not contain a single discernible structure in which all concepts fit into a coherent, unified network. There may be several, perhaps competing, structures that cannot be reconciled. Determining the structure of theory will be difficult if the network of relationships is unclear or very complex. Figure 8-1 illustrates a sample of four structural forms and the ideas they suggest. Some theories may reflect one or more of these structures, whereas others will not. Sometimes individual concepts within theories may be structured in these forms. Structural forms are powerful devices for shaping our perceptions of reality. As you describe theory, do not expect that it will fit into one of these four structures. It may, but many more are possible. Conversely, in the process of theory development these are only examples of various structures that might evolve in the process of relationship structuring.

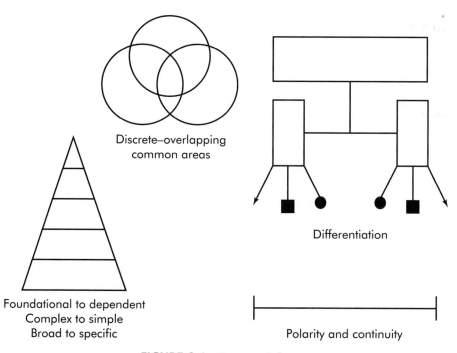

Discrete–overlapping
common areas

Differentiation

Foundational to dependent
Complex to simple
Broad to specific

Polarity and continuity

FIGURE 8-1 Structural forms.

Consider how you might structure the following relationship statement: "Individuals are composed of component parts." This statement only suggests a structure in which parts are perceptible, and any image on Figure 8-1 could easily represent it except the one that suggests polarity. Suppose each of these structures represents the broad theory of health. The triangular drawing suggests that health is composed of a series of related subconcepts that vary in breadth or simplicity. It also suggests foundational concepts on which other subconcepts are built. The base level might be genetic integrity, followed by organ-system health, and finally health of communities or societies. A theory that deals with how genetic health forms the basis for individual, collective, and societal health might be structured this way.

The overlapping circles depict discrete components that have common areas between and among them. Health might be viewed as having biophysiologic, psychoemotional, and sociocultural aspects. If a person is biologically well but psychoemotionally unwell, the diagram suggests that illness will affect biophysiologic wellness. Psychoemotional ill health could result in biophysiologic consequences. Basically the overlapping circles illustrate that health is composed of separate components, but there is sharing between any two components, as well as among all three. The structure, as illustrated, suggests an equality in importance, overlap, and sharing among the three subunits.

Applying this idea to the horizontal line drawing on the figure shows health represented as a continuum—in a linear relationship with illness. When health is placed on a continuum with illness on the opposite end, health and illness are conceptualized as a continuous variable, and degrees of health and illness are possible. The extremes of a continuum also suggest that health is the absence of illness and illness is the absence of health. If health is viewed as a concept that is continuous with illness, health and illness can be represented by a continuum. If health and illness are considered as not continuous concepts, they do not fit this structural form.

The fourth structural form conveys the idea of differentiation, dividing major concepts into subconcepts. For this structural form, health might be differentiated into its mental and physical aspects. Physical health could be further divided into bodily or anatomic health and functional or physiologic health, with some comparable division such as emotional and spiritual for mental health. Differentiation can proceed indefinitely. Some concepts lend themselves to differentiation more easily than others. *Needs* is a concept that can be easily differentiated, whereas the concept of *wholism* cannot.

Conceptually unrelated or distinctly different concepts cannot be structured as a continuum. A relationship between gender and society could not be represented on a continuum. Gender and society could be structured as overlapping circles, as two conceptual entities that influence one another, or in a structure in which society shapes gender. As you study the examples of structure, note how different concepts fit some structures more easily than others and how some concepts such as *wholistic health* cannot be represented well by any of them. In fact, none of these structures for representing health may make sense for you because the structures are inconsistent with your personal ideas about the nature of health.

As relationships are explored, the overall theoretic structure and the structures of individual components begin to emerge. To address questions of structure, begin by asking the following questions: What are the most central relationships? What are the direction, strength, and quality of relationships? Can I draw a model that shows the structure of the theory? What is the order of appearance of relationships within the narrative? Do relationships appear to move toward or away from the theoretic purpose? Do relationships coalesce concepts or differentiate them? Does the theorist diagram the structure?

Once the structure of the major or central relationships is identified, other aspects of structure can be described. How are other structures united with central or core relationships? Can all relationships be structured? Do the structures take multiple forms? Are competing or partial structures suggested? Does the theorist provide diagrams that illustrate aspects of structure?

After you have linked together concepts and purposes in relationships, describe the entire structural form. Notice how the relationships move as the theory unfolds. A theory that defies structuring can sometimes be approached by simply outlining the order in which concepts are presented. Outlining can provide insight about how ideas are organized. Some recognizable structure is essential to theory because structure flows from relationships.

What Are the Assumptions in This Theory?

Assumptions are those basic givens or accepted truths that are fundamental to theoretic reasoning. To uncover assumptions, a central question is: "What is the author taking as an accepted truth?" This question can be asked once the purposes are determined, the concepts are structured by relational statements, and the definitions are described.

Sometimes the theorist states assumptions explicitly. If so, ask the following: "What are they?" and "What do they assume?" Statements explicitly labeled as assumptions may not be the same as the assumptions that are basic to the theory. The extent to which explicitly labeled assumptions are assumptions and not something else must be examined. It often is difficult to separate assumptions that are implicit or integrated into the narrative of the theory from relationship statements, but they can be identified. As with explicit assumptions, ask the following: "What are the implicit givens?" and "What do they assume?"

Explore your ideas about the assumptions of the theory further. What individual, environmental, nursing, and health-related assumptions are made? Are assumptions competing or compatible? Are there several assumptions about one phenomenon and few about another? Are assumptions made at the outset, between and within relationships, or in relation to the purposes of the theory?

Assumptions may take the form of factual assertions, or they may reflect value positions. Factual assumptions are those knowable or potentially knowable through perceptual experience. Value assumptions assert or imply what is right, good, or ought to be. Often an empirically knowable assumption, such as "It is assumed for the purposes of this theory that people want information," contains important underlying value assumptions. The assumption that people want information (which could be empirically verified) may further imply that information is good, which cannot be verified empirically. The value assumption that it is good to have information leads to further questions about what sort of information is good. It is important to examine factual assumptions by asking the following: "What value does this factual assumption reflect?" It also is important to examine all other components of theory. What does this concept, definition, relationship, structure, or purpose assume?

Once you discern assumptions, the values held by the theorist can be explored. What does the theorist assume to be valuable, good, right, wrong, or worthwhile? Are there value-laden terms and phrases in the definitions of concepts and in the supporting narrative of the theory? Who is assumed to be responsible for the experiences or circumstances of the theoretic reality? Who benefits from the circumstances or experiences of this theory? These questions often give clues to values that form fundamental assumptions. For example, the Freudian theoretic notion of *penis envy* implies that penises are body parts that are so valued as to be enviable and that a person who does not have a penis will experience this value-laden emotion. A useful approach to uncovering hidden values is to imagine possibilities other than that presented in the theory. If these alternative possibilities are plausible but unconventional, you have uncovered important value assumptions. Imagining the idea of *womb envy,* which is not a part of Freudian thinking but is a plausible alternative possibility, indicates that you have uncovered an important androcentric assumption from which the theory builds.

The descriptive component of assumptions often is based on ideas taken so much for granted that they are difficult to recognize. An example of such an obvious assumption is that empiric knowledge is dependent on perceptual experience. This assumption is fundamental to empirics, but it is not an assumption of other patterns of knowing.

Sometimes it is not possible to personally agree with and accept a theory because it is unusual or unfamiliar. Uneasiness or discomfort with a theory sometimes is a clue to assumptions that are unlike your own beliefs or values. Once assumptions are recognized, the theory containing them can be understood on its own terms.

Forming a Complete Description

In summary, the six questions we propose for describing theory are as follows:

1. *What is the purpose of this theory?* This question addresses why the theory was formulated and reflects the contexts and situations to which the theory can be applied.
2. *What are the concepts of this theory?* This question identifies the ideas that are structured and related within the theory. It questions the qualitative and quantitative dimensions of concepts.
3. *How are the concepts defined?* This question clarifies the meaning for concepts within the theory. It questions what empiric experience is represented by the ideas within the theory.
4. *What is the nature of relationships?* This question addresses how concepts are linked together. It focuses on the various forms relationship statements can take and how they give structure to the theory.
5. *What is the structure of the theory?* This question addresses the overall form of the conceptual interrelationships. It discerns whether the theory contains partial structures or has one basic form.
6. *On what assumptions does the theory build?* This question addresses the basic truths taken to underlie theoretic reasoning. It questions whether assumptions reflect philosophic values or factual assertions.

A general approach to describing theory is to read the work and then begin to consider the descriptive questions. All questions are not necessarily answerable for a single theory. However, as you answer the questions that apply to the theory under consideration, concepts will be tentatively identified and the purpose of the theory will emerge. As definitions become evident, you will begin to see relationships. From the nature of the relationships, you will be able to address questions concerning the structure of the theory. Responses to questions concerning assumptions provide a level of awareness of meanings and will help you form an understanding of the theory. After an initial description of components, each component can be re-examined and revised.

For any theory, it often is not easy to describe theoretic purpose and assumptions. Concepts and their definitions may be more readily identifiable, especially if they are fairly explicit. Discerning relationships and structure often is a problematic area in describing theory, but these traits, too, will be present in theory.

Forming a complete description of theory requires systematic and critical examination of the work. When approached seriously, every word, phrase, and sentence must be examined and reexamined for meaning. Ideas that emerge in response to the descriptive questions often lead to uncertainty and revisions of earlier ideas. After a time, the description does begin to take shape, and fewer changes occur. There always will be some tentativeness in your descriptions because your description requires your own interpretive insights with respect to the theorist's ideas, and these insights change. If you are not able to reach a tentative resolution with respect to the fundamental nature of a theory after reasonable study and thought, the best course of action is to propose your ideas for revision and further development of the theory. Your continuing uncertainty indicates that further theoretic development must occur. Box 8-1 summarizes the questions that form a complete guide to the description of theory.

HOW DOES IT WORK? THE CRITICAL REFLECTION OF THEORY

Once theory is described, critical questions can be addressed to develop information about how well developed a theory is or how adequate it is in relation to its purposes. Note that describing and critically reflecting theory are fundamentally different processes. Description can be compared with a more objective process of setting forth facts about the theory by asking the following: "What is this?" Critical reflection, by contrast, involves ascertaining how well a theory serves some purpose. In the section that follows, we identify questions that can be used in critical reflection. As you question the worth of the theory, you will form insights that will help you know how theory might be used and how it might be further developed.

As you study and read different nursing theories, you may think, "This does not seem right," "Maybe I could change my practice along this line," or "This is really exciting." When these types of thoughts occur, you are comparing the theory with some personal and perhaps unrecognized ideas about

---

Box 8-1
Guide for the Description of Theory

1. PURPOSE

- Why was this theory formulated?
- Is there an overall purpose for the theory? A hierarchy of purposes? Separate numerous purposes?
- Is there a purpose for the nurse? The person receiving care? Society? Environment?
- How broad or narrow is the purpose?
- What is the value orientation of the purpose? Positive, negative, neutral?
- Does achieving the theoretic purpose require a nursing context?
- Does (do) the purpose(s) reflect understanding? Creation of meaning? Description, explanation, and prediction of phenomena?
- When would the theory cease to be applicable? What is the end point?
- What purpose not explicitly embedded in the matrix of the theory can be identified?

2. CONCEPTS

- Is there one major concept with subconcepts organized under it?
- How many concepts are there?
- How many major ones?
- How many minor ones?
- Can the concepts be ordered, related? Arranged into any configuration?
- Are there concepts that cannot be interrelated?
- Are concepts broad in scope? Narrow?
- How abstract or empiric are the concepts?
- What is the balance between highly abstract and highly empiric concepts?
- Do concepts represent objects, properties, events? Can you say? Are there concepts that are closely related?

3. DEFINITIONS

- Which concepts are defined? Which are not?
- Which concepts are defined explicitly? Which are implied?
- How much meaning needs to be inferred?
- Which concepts are defined specifically? Generally?
- Are there competing definitions for some concepts? Are there similar definitions for different concepts?
- Do any explicitly defined concepts not need definition?
- Are any concepts defined contrary to common convention?

4. RELATIONSHIPS

- What are the major relationships within the theory?
- Which relationships are obvious? Which are implied?
- Do relationships include all concepts? Which are not included?
- Are some concepts included in multiple relationships?

Continued

Box 8-1

Guide for the Description of Theory—cont'd

4. RELATIONSHIPS—cont'd

- Is there a hierarchy of relationships? Do relationships create meaning and understanding? Do they do this by describing, explaining? Predicting? What mix of each?
- Are relationships directional? What is their direction? Are they neutral?
- Are there mixed, competing, or incongruous relationships?
- Are relationships illustrated?

5. STRUCTURE

- How are overall and individual ideas organized?
- If outlined, what would the theory look like?
- Do relationships expand concepts into larger wholes or vice versa? Do they link concepts in a linear fashion?
- Does the structure move concepts away from or toward the purposes?
- Are there several structures that emerge? What is their form? Do they fit together?
- Could more than one structure represent the overall structural relationships?
- Where is there no structure?

6. ASSUMPTIONS

- What assumptions underlie the theory? Are assumptions explicit, implicit, or derivable from context and meanings?
- What are the individual, nurse, society, environment, and health assumed to be like?
- Do assumptions have an obvious value orientation? What is it?
- Could assumptions be factually verified?
- Where are assumptions located within the structure—before, within, or after theoretic reasoning?
- Can assumptions be hierarchically arranged or otherwise ordered?
- Do assumptions have any identifiable relationship to theoretic relationships or structure?
- Are there competing assumptions?

---

what is important for theory. Each person's ideas of the adequacy of a theory are influenced by a personal perspective of what is valuable or good. For research, you might agree, "This could be helpful." For practice, you might think, "Maybe I could use this." For idea stimulation, you might think, "This really gives me some exciting new ideas." In these instances, you have formed an impression of the value of the theory from your personal values about practice, research, and critical thinking. Your values are important components that are integrated into a more formal critical reflection process.

Critical reflection contributes to understanding how well the theory relates to practice, research, or educational activities. Members of a discipline form ideas about what questions to ask and what responses generally are accepted if a theory is to be seen as valuable for the discipline. Just as there are many ways to describe theory, there are many critical questions that can be asked about the functional value of theory and many responses to these questions. Once the questions are asked, members of a discipline can consider what responses they tend to value and why. The questions we pose are consistent with generally accepted methods for evaluating theories that have been described in the nursing literature (Barnum, 1998; Ellis, 1968; Fawcett, 2004; Hardy, 1974; Tomey & Alligood, 2006). However, our approach differs from accepted methods in that normative criteria are not implied.

The questions for critical reflection are as follows:

- How clear is this theory?
- How simple is this theory?
- How general is this theory?
- How accessible is this theory?
- How important is this theory?

Because these are not normative criteria, there are no correct answers to these questions, and the questions do not imply the responses. For example, "How clear is this?" does not necessarily mean that a theory should be perfectly clear or "the clearer, the better." Rather, when you address this question you are using it as a tool to examine whether the level of clarity of the theory is adequate for the theory's purpose. As you engage in discussions that are centered around the questions, you can form a consensus with your colleagues as to where to go next with the theory. These insights can best be formed in discussion among people with diverse perspectives. For example, even though a theory that challenges assumptions about practice is somewhat unclear, it may be an important theory for changing nursing practice and for providing new concepts with which to work. The fact that it is not perfectly clear leaves room for imagining new possibilities, which may be part of the theory's strength.

Although each of the five critical reflection questions is fundamentally different, the questions are interrelated. For example, one question addresses accessibility, and another addresses generality. If a theory is seen as general or broad in scope, it may be less accessible (less related to perceptual experience) than a narrower (less general) theory.

Responses to the questions used in creating a description affect your responses to the critical reflection questions. For example, to decide how clear, accessible, or general a theory is, you need to describe the purpose of the theory, what concepts are included, and how those concepts are structured. As your description of the theory is formed, you can begin the process of critical reflection. The ideas you develop from this process contribute to your own critical insights and to substantive discussion that gives direction for further theory development. The issues to consider as you address each of the questions for critically reflecting theory are described in the following sections.

How Clear Is This Theory?

In determining how clear a theory is, you will be considering semantic clarity, semantic consistency, structural clarity, and structural consistency. Clarity, in general, refers to how well the theory can be understood and how consistently the ideas are conceptualized. Semantic clarity and consistency primarily refer to understanding the intended theoretic meaning of the concepts. Structural clarity and consistency reflect understanding the intended connections between concepts within the theory and the whole of the theory.

Semantic Clarity. The definitions of concepts in the theory are an important aspect of semantic clarity. Definitions help to establish empiric meaning for concepts within the theory. If concepts are not defined or are incompletely defined, the empiric indicators for the idea become less clear. When concepts are clearly defined, empiric indicators can be more easily identified. Clarity implies, in part, that when different nurses read the theory, a similar empiric reality comes to mind when the word for the concept is used. If there are no definitions or if only a few of the concepts are defined, clarity is limited.

The types of definitions that are used within theory affect semantic clarity. Definitions that reflect both specific and general traits enhance clarity, whereas a general or a specific definition alone often limits clarity. Specific definitions usually lend clarity because they provide clear and accurate guidance for the intended empiric indicators for a concept. General definitions contribute a contextual sense of meaning for concepts and lend a richness of meaning that is not possible with specific definitions. Considering the extent to which each type of definition contributes to clarity of meaning can help you form your own ideas about the adequacy of the theory for your purpose.

Clarity may be obscured by borrowing terms from other disciplines or by using common-language terms that carry broad general meanings. Words such as "stress" and "coping" have general common-language meanings, and they also have specific theoretic meanings in other disciplines. If words with multiple meanings are used in theory and not defined, a person's everyday meaning of the term, rather than what is meant in the theory, often is assumed; therefore, clarity is lost. Clarity is enhanced when the concept's definition is consistent with common meanings of the term within the profession.

Clarity is affected when words that have no common meaning are used or when the theorist invents or coins words to represent some idea. Coined words can help to convey a meaning for which there is no word, but they also can detract from clarity, especially when a more familiar word or phrase would suffice. It would be possible to generate an entire theory about quizzendroids, plankerods, and ziots. The theory could be logical and consistent but unclear because the words are invented and have no meaning. Although this example is exaggerated, it demonstrates the effects on clarity when vague or strange words are used, when words are not defined, or when words with many possible meanings are used and not defined.

Semantic clarity also can be affected by excessive verbiage. Normally, varying words to represent similar meanings is a writing skill that can be used to avoid overuse of a single term. But, in theory, if several similar concepts are used interchangeably when one would suffice, there is excess verbiage, and the clarity of the theory's presentation is reduced rather than improved. In theory, varying the word for an important concept interjects subtly different meanings. For example, interchanging the words "restoration," "rehabilitation," and "recovery" for the same concept changes clarity because each word has a slightly different meaning and suggests different contexts of use.

Clarity also is affected when excessive narrative is included. Semantic clarity may be decreased by excessive examples; however, the judicious use of examples usually aids clarity. Diagrams can enhance or obscure clarity. To enhance clarity, diagrams should be self-explanatory and simple in expression because overly complex illustrations discourage comprehension. In general, the alternative mode of providing information in the form of diagrams helps to make the ideas in the theory clearer.

Economy of words, key definitions, and wise use of examples and diagrams lend clarity. Absolute semantic clarity can never be achieved, nor is it necessarily desirable. Because of the limitations of language, no matter how clearly the theorist represents theoretic meaning, it will not be perceived uniformly by all readers.

Semantic Consistency. Semantic consistency is a second feature to consider with respect to the question of clarity. A theory that implicitly or explicitly defines concepts inconsistently gives competing messages around meaning. Semantic consistency means that the concepts of the theory are used in ways that are consistent with their definition. Sometimes a definition is explicitly stated, and somewhere within the theory another meaning is implied. When key words are not explicitly defined, their implied meanings may be inconsistent from one usage to the next. Occasionally, words are explicitly defined but in different ways. Inconsistencies that occur when terms are defined explicitly are fairly easy to uncover, but other types of inconsistencies may be more covert.

The consistent use of basic assumptions is also important in achieving consistency. The theory's purpose, definitions of concepts, and relationships need to be consistent with the stated assumptions of the theory. Examples and diagrams also can be considered in light of the assumptions of the theory. Suppose, for example, a basic theoretic assumption is the unity of persons and environment and that both change simultaneously and irreversibly through time and space. This assumption is consistent with a definition of health as expanding consciousness but inconsistent with a theoretic conceptualization of health as a state of adaptation. Adaptation typically implies conforming or adjusting to environmental stimuli to fit within the environment. The concept of *adaptation* tends to suggest the assumption that events external to the person are primary as a determinant of health and that the person and the environment are separate entities. Unity of person and environment is a concept that can be used to convey an assumption that humans and environment are interconnected and change simultaneously. Simultaneous change negates the idea of conforming or adjusting to stimuli as health; rather, it implies incorporating change, becoming a different person, and increasing options and awareness of choice.

For clarity, the purposes of the theory must be consistent with all other components. A purpose of health, achieved by deliberate nursing actions, may be at odds with the basic assumption that health is deterministic. As you become aware of inconsistencies, you will uncover other meanings that are conveyed in the definitions and other components of the theory.

In reflecting on consistency, examine your descriptions for each component of theory and consider where there are consistencies and inconsistencies within the descriptive elements of the theory, as well as between them. Definitions must be examined for consistency with one another and in relation to assumptions. Structure is sometimes inconsistent with relationships. If a theory is extremely inconsistent, it is difficult to continue the process of critical reflection concerning the theory. Some semantic inconsistencies within theory are more common early in their development and leave room for new possibilities for further development. However, inconsistencies at the basic roots of theory, such as between assumptions and goals, have implications that will affect the entire theory and must be addressed.

Structural Clarity. Structural clarity is closely linked to semantic clarity. Structural clarity refers to how identifiable and apparent the connections and reasoning within theory are. The descriptive elements of structure and relationships provide important information for addressing this dimension of clarity.

In a theory with structural clarity, you can readily identify and recognize the underlying conceptual network. With structural clarity, concepts are interconnected and organized into a coherent whole. If you cannot discern the structure of the theory, you begin to search for those structural elements that are related and for gaps that occur in the flow of the theory. If all major relationships are included within a single structure, clarity is enhanced. Clarity is lost when significant relationships are not contained within a coherent structure. Pieces of relationships, rudiments of structure, or concepts that stand alone are evidence that parts have not yet been integrated into the whole during the development of the theory.

Structural Consistency. Structural consistency refers to the consistent use of structural form within theory. Often theory, especially more middle-range theory, is built around one predominant structural form, such as forms that differentiate concepts, structure concepts linearly, or structure concepts in a hierarchy. Sometimes one structural form provides an overall, general profile for major relationships within theory, and more minor components of the theory take a different structural form. Whatever the structure or structures used to link together concepts and relationships, their consistent use throughout the theory serves as a structural map that enhances clarity. A theorist may begin with a structural movement that is linear. If this structure is reflected in the linkages among elements in the theory, you will observe a high level of structural consistency. A shift in reasoning to a structure that integrates concepts, such as the Venn diagram of overlapping circles, may be confusing, or the structure might function well within a structural scheme that is linear in nature.

In summary, "How clear is this theory?" can be asked to explore in what ways a theory is clear and comprehensible, how it is not, and what its level of clarity means for the development and use of the theory. The ideas of semantic and structural consistency and clarity can be used to guide discussion of issues of clarity because inconsistencies provide double messages that confound clarity. A very general (broad-scope) theory may be quite ambiguous but useful in stimulating new ideas. A middle-range theory of hopelessness, for example, may have aspects that are vague but still be important in helping nurses understand the experience. However, the ambiguity of that same theory may affect its usefulness for guiding research. Becoming aware of the ways in which clarity is obscured in light of your purpose makes it possible to design ways to further develop the theory's clarity. The degree to which a theory must be clear depends on how the nurse intends to use it.

How Simple Is This Theory?

Simplicity means that the number of elements within each descriptive category, particularly concepts and their interrelationships, are minimal. Complexity implies many theoretic relationships between and among numerous concepts. The following example illustrates theoretic simplicity. Suppose that a theory contained the following three major concepts: A, B, and C. A theory interrelating these as discrete concepts would be quite simple because only three interrelationships would be possible: A and B, A and C, and B and C. Adding subconcepts 1 and 2 to A, B, and C (for example, A1, A2) would leave the theorist with three major concepts (A, B, and C) and six subconcepts, for a total of nine concepts. A theorist working with nine concepts has significantly greater theoretic complexity than a theorist working with only three concepts. Adding even one or two concepts to a theory greatly increases the potential for theoretic interrelationships and, subsequently, complexity.

The desirability of simplicity or complexity can vary with the stage of theory development. In grounded theory or phenomenological descriptions for example, there may be considerable complexity as the theory begins to emerge, but, as it develops, relationships and concepts are coalesced, and the theory becomes more simple. Regardless of the approach to theory development, some concepts created early in the process eventually may be deleted or changed. In the previous example, suppose concepts A, A1, and A2 came to be seen as unimportant in relation to the theory's purpose. The theoretic complexity added by A and its subconcepts could be removed, and only the simpler relationships between B and C and their subconcepts would remain.

Theories reflect varying degrees of simplicity. In nursing, some situations suggest the need for relatively simple and broad theory that can be used as a general guide for practice. Other situations suggest simple but more empirically accessible theory to guide research. Still other situations suggest the need for theory that is relatively complex because of the value such theory has for enhancing understanding of extremely complex practice situations.

How General Is This Theory?

The generality of a theory refers to its breadth of scope and purpose; a general theory can be applied to a broad array of situations. *Parsimony* sometimes is used as a synonym to describe the trait of theoretic simplicity, but the concept of parsimony also includes the idea of generality. A parsimonious theory is conceptually simple (contains few structural elements) but accounts for a broad range of empiric experiences.

The scope of concepts and purposes within the theory provides clues to its generality. A theory containing broad concepts will encompass more empirical indicators than one containing very narrow concepts. Concepts of *humans* and *universe* could be interpreted as organizing almost every empirical indicator possible. A comprehensive theory with these two concepts would be highly general. A theory interrelating the individual and the physical environment is less general, although still fairly broad in scope. The concept of *individual* implies that the theory is concerned with a single person. The use of *physical* as a modifier for *environment* conveys the notion of environment in part only. Information about individuals in communities could not be understood within this theory. A theory relating characteristics of acutely ill people in the intensive care unit environment is even less general, and the scope of concepts narrows.

Questions that address the generality of theory include the following: To whom (or what) does this theory apply, and when does it apply? Does the purpose pertain to all health care professionals? To people in general? Does the purpose apply to specific specialties of nursing and only at given times? The more limited the scope of application of the theory, the less general the theory.

Whether generality is viewed as desirable depends on your purpose for the theory. General theory is quite useful for generating ideas or hypotheses. Nursing theories that address broad concepts, such as *individuals, society, health*, and *environment*, have a high degree of generality and are useful for organizing ideas about universal health behaviors. Theories that address a specific human experience such as *pain* are less general and, because of their relative specificity, are useful for guiding practice in a clinical setting.

How Accessible Is This Theory?

Accessibility addresses the extent to which empiric indicators for the concepts can be identified and to what extent the purposes of theory can be attained. If a theory is to be used for explaining some aspect of practice, its theoretic concepts must be linked to empiric indicators available in practice. Empiric indicators are perceptually accessible experiences that can be used in practice to assess the phenomena that the theory describes and that can be used to determine whether the purposes of the theory are realized in a way that the theory suggests.

Only selected dimensions of highly abstract concepts may be empirically accessible. If the concepts of a theory do not reflect empiric dimensions or if the empiric dimensions are very obscure, they may be ideas that cannot be explored or understood empirically.

Consider the example of a theory about rehabilitation and interaction. The theoretic definitions of the concepts are clues to the accessibility of the theory. Without definition, the words "rehabilitation" and "interaction" can assume many dimensions of meaning. If the concepts are defined, how they are to be empirically accessed is clearer. If the definitions point to the measurements or observable behaviors that can be associated with rehabilitation and the specific kinds of interactions that promote rehabilitation, then the theory can be judged to be relatively accessible in a clinical context.

Increasing the complexity within theories often increases empiric accessibility. As subconceptual categories are clarified, empiric indicators become more precise. Suppose that the concepts of *rehabilitation* and *interaction* are related within the same theory. The theory is judged to have a high degree of generality and simplicity because the concepts are broad and few in number. Complexity would be increased by designating five subconcepts for each. Those five subconcepts are likely to have more precise empiric bases than are the broader concepts. With empirically accessible subconcepts, the empiric accessibility of the theory increases. If a concept does not have an empiric basis at the outset, specifying subconcepts for larger wholes does not increase empiric accessibility.

Research testing requires the empiric accessibility of concepts. It also confirms which concepts are clinically relevant and accessible. For example, if *rehabilitation* is defined in a research project as "able to complete activities of daily living independently," you have established a clear link between the idea—rehabilitation—and a reasonable clinical observation. If the research supports the hypothesis derived from the theory, it also provides evidence of empiric accessibility for the concept of rehabilitation.

Empiric accessibility of concepts contained within theory is basic to validating theoretic relationships and using the theory in practice. Although grounded approaches to generating theory assume empiric accessibility, the extent to which empiric accessibility is important can vary. Considering the theory's purpose will help you make judgments about how empirically accessible a theory should be. Theory that provides a conceptual perspective of clinical practice may not need much empiric accessibility. If a theory is to be used to guide research, empiric accessibility is important. If a theory is to be used to shape nursing practice, concepts need to be empirically accessible in the clinical area. If concepts are not empirically grounded, creating conceptual meaning may provide direction for empiric indicators needed for research.

How Important Is This Theory?

In nursing, the importance of a theory is closely tied to the idea of its clinical significance or practical value. An important theory is forward-looking, used in practice, education and research, and valuable for creating a desired future. The central question is, "Does the theory create understanding that is important to nursing?" Some nursing theories guide research and practice, some generate radically new ideas about health and caring, and some differentiate the focus of nursing from other service professions.

If a theory contains concepts, definitions, purposes, and assumptions that are grounded in practice, it will have practical value for enhancing theory-based research that can become research evidence that is integrated into evidence-based clinical decisions. A theory that has limited empiric accessibility may not have practical value for research but can stimulate ideas and spark political action that improves practice.

One approach to addressing the question of importance is to reflect on the theory's basic theoretic assumptions. If underlying assumptions are unsound, the importance of the theory is minimal. If, for example, a theory is based on a view of the individual as parts, its importance for wholistic nursing is minimal. If a theory is based on an assumption of wholism and it moves understanding of wholism to a new dimension, it likely is to be highly important to nursing.

Theories that have extremely broad purposes may be essentially unattainable and therefore have limited value for creating clinical outcomes. This same theory may be important for generating ideas and challenging practice.

The importance of theory depends on the professional and personal values of the person who is addressing the question. Asking the questions "Do I like this theory?" and "Why?" will help you identify the values you hold for yourself, your practice, the profession, and the theory. Contributing your ideas about what is important for nursing through careful deliberation and discussion among nurse colleagues will help clarify the direction for a theory to achieve important professional purposes.

Forming a Complete Critical Reflection

The summary of critical reflection questions presented in Box 8-2 provides a guide for forming a critical reflection of theory.

Box 8-2

Guide for the Critical Reflection of Theory

HOW CLEAR IS THIS THEORY?

Semantic Clarity

- Are major concepts defined? Are definitions explicit? Implicit? Inferable?
- Are significant concepts not defined? Are definitions clear?
- How general are definitions? How specific?
- Are words coined? Are coined words defined?
- Is the amount of explanation appropriate and useful? Too much? Not enough?
- Are examples meaningful and helpful? Needed and not present?

Semantic Consistency

- Are definitions consistent with one another?
- Are the same terms defined differently?
- Are different terms defined similarly?
- Are implied or inferred meanings different from explicit meanings?
- Is the view of person and environment compatible?
- Are words borrowed from other disciplines and used differently in this context?
- Are assumptions and purposes compatible with other elements in the theory?
- Are competing assumptions or purposes present?
- Are examples consistent with one another?

Structural Clarity

- Do all relationships fit within the structure of the theory?
- Can the order of the theory be comprehended?
- Can an overall structure be diagrammed?
- Where, if any, are gaps in the flow? Do all concepts fit within the theory?

Structural Consistency

- Do diagrams and visual structures provide support, or compete with one another?
- Is there one structural form or several? If more than one form, do they complement, or compete with, one another?
- Are examples consistent with one another?
- Are basic assumptions consistent with one another? With purposes?
- Are compatible and coherent structures suggested for different parts of the theory?
- Are there any ambiguities as a result of sequence of presentation?

HOW SIMPLE IS THIS THEORY?

- How many relationships are contained within the theory?
- How are the relationships organized?
- How many concepts are contained in the theory?
- Are some concepts differentiated into subconcepts and others not?

Box 8-2
Guide for the Critical Reflection of Theory—cont'd

- Can concepts be combined without losing theoretic meaning?
- Is the theory complex in some areas and not in others?
- Does the theory tend to describe, explain, or predict? Impart understanding? Create meaning?

HOW GENERAL IS THIS THEORY?

- How specific are the purposes of this theory? Do they apply to all or only some practice areas? When?
- Is this theory specific to nursing? If not, who else could use it? Why?
- Is the purpose justifiably a nursing purpose?
- If subpurposes exist, do they reflect nursing actions? How broad are the concepts within the theory?

HOW ACCESSIBLE IS THIS THEORY?

- Are the concepts broad or narrow?
- How specific or general are definitions within the theory?
- Are the concepts' empiric indicators identifiable in experience? Are they within the realm of nursing?
- Do the definitions provided for the concepts adequately reflect their meanings?
- Is a very narrow definition offered for a broad concept? A broad meaning for a narrow concept?
- If words are coined, are they defined?

HOW IMPORTANT IS THIS THEORY?

- Does the theory have potential to influence nursing actions? If so, to what end? Is that end desirable?
- Is the theory used? Does the theory guide nursing education? Nursing research? Nursing practice? All three? If so, to what end? Is that end desirable?
- How specific are the purposes of the theory? Do they provide a general framework within which to act or a means to predict phenomena?
- Is the theory's position about people, about nursing, and about the environment consistent with nursing's philosophy?
- Given the purpose of the theory and its orientation, what significant factors for nursing or health care have been omitted?
- Is the stated or implied purpose one that is important to nursing? Why?
- Will use of the theory help or hinder nursing in any way? If so, how?
- Will application of this theory resolve any important issues in nursing? Will it resolve any problems?
- Is the theory futuristic and forward-looking?
- Will research based on the theory answer important questions?
- Are the concepts within the domain of nursing?
- Do I like this theory? Why?

In summary, the five questions for critically reflecting a description of theory are as follows:

1. *Is this clear?* This question addresses the clarity and consistency of presentation. Clarity and consistency may be both semantic and structural.
2. *Is this simple?* This question addresses the number of structural components and relationships within theory. Complexity implies numerous relational components within theory; simplicity implies fewer relational components.
3. *Is this general?* This question addresses the scope of experiences covered by theory. Generality infers a wide scope of phenomena, whereas specificity narrows the range of events included in theory. Generality combined with simplicity yields parsimony.
4. *Is this accessible?* This question addresses the extent to which concepts within the theory are grounded in empirically identifiable phenomena.
5. *Is this important?* This question addresses the extent to which a theory leads to valued nursing goals in practice, research, and education.

REFLECTION AND DISCUSSION

This chapter discusses processes for describing and critically reflecting theory. Questions that objectively describe theory are followed by questions useful to evaluate theory's utility for a specific purpose. A central message of this chapter is that the processes of description and reflection are critically important if theory is to be utilized in a practical way in practice and research. Description and critical reflection of theory are also necessary for efficiently extending existing theory.

To deepen your appreciation of description and critical reflection, consider the following related to the content of this chapter:

1. Create several structural forms for the concept of your choice. What do each suggest about the concept?
2. Name a concept of interest to nursing that defies structuring and think about why it is so difficult to structure.
3. Identify a theory that you find likable or workable. What is it about the theory that you like? Which particular component(s) of the theory have contributed to your feelings?

4. Conversely, name a theory you dislike or find not workable. What is it that you dislike? And which particular component(s) of the theory have contributed to your feelings?
5. If you were going to describe the features of theory that would be most useful for nursing, what would you say? What would the components of such a theory look like?
6. For a theory used in nursing that you find not workable, or really don't like, describe at least three things it would be important for in nursing.

Reference List

Abdellah, F. G., Beland, I., Martin, A., & Matheney, R. V. (1960). *Patient-centered approaches to nursing*. New York: Macmillan.

Barnum, B. J. S. (1998). *Nursing theory*, (5th ed.). Boston: Lippincott-Raven.

Ellis, R. (1968). Characteristics of significant theories. *Nursing Research, 17*(3), 217–222.

Fawcett, J. (2004). *Contemporary nursing knowledge: Analysis and evaluation of nursing models and theories*. Philadelphia: FA Davis.

Hall, L. E. (1966). Another view of nursing care and quality. In K. M. Straub & K. S. Parker (Eds.), *Continuity in patient care: The role of nursing*. Washington, DC: Catholic University Press.

Hardy, M. E. (1974). Theories: Components, development, evaluation. *Nursing Research, 23*(2), 100–107.

Koltoff, N. (1967). The use of the laboratory. *Nursing Research, 16*, 122.

Tomey, A. M., & Alligood, M. R. (2006). *Nursing theorists and their work*, (6th ed.). St. Louis: Mosby-Elsevier.

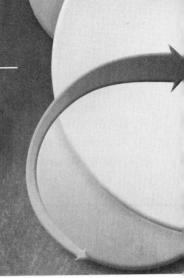

CHAPTER 9

Validating and Confirming Empiric Knowledge Using Research

Research extends knowledge through application of scientific methods—
not with absolute certainty—but with minimal misinformation.
Skepticism, alert self-criticism, constant testing of hypotheses by
empirical research and awareness of limitations of science make research
a most dependable source of information.

Laurie M. Gunter (1964, p. 231)

In this chapter we focus on research methods for validating and confirming empiric phenomena. Figure 9-1 shows the empiric quadrant of our model for nursing knowledge development, highlighting the role of validating and confirming theories and formal descriptions. These processes authenticate what is expressed in the formal knowledge of the discipline, which in turn strengthens scientific competence in practice. Validation and confirmation of theories and formal descriptions, as well as other forms of empiric knowledge, also draw on practice-based methods, which we present in Chapter 10. The research and practice-based methods, taken together, provide a strong foundation for nursing practice.

Development of empiric knowledge depends on systematic methods of inquiry. Research can be used as a means to test empiric knowledge and as a method to generate the concepts and relationships for empiric

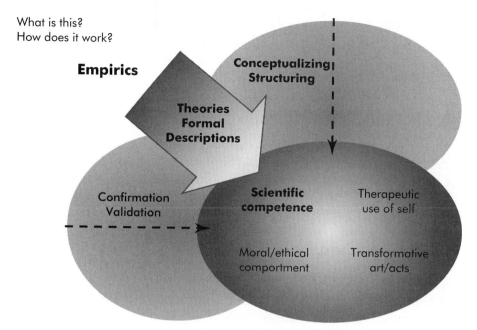

What is this?
How does it work?

Empirics

Conceptualizing
Structuring

Theories
Formal
Descriptions

Confirmation
Validation

Scientific
competence

Therapeutic
use of self

Moral/ethical
comportment

Transformative
art/acts

FIGURE 9-1 The empiric pattern of knowing: validation and confirmation of formal expressions of empiric knowledge to develop scientific competence.

knowledge structures that are being developed. Sound empiric knowledge development requires that the researcher make deliberate choices that link the underlying philosophy about science and nursing, research methods, theory, and practice.

Of all of the processes of empiric knowledge development, research-related activities are more visible to the casual observer than are the cognitively based theoretic processes. The concept of research often is associated with the image of a laboratory where experiments are conducted or some other activity occurs that involves discovering facts. Actually, creating empiric knowledge is more related to abstract theoretic processes than it is to uncovering isolated facts that can be reported in great detail and with numbers. Factual knowledge is useful, but facts alone are insufficient for developing useful empiric knowledge. To develop empiric knowledge that is valuable for practice, facts and observations must be interpreted, or made meaningful, in relation to one another. It is theory that helps locate facts and isolated observations into meaningful interrelationships.

In the next section we distinguish between theory-linked and isolated research. The remainder of the chapter reviews the processes required to refine concepts and theoretic relationships using empiric research methods, and we review approaches that will help ensure that any given research project fulfills sound standards of theoretic adequacy. Throughout the remainder of the chapter we use the term *theory*, consistent with our broad definition, to include a wide range of empirically grounded knowledge structures.

THEORY-LINKED RESEARCH AND ISOLATED RESEARCH

Research, like theorizing, can be conducted in a variety of ways and with many motivations. There are many types of research, and each research text presents a somewhat different way of viewing the total process. The traits that are common for each approach reflect certain basic standards that have been established to obtain results that are considered valid and confirmable, that is, accurately representative of empiric phenomena.

Any of the accepted research methods that are described in methods textbooks can be used with a theoretic link. The major trait that distinguishes theory-linked research from research that is not theory linked, which we call isolated research, is that theory-linked research is designed to develop, refine, or test theory. This quality sets the stage for research studies to contribute to the larger knowledge of the discipline. Isolated research, by contrast, is not linked to the processes of theory development.

From a research point of view, theory-linked and isolated research can both be of excellent quality. Both types of research ultimately can contribute to knowledge, although isolated research is much more limited in the contribution it can make to a discipline. Because theory-linked research is conceived and conducted to create, examine, or extend theory, the findings of research imply significance at an abstract level of understanding. The research findings not only are useful in relation to the research problem or question, but also are valuable in developing the theory or in speculating about other situations in which the theory might be tested or applied.

In isolated research, the research problem is not linked to theory in any deliberate way. Rather, the investigator formulates questions or hypotheses and uses accepted methods to refute or support the hypotheses or to answer the questions. When theory is used as a loose guide to spark ideas for research questions, we would consider the research to be isolated. For it to be theory-linked, the researcher must intend to extend, examine, develop, or validate theory, and deliberate linkages to the theory must occur in the process of research development. Questions or hypotheses may come from the practical circumstances surrounding the investigator's work, the imagination, an idea that occurred as the investigator read other research results, or any number of other sources. These same factors also can provide direction for the development of theory-linked research.

All research is confined to a particular place and time in history. Because theories are constructions of the mind, they can transcend, to a certain extent, the limitations of time and space. The cultural and historical circumstances of the theorist influence the mental construction of the theory, but because the theory is an abstraction, it is possible to move beyond the limits of particular circumstances. Isolated research that neither begins from nor ends with a relationship to theory often focuses on the particulars of a specific problem and offers little potential for speculating about the significance of the research beyond what can be justified by the method, design, and analysis of study results. The results of isolated research can provide new insights that prompt the researcher, or someone reading a report of the research, to speculate about larger implications of the research, which in turn can lead to developing theory that has broader meaning for the discipline.

Theory-linked research has advantages that overcome the limitations of the specific place and time in which the research occurs. Theory-linked research hypotheses that are developed from abstract statements of the theory represent a translation of the theory's statements to the circumstances of the specific study. Theory-generating research studies culminate with a linkage to theory by organizing study data into a more abstract theoretic structure. Theory-linked research findings can be generalized only within limits, just like those reported in isolated research. However, the study findings in theory-linked research can be retranslated to theoretic terms and implications discussed in relation to the theory.

Challenges Related to Theory-Linked Research

Although theory-linked research has definite advantages over isolated research in its ability to contribute to the development of knowledge, certain hazards and challenges are unique to this type of research.

Inappropriate Use of Theories. It is possible to use a theory inappropriately in conducting research. For example, if a theory is designed to explain animal behavior, it may not be appropriate as a basis for explaining or understanding human behavior, and vice versa, without sufficient conceptual examination. Theory and theoretic concepts that are used inappropriately lead to erroneous conclusions. Reed (1978), for example, described how some theories in behavioral sciences have resulted in erroneous information concerning primate behavior. Using theories of human behavior, researchers categorized primate sexual behavior as monogamous or polygamous, consistent with the normative expectations for human behavior. On the basis of limited observations of animal behavior, it became common practice to describe animal behavior by these terms. Reed pointed out that in reality, animals seldom cohabit on the basis of sex differences and that segregation of male and female primates is more pronounced than cohabitation. Theories sometimes provide a mental set that clouds observations or skews interpretations of meaning, especially if the theory is assumed to be true or consistent with prevailing values.

Theories as Barriers. Theories can obscure a researcher's ability to notice certain features of data or events. The mindset provided by theory, whether appropriate or not, may preclude recognition of other possibilities. When the focus is on expected outcomes, unless something startling or drastically different occurs, some elements may not be noticed. For example, you can view a child's behavior and because of a certain theory assume that what you observe is problem-solving ability. At the same time, you might fail to notice other things about the child's behavior that are not brought to your attention by the theory. These other behaviors might include less obvious and therefore easily overlooked actions such as body posture, facial expressions, or eye motion. It is possible that qualities of these behaviors relate to problem-solving ability, but the mental set that you acquire from the theory focuses your attention on limited behaviors, and something potentially important in understanding the child's experience is overlooked. If you are conducting a grounded-theory study with the purpose of uncovering the parental processes of attributing blame when teenaged children join gangs, your background knowledge of socialization patterns of adolescents will influence how you interpret and understand interview data.

Paradoxically, although a theory may be useful and appropriate for understanding phenomena, it may limit your thinking about the range of possibilities and experiences. Overcoming this difficulty requires you to constantly question what you read, think, and observe. Theory is not intended to represent phenomena and events exactly; it is intended to be an approximation and a tool to see possibilities. The purpose for using research to develop theory is to discover to what extent a theory can be regarded as sound and to what extent it functions to open new possibilities.

Ethical Considerations. Theories also can exceed acceptable limits of reality; theories as mental constructions may relate ideas that cannot or should not be tested, out of respect for human and animal rights and dignity. For example, given the threat of nuclear accidents, you might imagine that it would be useful to predict events in a large population of people who could experience a significant exposure to radiation. This knowledge might help in preparing for this circumstance. In reality, however, it is not ethical to subject humans or animals to such an experience to develop theory. It also is not feasible to test imagined theoretic ideas that claim to predict the consequences of exposure to radiation. Ethical considerations also may be much subtler and need to be examined. For example, certain approaches to the study of cultures outside the mainstream (for example, persons who are hearing impaired, ethnic minority groups, gay or lesbian cultures) undermine those cultures and provide avenues for further discrimination. Also, ethical considerations may curtail a study when interim findings suggest that its continuation is likely to harm participants.

Occasionally, historical circumstances provide evidence that is used to develop useful theory, but further development is limited by concern for human and animal welfare. Theories of mother–infant attachment and separation grew out of the experiences of wartime children separated from their mothers for extended periods. Subsequent to the destruction of the World Trade Center on 9/11, the effects of exposure to toxins in the rubble on rescue personnel are being studied. The evidence that grows out of historical disasters can demonstrate their harmful effects, but research that replicates similar circumstances is ethically indefensible.

REFINING CONCEPTS AND THEORETIC RELATIONSHIPS

A particular type of theory-linked research is research designed specifically to refine concepts and theoretic relationships. These types of investigations are crucial early in the stages of a theory's development but can be used at any point of theoretic development. Refining concepts and theoretic relationships involves a focus on the correspondence of the ideas of the theory with perceptible sensory experience (Dubin, 1978; Glaser & Strauss, 1967; Newman, 1979; Reynolds, 1971). Because empiric concepts and theories are abstractions of what can be observed or perceived in experience, a translation is made from the theoretic to the empiric (deductive approach) and from the empiric to the theoretic (inductive approach).

To function as viable structural elements of theory, concepts must adequately represent experience. Descriptive approaches, both quantitative and qualitative, typically are used to obtain empiric evidence that the concepts, as created within the theoretic structure, have adequate empiric indicators. The evidence from the investigations may suggest using processes of creating conceptual meaning in order to better represent the experience. Investigations designed to develop and refine empiric indicators and operational definitions for concepts are crucial for adequate research to refine and test theoretic relationships.

Theoretic relationships, which connect two or more concepts in a specific structure, are directly influenced by the nature of the empiric indicators for the concepts being related. The activities of refining concepts and theoretic relationships involve both qualitative and quantitative approaches. Replication requires repeating the validation or confirmation activities in other contexts. Theoretic relationships cannot be proven, but it is possible to show empiric support for proposed relationships. If the evidence does not support theoretic relationships, the ideas of the theory cannot be sustained. Alternative theoretic explanations are then considered based on the empiric evidence.

Refining concepts and theoretic relationships draws on one or more of the following subcomponents: (1) identifying empiric indicators for the concepts, (2) empirically grounding emerging relationships, and (3) validating relationships through empiric methods.

Identifying Empiric Indicators

Empiric indicators and operational definitions are used to represent concepts as variables in empiric research and are empirically formed for concepts as an outcome of some inductive research approaches. Formally structured theory can propose empiric indicators, but until they are put into operation in research, they remain speculative. Using the ideas in actual research makes it possible to refine the theory.

Consider the following abstract relationship statement:

As the adult's eye contact increases, the infant's eye contact will increase.

Imagine that a research project is designed to obtain empiric evidence about the use of eye contact as an empiric indicator of mothering. Details such as length of gaze and frequency of eye contact could be specified for the relatively abstract concept of *eye contact*. To use these indicators, the researcher would create a method for observing and timing the length of gaze and the frequency of eye contact.

Part of the process for identifying empiric indicators, especially when primarily deductive processes are used, is to state operational definitions. Operational definitions specify the standards or criteria to be used in making the observations. For example, an operational definition of the term *gaze* might be "a steady, direct, visual focusing on an object that lasts at least 3 seconds." This definition indicates what gaze is (the empiric indicator for visual contact), characteristics that are to be used in calling a behavior a gaze (direct visual focusing on an object), and a standard time parameter that distinguishes a gaze from other related behaviors such as a glance or a look.

It is difficult to identify empiric indicators for concepts that are more abstract than the concept of *eye contact*. Many concepts related to nursing (for example, *anxiety, body image,* and *self-esteem*) are highly abstract and cannot be directly measured. Tests and tools have been constructed to provide an indirect estimate of traits such as these. The fact that they cannot be measured directly does not mean they are nonexistent or cannot be assessed. The empiric challenge is to refine ideas about and evidence for empiric indicators so that strength of relationships can be explored.

The difficulties of finding adequate empiric indicators for abstract concepts can be compared to trying to describe the taste of a tomato. Once a person bites a tomato, that person knows how it tastes. Or, once a nurse smells a purulent wound, that nurse recognizes that smell as associated with a wound that is not healing well. The descriptions of that taste or smell are not at all adequate in comparison with the actual taste or smell experience. Many of the concepts that are important for nursing are highly abstract, and even the actual experience is not clearly perceived. Subsequently, the problem of finding reliable empiric indicators becomes complex and difficult. For example, *anxiety* is an abstract concept that can be theoretically defined, but when we explore the experience of anxiety, we find that people recognize what we mean by the term *anxiety* but that their actual experiences are as elusive as the taste of a tomato, and the experience of anxiety is not as clearly perceived as the perception of a taste. However, if the concept is important for nursing, empiric knowledge development depends on diligent efforts to make visible, as accurately as possible, the link between the abstract concept and the contextualized human experience. These examples underscore the value of creating conceptual meaning for adequate theory in nursing.

One approach that can be used to derive empiric measures for abstract nursing concepts is to use multiple empiric indicators to form useful research definitions. For example, anxiety might be measured with a self-report tool. The tool can be constructed to include many sensations that generally are indicative of anxiety. An operational definition of the concept of *anxiety* then becomes "what is assessed with the use of the tool." Anxiety also might be assessed empirically by observing a person's behavior and the physiologic indicators of neuroendocrine function. In this case, operational definitions would include specific ways to measure the behaviors observed and the specific range of laboratory test results associated with anxiety. All of these empiric indicators are possible. If they are used together in situations in which anxiety is likely to occur, the study will provide substantive evidence about the usefulness of each measure as an empiric indicator.

It is important to recognize that the empiric indicators identified for concepts must consider the theory to be validated. For example, if the concept of *caring* in the context of Madeleine Leininger's theory needs to be empirically assessed, it would be counterproductive to use a tool to assess caring developed for use in Jean Watson's theory. Also, dictionary definitions are generally not a good source of empiric indicators for concepts. In other words, when concepts are operationalized, they must be defined and measured in concert with the meaning of the theory in which they are embedded, and not any approach to measurement will do.

When inductive research processes form the basis for refining empiric indicators, the indicators are directly or indirectly observed and are used to form concepts. Knowing the empiric indicators used in generating the concepts would assist the deductive testing and extension of the theory into other contexts.

The work of Ferrans (1997) and Ferrans and Powers (1992) in developing the concept of *quality of life* is an example of the use of several different research approaches to develop and refine a conceptual model. *Quality of life* is a complex construct requiring a complex set of empiric indicators and operational definitions. Ferrans used qualitative research methods to find out what indicators people from different cultural groups associated with the idea of quality of life. Ferrans and Powers also used the statistical technique of factor analysis to identify how various indicators clustered together within domains. Using factor analysis they identified four domains (factors) associated with quality of life: health and functioning, psychologic-spiritual, social and economic, and family. They then developed a tool, the Quality of Life Index, to assess and measure the concept of *quality of life* within these four domains.

Empirically Grounding Emerging Relationships

The process of empirically grounding emerging relationships involves connecting experiences with representations of those experiences. When an abstract theoretic relationship is taken as the starting point, the investigator designs a study in which the hypothetic relationship, framed in terms of the empiric indicators for the concepts, can be studied. Several investigations may be required to confirm that the relationship proposed is accurate. When the investigations provide sufficient empiric evidence that conclusions can be drawn about the relationship, the investigator can return to the theoretic ideas and refine the theoretic statements to reflect what has been supported empirically. These conclusions often are presented as examples, citing the empiric investigations, within the narrative explanations of the theory.

An investigator can begin by exploring a selected empiric situation as the starting point, with the goal to find the concepts and relationships that accurately represent a situation that is not yet clearly understood but is recognized as important to the discipline of nursing. The investigator selects a social context in which the phenomenon under consideration is likely to occur and observes the interactions and circumstances of that context. From the observations, the investigator derives relationship statements that are grounded in the available empiric evidence. A variety of inductive approaches can be used to ground emerging relationships (Glaser & Strauss, 1967; Lincoln & Guba, 1985).

Validating Relationships Through Empiric Methods

Validating theoretic relationships requires creating a design that tests the descriptive and explanatory powers of a designated relationship. Designs may be proposed after theory is structured (deduction). When the purpose of the research design is to use inductive methods to generate theoretic relationships, the relationships are considered to be confirmed and ready for replication and validation in other settings.

A key to deductive validation of theoretic relationships is to use a design that ensures that the proposed relationship is actually the one that accounts for the study findings. For example, if a study concludes that a mother's gaze prompts an infant's gaze in return, the researcher needs to consider ways to be sure that it is actually the mother's gaze that accounts for the infant's behavior. Typically the researcher designs the study so that other factors that could influence the behavior of the infants in the study (for example, sensory experiences such as noise, touch, or visual distractions that might affect the process of visual interaction) are accounted for or held constant.

The purpose of deductively refining any relationship statement is to provide empiric evidence that the relationships proposed in the theory are adequate for a specific situation. With each approach to design that is used, the research question or hypothesis is revised to suit the type of design selected. Empiric evidence based on many different approaches to research design provides a basis for judging the adequacy of the theory. If theoretic statements are deductively tested and not supported by empiric evidence, one or more of the following four possibilities can account for the disparity between the theory and empiric findings:

- *The meaning of the concepts is not adequately created.* The process of creating conceptual meaning can be used to determine whether the definitions and meanings of the concepts under study are clear and whether they are well differentiated from related concepts. If they are not, theoretic revisions can be made, resulting in new approaches to empiric study.

- *The relationship statement is not adequately structured.* The processes of theory structuring and contextualizing can be used to examine the logic or form of the statements. Given the benefit of the empiric evidence, new insights into the form and structure of the theory might emerge. The theorist can revise the theoretic relationship statements on the basis of these insights.
- *The empiric indicators for the concept are not adequate.* The empiric evidence might point to new possibilities for empiric indicators or suggest revisions in the existing indicators. This process is particularly important when the empiric indicators represent highly abstract concepts and are constructed out of speculative ideas about how the concepts can be observed empirically.
- *The definitions are inadequate or inconsistent.* Typically, conflicting research results are attributed to faulty definitions and the related measurement problems of empiric research. This is a possibility, but accurate assessment depends on adequately conceived concepts, sound theoretic statements, and adequate empiric indicators. If these are all in place, it is then reasonable to consider problems in measurement or assessment of the concept.

When inductive methods are used to refine concepts and theoretic relationships, the relationships may be considered valid and confirmed if sound research procedures and processes are used for generating them. When relationships are deduced from inductively generated theory, they can be explored in similar settings or extended into new contexts. When this occurs, problems with faulty concepts, relational statements, empiric indicators, and operational definitions will become evident.

DESIGNING THEORETICALLY SOUND EMPIRIC RESEARCH

Investigations that are linked to theory can take one of the following two forms: theory-generating and theory-validating. In the following sections, we explain each type of approach and provide guidelines that you can use as a frame of reference for designing investigations in planning a study, or to assess the theoretic adequacy of a completed investigation.

Theory-Generating Research

Research that generates theory is designed to clarify and describe relationships without imposing preconceived notions of what the relationships mean. This approach usually is thought of as inductive. It is impossible to observe or interpret events or phenomena in the world without some pre-conceived idea of what they mean. Preexisting ideas are inherent in the experience of being socialized in a human culture, and the process of learning the theories of a discipline conveys meanings. A researcher who designs a study to generate theory observes with as open a mind as possible to see things in a new way.

As an example, suppose that a graduate nursing student, Carson, is com-pleting his master's thesis around what motivates elders to purchase nutri-tional supplements. Carson has noticed that lately advertising of nutritional supplements has been intentionally directed at the elderly. His knowledge of gerontologic nursing suggests that much of this advertising is promoting supplements that have limited, if any, benefit. Carson has just completed a course in nursing theory and decides to use a theory-generating approach for his thesis research. He might begin by observing the shopping behavior of elderly persons in stores where a variety of nutritional supplements are sold, including those supplements that are heavily advertised. Carson proba-bly would have some belief, based on theories of marketing and vulnerabil-ity, that aging elders who feel vulnerable to the effects of aging demonstrate purchasing behaviors that are linked to television advertising. Carson's perceptions during the observation would not be really pure but would be influenced by theoretic notions about marketing and vulnerability of elders. However, if Carson intends to be open to previously unaccounted-for variables or features of shopping behavior that are potentially useful but have not been described, preconceived ideas must be recognized and set as far aside as possible.

One approach to theory-generating research that has been used in nursing is grounded-theory (Glaser & Strauss, 1967). This form of field methodology requires the simultaneous processes of collecting, coding, and categorizing empiric observations and forming concepts and relation-ships based on the data obtained. Grounded-theory methodologies also use deductive approaches to examine developing propositions of theory. However, it initially is an inductive method.

Other forms of theory-generating research include field observations, as used in anthropology, and participant observation, as used in sociology. The investigator attempts to minimize any intrusion or effect on events observed and seeks to view and describe things occurring as they would if the observer were not present. The investigator attends to clues about how one event affects another and explains the things observed by develop-ing theoretic relationship statements about those observations (Coffey & Atkinson, 1996; Eaves, 2001; Strauss & Corbin, 1998).

Because many phenomena cannot be observed directly, theory-generating research sometimes must use indirect ways of gathering data. Phenomenology is one example of this approach. Phenomenology as a research method is designed to describe or interpret the subjective, lived experiences of people and to comprehend the meanings that people place on these experiences (Benner, 1994). These experiences cannot be observed; they are directly accessible only to the person who has the experience. Indirect ways of observing include interviewing or questioning individuals about what they feel or remember or how they respond to certain situations. Feelings, thoughts, memories, dreams, and private human experiences can be known only through how people choose to relate them.

Different inductive methodologies produce different types of knowledge and different forms of descriptive statements or theories. Grounded-theory methods generate a structure of relationships and core variables that the researcher has observed. Phenomenology results in interpretive narratives that describe meaning as fully as possible. Phenomenology as a research method is not intended to generate formal theory, but the processes utilized are rigorous and systematic. We believe the products of phenomenologic inquiry fall within our broad definition of theory. Regardless of how the products generated by phenomenologic inquiry methods are classified, the insights that they yield can contribute to conceptual clarity and theoretic thinking. Regardless of the approach, inductive investigators whose purpose is to contribute empiric knowledge for the discipline address issues of soundness by systematically organizing and describing their research results.

Theory-Validating Research

Once theory is constructed, by whatever means, it is possible to use research methods for validation. The methods are designed to ascertain how accurately the theory depicts empiric phenomena and their relationships. Theoretic statements can be translated into questions and hypotheses so long as the abstractions of the theory can be directly or indirectly represented with empiric indicators. A single study usually is based on one or two relational statements from among several that might possibly be extracted from a theory. No one study can test the entirety of a theory. Some theories contain relationship statements that can be tested and other relationship statements that cannot be tested by research because empiric indicators cannot be identified.

Even though a theory has been incompletely tested, it is regarded as relatively sound if several research studies conducted over time in different settings demonstrate a degree of confidence in the theory. If some statements are supported by research, whereas others are unsupported or refuted by research, the research provides a basis for revising the theory or developing new theory.

Theory-validating research usually is considered a deductive approach. The research starts with an abstract relational statement derived from theory. From the theoretic statement, hypotheses or research questions are created for a specific research situation.

Research questions also may be used in theory-validating research. This type of research typically uses descriptive and correlational designs. The concepts in the research questions are empirically represented, and observations are made. The data are collated and described in such a way that the questions are addressed and the implications related to the development of the theory are stated.

Because hypotheses must contain a relationship between at least two variables, the research design usually is an experimental, quasi-experimental, or correlational approach (Polit, Beck, & Hungler, 2001). In theory-validating research, the investigator deliberately changes or controls conditions so that the study clearly focuses on the nature of the relationship between the variables that have been selected for study. Several descriptive and relationship-validating studies usually are needed to validate and extend a theory because only a limited number from among all possible relationships can be included in one study. A single study can contribute appreciably to the validation process if it is theoretically sound.

In the following sections we examine the general research process and identify how both theory-generating and theory-validating research can be designed and therefore evaluated to achieve the most value from the research effort.

DEVELOPING SOUND THEORETIC RESEARCH

The research process can be examined for theoretic soundness at each stage. The following descriptions of each stage can serve as a guide for developing or evaluating the theoretic soundness of a research study. Examples are given in each section from two research studies to illustrate features of theory-validating and theory-generating research. The example of theory-generating research used a grounded-theory method to develop a theory of mothering with serious mental illness (Montgomery, Tompkins, Forchuk, & French, 2006). The example of theory-validating research used a correlational, causal modeling study to examine the relationships between racism, chronic stress emotions, and blood pressure in African Americans (Peters, 2006).

The Clinical Problem, Research Purpose, Research Problem, and Hypotheses

In *theory-linked* research, the clinical problem statements, research purpose, and hypotheses are designed to show the relationships between the chosen theory base and the particular study being conducted. In *theory-validating* research, each of these statements should be explicitly formulated because each guides the process as it moves from the broad, general intent to the empiric specifics of the study. In descriptive and exploratory theory-validating research, hypotheses may not be stated or labeled as such, and research problems (questions) are developed. Although not necessarily stated in relationship form, the questions imply underlying relationships of significance to the developing theory.

In *theory-generating* research, only the clinical and research problems are required; the other statements may or may not be developed explicitly in the course of the research process. They are not necessarily explicitly stated in published reports of completed research, but in well-reported studies the statements appropriate to each approach can be inferred from the text of the published article.

In *theory-validating* research, statements of purpose, problem, and hypotheses or questions are formulated in advance of conducting the data-gathering activity. In *theory-generating* research, the purpose and problem statements are formulated in advance; if relationships are stated, they are derived from the data. Table 9-1 describes the purpose served by each type of statement and shows how the clinical problem, research purpose, research problem, and hypotheses follow from each other and provide a conceptual link between the theory and the research study. As the table shows, there are two types of problems: clinical and research.

The clinical problem is a question that reflects the general experiential concern that generated or influenced the study and suggests the study context. The clinical problem clearly reflects the experiential questions that are fundamental to developing empiric knowledge: What is this? How does it work?

The research purpose indicates whether the study is theory-generating or theory-validating in nature and whether the study focuses on description, explanation, or prediction. If the study is *theory-generating,* the purpose further states the empiric observations to be made. If the study is *theory-validating,* the purpose states the theoretic frame of reference for the study.

For both *theory-generating* and *theory-validating* research, the research problem is less general than the statement of purpose and directs the more specific, circumstantial focus of the study. The research problem is phrased in the form of a question that implies how the purpose of the study is to be achieved. It reflects the variables or events to be studied and implies that

TABLE 9-1 Comparison of Clinical Problem, Research Purpose, Research Problem, and Hypothesis Statements in Theory-Linked Research

Type of Statement	What the Statement Conveys	Theory-Generating*	Theory-Validating†
Clinical problem	Specifies the experiential observations that generated or influenced the study	Little is known about mothering for women with serious mental illness, but despite this lack of knowledge it is viewed as a pathologic problem by health care professionals	Is there a relationship between stressors of racism and blood pressure in African Americans?
Research purpose	Specifies whether the research is theory-generating or theory-validating	To describe the experiences of mothers with serious mental illness and develop explanations of how they manage mothering	To test a middle-range theory of chronic stress emotions as an explanation of the psychological and physiological consequences of racism in African Americans.
Research problem	Poses a question to be answered Is less general than the purpose and makes clear how the purpose is to be achieved Expresses the nature of the variables or events to be studied Implies the empiric possibilities for the abstract concepts given in the purpose Expresses the relationships between concepts if the relationships are the focus for the study	What is the experience of mothers with serious mental illness? How do mothers with serious mental illness attempt to manage their mothering circumstances?	Does the experience of racism contribute to the development of negative psychologic outcomes? Do people with lesser skill in emotional regulation experience greater levels of chronic stress emotions? Does the chronic stress of racism contribute to hypertension?

*Data from Montgomery, P., Tompkins, C., Forchuk, C., & French, S. (2006). Keeping close: Mothering with serious mental illness. *Journal of Advanced Nursing, 54*(1), 20–28.
†Data from Peters, R.M. (2006). The relationship of racism, chronic stress emotions, and blood pressure. *Journal of Nursing Scholarship, 38*(3), 234–240.

Continued

TABLE 9-1 Comparison of Clinical Problem, Research Purpose, Research Problem, and Hypothesis Statements in Theory-Linked Research—cont'd

Type of Statement	What the Statement Conveys	Theory-Generating*	Theory-Validating†
Hypothesis	Identifies the specific choices made in relation to the variables for the study Implies the design of the study Implies the type of analysis used	Developed from the study findings The core concern of mothers with serious mental illness is "keeping close," which consists of three categories: appearing normal, creating security, and being responsible. Subcategories of strategies used to keep close were pretenses intended to imitate ideal representations of "mother." These pretenses included masking, censoring speech, doing motherwork, and seeking help.	Posed at the outset to guide the research methodology There is a significant positive correlation between perceived racism and chronic stress emotions. There is a significant positive correlation between perceived racism and hypertension. There is a significant relationship between emotional regulation of stress and somatic health.

empiric possibilities for abstract concepts to be developed are embodied in existing theoretic relationships.

In *theory-validating* research, hypotheses may or may not be stated. When hypotheses are stated, they indicate the circumstantial restrictions of the study, reflect the study design, and suggest the analysis to be made of data. Hypotheses usually provide specific guidance for statistical analysis of quantitative data. If the analysis of the research data does not depend on statistics for drawing conclusions, hypotheses might not be stated; rather, research questions are used to guide data analysis.

In *theory-generating* research, hypotheses also may or may not be stated. Problem statements or research questions may be appropriate for guiding a study intended to generate theory, and hypotheses are formulated at the conclusion of the study, if at all. When formulated, hypotheses provide specific direction for future research.

Background of the Study and Literature Review

In all research, the literature review surveys research findings that are pertinent to the study that is being conducted. In theory-linked research, the literature review also includes a summary evaluation of the theoretic background for the study.

For *theory-generating* research, the background for the study includes a review of previous work pertinent to the area of concern. The author's thinking and experience are important as background for the study. The literature review is comprehensive and continues throughout the data-gathering and analysis phases. As the ideas and concepts emerge from the data, the researcher uses the data to guide explorations in the existing literature. The empiric observations remain the primary source for analysis and interpretation, but in some instances the literature provides a basis for refining and delineating central concepts and the relationships between them.

In the theory-generating study that explores mothering with serious mental illness (Montgomery et al., 2006) the authors summarized the scant evidence that has been published in the literature concerning mothering with serious mental illness. There are an abundance of studies that support a negative relationship between mental illness in mothers and their children's well-being, but no causal relationship has been established from the published research which emphasizes maternal characteristics and neglect-related variables of stigma, poverty, lack of support, inadequate living accommodation, symptomatology and medication side effects, and interactions of mothers and legal protection services. There is a primary gap in knowledge about the experience of mothers with serious mental illness.

In *theory-validating* research, previous studies based on the theory form a substantial portion of the literature review. The review also contains a critique of previous research based on alternative theories and on concepts or variables related to the study's central purpose. The review traces how the study has been conceived and summarizes the theoretic ideas that are being tested. It clarifies how and why specific relationships within the theory are being tested.

In the theory-validating study of the relationships between racism, chronic stress emotions, and blood pressure (Peters, 2006), the author confirms the demonstrated fact that hypertension is a disproportionate problem for African Americans, that no evidence has been found of a genetic variant that is unique to African Americans, and that there has been scant research on the effect of racism on blood pressure. Based on Lazarus' theory of stress and emotion, the author constructed a middle-range chronic stress emotion theory.

The Research Methodology

The following concerns with regard to research method must carefully be considered when theory-linked research is undertaken: the means of obtaining the data, the selection of the sample for study, the design of the research, and the analysis of data and conclusions.

The Means of Obtaining Data. How the data are collected or recorded must be consistent with the purpose of the research design. For *theory-generating* research, the study usually is descriptive in nature and requires either directly or indirectly observing and recording empiric events that the investigator does not alter during the course of study. *Theory-validating* research also draws on these means of obtaining data. Because theory-validating research often relies on some type of experimental or correlational analysis, the tools and assessments used tend to be those that yield quantitative measures of the variables.

Direct observation requires being physically present. Data are recorded by some means, such as note taking, audiotaping, or videotaping. Examples include watching and making notations about behavior during the process of mother–infant interactions, about interactions between nurses and patients within an intensive care unit, and about the behavior of a person experiencing a crisis such as pain.

Indirect observation includes the following: interviews; questionnaires and standardized tools that elicit feelings, thoughts, or memories; and self-reports of experiences not directly observable. Tools and assessments that are designed to elicit reports about selected phenomena must be carefully examined to ensure that they can provide the evidence needed to achieve the purposes of the study. In *theory-generating* research, tools developed with a particular theoretic bias introduce a perspective that may not be desirable. In *theory-validating* research, the means of obtaining data must be carefully considered in relation to the theoretic adequacy of tools and assessment approaches. In both types of research, the problems of reliability and validity of both direct and indirect observations are considered. Tools that are designed to yield a numeric score are assessed for reliability and validity via statistical methods. Interview approaches that are designed to produce narrative descriptions are examined carefully to ascertain how well the approach will function to elicit the types of responses that are needed. The research report should include a discussion of the level of development for the tools used, what theoretic perspective underlies any tools used, and available evidence related to the tools' reliability and validity.

In Peters' (2006) theory-validating study, several instruments were used to measure variables that were linked to the theoretic concepts being tested. Perceived racism was measured using two instruments: the Racism and Life Experience Scales, and the Krieger Racial Discrimination Questionnaire. Taken together, these scales were judged to be reasonably adequate measures of perceived racism. Emotion-focused coping was judged to be a reasonable measure of the theoretic concept of emotional regulation. Three scales were chosen to measure emotion-focused coping: The Toronto Alexithymia Scale, the Emotional Approach Coping Scale, and the Anter Expression subscale of the State-Trait Anger Expression Inventory-2. Chronic stress emotions were measured using the trait anger, trait anxiety, and trait depression subscales from the State-Trait Personality Inventory (Peters, 2006).

Data were obtained in the theory-generating study of mothering with serious mental illness using an unstructured formal grounded-theory interview (Montgomery et al., 2006). The interviews of 20 participants were tape recorded. Field notes also provided data for the study.

The Selection of the Sample. The selection of the sample essentially is what limits the research to a particular time and place. It is a part of the research that links the abstractions of the theory with empiric phenomena. In *theory-generating* research, the investigator begins with the following assumption:

There is some phenomenon or event happening that will be evident if I observe this particular group of people. Furthermore, this particular group is sufficiently like other groups of people who have this experience to represent them.

The individuals chosen for the sample are purposely selected because they can contribute information and insight related to the phenomenon that is being studied.

In *theory-validating* research, sample selection requires the investigator to take the position that if the theory is empirically reasonable, it will be supported by what happens with the specific persons selected for study, or, if the theory is not empirically accurate, the responses of the sample studied will refute the theory. Because most theory-validating research relies on statistical analysis of quantitative data, sample selection is guided by the requirements of statistical analysis. Both the population to whom the theoretic relationship applies and the sample that is being tested must be specified. Drawing the conclusion of empiric accuracy of the relationship depends on the assumption that the statistical requirements for sampling from the identified population have been met.

In Peters' (2006) theory-validating study of the relationships between racism, chronic stress emotion, and blood pressure, a convenience sample of 162 African Americans ages 18 through 80 were recruited from two urban settings. Peters deliberately sought a wide age range to reflect varying levels of stressful life experience, and varying levels of blood pressure. In the theory-generating study of mothering with serious mental illness (Montgomery et al., 2006) both purposive and theoretic sampling was used. Twenty mothers were interviewed who had a range of major mental illness diagnoses and who identified as the mother of at least one child between the ages of 2 and 16 years.

The Research Design. The design of the research outlines the procedure and contingencies used for answering the research questions or testing the hypotheses. In *theory-generating* research, the design must be consistent with the theory-generating orientation of the research. It often involves observation of a particular kind of phenomenon of interest in given groups. Stern (1980) described the design of grounded-theory as a matrix in which several research processes are in operation at once. The investigator examines obtained data and begins to code, categorize, conceptualize, and write impressions about their meaning.

Sometimes research designs that typically are used in *theory-validating* research are needed for *theory-generating* research. This is the case when a sequence of ordinarily occurring events is an area of concern. For example, suppose something happens to create a sequence of events, such as the birth of a child or the death of a loved one. The research interest might be to describe the usual responses of individuals over a period of time, both before and after this event, to generate theory regarding how people live through these situations. In these instances, comparative assessments over time are needed. The investigator does not, as in classic experimental designs, impose the changes as a part of the design, but rather waits for the changes to occur. The investigator then describes the nature of outcomes that occur before and after the event to develop theory.

Theory-generating research also may require comparison groups that are typical of experimental designs to determine whether a phenomenon occurs only under certain circumstances. Suppose, for example, that an investigator wanted to determine whether body image formation is appreciably affected by chronic illness. The phenomenon could be studied by comparing body image formation in a group of people who have a chronic illness with body image formation in a group who do not have chronic illness. The comparison would determine whether aspects of the phenomenon of body image formation are unique to people with chronic illness. This information would contribute to the development of theory related to body image formation.

In some forms of *theory-validating* research, the researcher deliberately alters circumstances in some way to test the relationships expressed in the hypotheses. The design usually includes some intervention or investigator-created circumstances consistent with the theoretic basis for the study.

In Peters' (2006) theory-validating study of the relationships of racism, chronic stress emotions, and blood pressure, a descriptive correlational, causal modeling design was used. Montgomery and colleagues (2006) used a grounded-theory design following Glaser's grounded-theory approach in their theory-generating study of mothering with serious mental illness.

Analysis of the Data and Conclusions. The analysis of data in theory-linked research must be consistent with the purposes of the research and the research design. For *theory-generating* research, analysis of data involves narrative, descriptive, and other relatively qualitative types of analysis. Depending on the type of observation used, a quantitative, numeric, or statistical analysis of the data also can be presented, but it is accompanied by a theoretic analysis that includes the full range of observations and the ways in which the observations occurred.

In a grounded-theory approach, analysis of the data involves coding and categorizing the observations. In participant observation, the analysis may report sample observations that typify the characteristic events or the sequence of events that were observed. Whatever the form of data presentation, the investigator proposes concepts generated from the data and, if possible, a description of theoretic propositions that emerge from the data. The extent to which concepts and theoretic propositions are formulated depends on how well the evidence supports making conceptual and theoretic formulations and on the extent to which previous studies support such conceptual and theoretic development.

Montgomery and colleagues (2006) used the constant comparative analysis of incidents and categories to develop higher levels of abstraction required to theoretically explain the experience of mothering with serious mental illness. The study resulted in core categories and subcategories that explained the mothers' experiences.

In *theory-validating* research, analysis of the data should present sufficient quantitative and qualitative evidence to support or reject the hypotheses or to address the research questions. The conclusions of the study should include an interpretive analysis of the findings in relation to the theory being tested. The analysis of data focuses on the specific study findings, whereas the conclusions focus on the theoretic significance of the study.

Peters (2006) used structural equation modeling to examine the hypothesized causal and correlational links among racism, chronic stress emotions, and blood pressure. She concluded that the proposed mid-range theory of chronic stress emotion fit the sample data.

Generalizability and Usefulness of the Study

In theory-linked research, one of the important considerations for a single study is how it contributes to theory development. In most instances, a single study raises more questions than it answers, and questions raised must be presented to provide a basis for future study. *Theory-generating* research should result in relationship statements that can be studied and used in further developing the theory. *Theory-validating* research may result in evidence that suggests revision or extension of the theory tested, or it may suggest an entirely new avenue for the development of theory.

Theory-generating research can be useful for practice because of its grounding in the experience for which the theory is designed. Theory-generating research also often provides a basis for further theory-related work based on new insights and new questions. *Theory-validating* research also can have immediate practice application. If the research design is valid and the findings are generalizable and consistent with related research findings, the investigator may conclude that certain approaches in the realm of practice might be useful. However, immediate use in practice cannot always be expected. The primary value of theory-validating research is to stimulate further study and theory development that will add to empiric knowledge on which practice can be based.

REFLECTION AND DISCUSSION

This chapter reviews the characteristics of theory-linked and isolated research and provides an example of each. It also describes processes for validating and confirming theory using research. Processes described are identifying empiric indicators, grounding relationships empirically, and validating relationships using empiric methods. A centrally important message of this chapter is that validation and confirming processes depend on purpose-appropriate conceptual meaning and empiric indicators that adequately represent concepts. To deepen your appreciation of confirming and validating theory through research, consider the following related to the content of this chapter.

1. Identify a study you consider to be "isolated" from theory. How is its value limited because a deliberate linkage to theory is absent?
2. Locate a research study where hypotheses were not confirmed, or expected findings were not supported. Do you believe that

conceptual definitions and empiric indicators (operational definitions) for concepts contributed to errors in measurement that accounted for the findings? Why or why not?

3. Choose a substantive concept of interest to nursing that you believe is in the middle range. Create an operational definition for the concept. Does the definition "leave out" any ideas of importance? Is it possible to create an operational definition for the concept that fully contains the concept?

4. For the concept chosen in the preceding exercise, create subconcepts that you believe fairly represent it and propose operational definitions for the subconcepts. What impact does the creation of subconcepts have on your ability to formulate operational definitions?

5. Choose a theory—of whatever scope—and propose a relationship for validation. How might validation of the relationship proceed? Where could validation occur? If the relationship is validated, what might be a next step in relation to the theory?

6. Identify a theory developed using inductive methods such as grounded-theory. Would you consider this theory confirmed? If you were to extend the theory using research, how would you proceed? That is, what might be a "next step"?

Reference List

Benner, P. A. (1994). *Interpretive phenomenology: Embodiment, caring and ethics in health and illness.* Thousand Oaks, CA: Sage.

Coffey, A., & Atkinson, P. (1996). *Making sense of qualitative data.* Thousand Oaks, CA: Sage.

Dubin, R. (1978). Theory building (Rev. ed.). New York: Free Press.

Eaves, Y. D. (2001). A synthesis technique for grounded theory data analysis. *Journal of Advanced Nursing, 35*(5), 654.

Ferrans, C. E. (1997). Development of a conceptual model of quality of life. In A. G. Gift (Ed.), *Clarifying concepts in nursing research.* New York: Springer.

Ferrans, C. E., & Powers, M. (1992). Psychometric assessment of the quality of life index. *Research in Nursing and Health, 15,* 29–38.

Glaser, B., & Strauss, A. (1967). *The discovery of grounded theory.* Chicago: Aldine.

Gunter, L. M. (1964). Research techniques applied to nursing. *Nursing Research, 13,* 230.

Lincoln, Y. S., & Guba, E. G. (1985). *Naturalistic inquiry.* Newbury Park, CA: Sage.

Montgomery, P., Tompkins, C., Forchuk, C., & French, S. (2006). Keeping close: Mothering with serious mental illness. *Journal of Advanced Nursing, 54*(1), 20–28.

Newman, M. A. (1979). *Theory development in nursing.* Philadelphia: FA Davis.

Peters, R. M. (2006). The relationship of racism, chronic stress emotions, and blood pressure. *Journal of Nursing Scholarship, 38*(3), 234–240.

Polit, D. F., Beck, C. T., & Hungler, B. P. (2001). *Essentials of nursing research: Methods, appraisal and utilization* (5th ed.). Philadelphia: Lippincott Williams & Wilkins.

Reed, E. (1978). *Sexism and science.* New York: Pathfinder Press.

Reynolds, P. D. (1971). *A primer in theory construction.* Indianapolis, IN: Bobbs-Merrill.

Stern, P. N. (1980). Grounded theory methodology: Its uses and processes. *Image—The Journal of Nursing Scholarship, 12*(1), 20–23.

Strauss, A., & Corbin, J. (1998). *Basics of qualitative research* (2nd ed.). Thousand Oaks, CA: Sage.

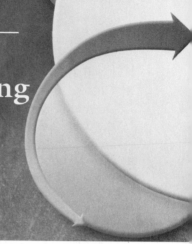

CHAPTER 10

Utilizing and Validating Empiric Knowledge in Practice

Practice is goal directed. Clinical testing of theory is therefore essential.
Choose your theory—it does not hold in all circumstances. The
professional must not be just a simple user of theory, but a developer,
a tester and expander of theory. Not for the purpose of scholarship,
but for intelligent practice.

Rosemary Ellis (1969, p. 1435)

Development of empiric knowledge, such as theories and formal descriptions for a practice discipline, requires the processes of deliberative utilization and validation in the practice setting to assess the value of theoretic knowledge for moving toward valued nursing goals. Research methods are used in these processes, and practice-based research findings contribute valuable information to the development of the theory being applied. Practice-based validation of theory contributes to the development of scientific competence among nurses and, in turn, contributes to improving the quality of nursing care. We use the phrase *deliberative utilization and validation* to refer to the use and evaluation of empiric knowledge for guiding practice and practice-oriented approaches that further contribute to empiric knowledge development. Deliberative utilization and validation of theory involve the use of practice to (1) refine conceptual meaning and (2) validate theoretic relationships and outcomes in practice.

By *practice*, we mean the experiences a nurse encounters during the process of caring for people. Some experiences are those of the client, others are those of the nurse; some are interactive, and some are environmental. These experiences occur in many settings, but when they occur in the context of providing nursing care, they are considered part of nursing practice.

In this chapter we address specific ways in which practicing nurses contribute to empiric knowledge development processes and ways in which empiric knowledge development processes contribute to practice. We discuss important dimensions of refining conceptual meaning that can be accomplished only in the context of practice. We present guidelines for validating theoretic relationships and outcomes of practice as well as guidelines for methodologic approaches to validating theoretic relationships and outcomes. The relationship between evidence-based nursing and the utilization and validation of theory in practice is considered.

REFINING CONCEPTUAL MEANING

Nursing concepts come from the experience of practicing nursing. Practicing nurses who reflect on the nature of their experiences and systematically communicate their reflections make significant contributions to validating empiric knowledge. Researchers who primarily are involved in knowledge development benefit from the ideas of many nurses who practice nursing clinically. Everyone does not participate equally in all processes required for the development of empiric knowledge. Some researchers, but not all, do engage in practice. Some practicing nurses, but not all, conduct research. Many who do engage in both practice and research find the experiences rewarding and beneficial. Regardless, each person participates in the collective endeavor to develop nursing knowledge.

Empiric concepts are formed from nursing practice by observing, naming, and making sense of what happens. The processes we described in Chapter 7 for creating conceptual meaning can be used to systematically document reflections concerning your experiences, from which you can derive a tentative conclusion about the experience you might want to study. Because your thinking will be grounded in nursing practice, you have a rich resource from which to explore conceptual meanings. Once you have tentatively described your phenomenon of interest, you can turn to activities for refining conceptual meaning. There are four practice-dependent activities required for refining conceptual meaning.

Identifying Empiric Indicators

Practice provides essential evidence that is used to select empiric indicators for abstract concepts. The experiences of practice can challenge existing theoretic conceptualizations, and they can reveal hunches that have not yet been linked to a particular concept or theory. The basic question is, "What have I experienced that can be linked to the abstract concept *X*?"

Anxiety is a good example of such an experience. Suppose that a wide range of behaviors observed in practice are described in a theory as manifestations of the concept of *anxiety*. These behaviors might include wringing of hands, silence and refusing to talk, excessive talking, laughing, crying, sweating, compulsive eating, not eating, or a lack of appetite. Tools have been constructed that assess the concept of anxiety using these empiric indicators. In your practice, you might observe that these ideas do not always fit, but indeed contradict one another. When you work with individuals who are anxious, you notice that they tend to behave in ways that are not consistent with the theoretic concept. There are some behaviors that you almost never observe, and others that are commonly experienced are not taken into account by the theory. Because *anxiety* as an abstract idea does convey something that you know exists, it might be helpful if you could better identify it, understand how it works, and determine how people experience it differently. As you draw on your experience, new ideas begin to emerge from the empiric behaviors you have noticed.

Differentiating Similar Concepts

Concepts that are similar yet different might share certain empiric indicators, and differentiating them may be difficult. If knowing the difference between them is important in practice, practice can provide the empiric information and conceptual insights required to distinguish them. This purpose becomes critical when you realize that errors can be made in assigning meaning to a person's experience. For example, you might have been taught that certain behaviors are manifestations of anxiety, based on a popular theory of anxiety. You have integrated research evidence, theory, and your experience to make expert clinical judgments about how to help anxious people reduce their anxiety and improve their function, but your approach does not seem to be as effective as you think it should be. One problem might be that the behaviors are not indicative of anxiety but are associated with fear. Your challenge is to begin to conceptualize anxiety more clearly, conceptualize what else might be happening, and begin to find ways to differentiate between the experiences of anxiety and fear. As you question and challenge the conceptualization and the conclusions that you draw from it, you will form a basis for restructuring the concepts and form new or revised concepts that better represent nursing experience.

Identifying New Concepts

Creating conceptual meaning is a process that can lead to identification of new concepts. Model, borderline, related, and contrary cases that come from practice reflect the richness and complexity of practice. As you reflect deliberatively on these situations, your insights can lead to new ideas that contribute to forming new concepts.

For example, suppose you begin to notice that something about how people learn in the postoperative period does not seem to be described in any of the literature you have read. Most learning theories have been developed and tested in classroom or laboratory settings, where learners are healthy students. In nursing situations, the learner often is experiencing health or illness unlike typical students in a classroom. The patterns of behavior that are the focus of learning in a nursing context may not have been addressed adequately in developing concepts and theories of learning in the classroom. As you reflect on your experience, you see meanings that are different from the meaning of learning in existing learning theories. As you discuss your ideas with other nurses, you find that they have made similar observations. From this awareness, you can build a new conceptualization that, once named, can be incorporated into theory and used in practice.

Identifying Conceptual and Diagnostic Criteria

Although criteria for nursing diagnoses are not the same as criteria for a concept in theory development, nursing diagnostic criteria can be partially derived from criteria for a concept, and vice versa. Nursing diagnostic criteria take into account generally accepted standards for practice, as well as knowledge and application of many areas of theory that are pertinent to the diagnosis. Consider, for example, the nursing diagnosis "impaired parenting" as defined by inappropriate and/or non-nurturing parenting behaviors and lack of parental attachment behavior (Carpenito-Moyet, 2006, p. 311). In practice, the purpose is to accurately identify this problem in order to provide effective nursing care. The diagnosis of "impaired parenting" implies knowledge of how certain factors affect non-nurturing parental behavior and parental-infant attachment. The observation of non-nurturing parental behaviors and lack of parental-infant attachment implies knowledge of human attachment theory and also suggests the focus for nursing actions. When criteria for nursing diagnoses are derived in part from a concept not yet well developed, the process of creating conceptual meaning can be used to form tentative diagnostic criteria that can be tested for empiric accuracy or validity.

The criteria for the nursing diagnosis of "impaired parenting" could include conceptual criteria for parenting. The diagnostic criteria also must address value qualifiers, such as the terms *impaired* and *non-nurturing* that convey the value that the practitioner assigns to a situation in the process of making clinical decisions. When the parent under consideration is the mother, the diagnostic criteria for impaired parenting might be as follows:

- Visual contact between mother and infant is minimal or absent.
- Physical touching of the infant by the mother is limited to necessary touch.
- There is minimal or no vocalization directed by the mother to the infant.
- The mother's verbal expressions focus on herself (that is, concerns for her own body or image or relationships with peers, rather than expressions focusing on the infant).
- Care of the infant is easily or passively given to another caretaker.

The diagnostic criteria just listed reflect but do not include all conceptual criteria for mothering used as an example in Chapter 7, which were as follows:

- Visual contact must be observed to be directed from the mothering person to the person who receives mothering.
- The person who receives mothering must be physically touched by the mothering person.
- Some positive feeling must be experienced by the mothering person and by the person who receives mothering.
- There must be a reciprocal interaction between the mothering person and the person who receives mothering.
- Vocalization by the mothering person must occur.

Notice that the diagnostic criteria specify an altered interaction, whereas the conceptual criteria point to observations that signify "mothering." The diagnostic criteria focus on those aspects that are relatively accessible to being empirically observed and assessed in practice. The conceptual idea of "some positive feeling" potentially could be operationalized and measured or otherwise assessed, but the many challenges in attempting to do so may not warrant pursuit of this line of development, particularly when more readily accessible indicators, such as visual contact and touch, are suggested and may be adequate for your purpose.

The diagnostic criteria may be adequate for creating standard approaches to practice and may be sufficient to use in formal testing of the theoretic concept. Evidence of the diagnostic criteria recorded in practice provides a basis for decisions about the adequacy of the criteria for research or practice, as well as direction as to how research should proceed. If the purpose of creating conceptual meaning is to form criteria useful for nursing diagnosis, then traits that are present in practice need to be emphasized.

VALIDATING THEORETIC RELATIONSHIPS AND OUTCOMES IN PRACTICE

Deliberatively utilizing theory involves employing research methods to demonstrate how a theory or other forms of empiric knowledge affect nursing practice. It involves processes that place a selected theory or formalized description within the context of practice to ensure that it serves the goals of the profession. Validation provides evidence of the theory's usefulness in developing nurses' scientific competence and in ensuring quality of care.

The essence of the theory-practice relationship is deliberatively utilizing and validating theory. Theory that addresses goals of practice provides a way to systematically develop substantial empiric knowledge within the discipline. Theory is not a quick-and-easy answer to a problem but rather provides knowledge and understanding to ultimately enhance the practice of nursing.

A first step is to ascertain whether the theory can be used in practice. Some theories that hold promise may not be sufficiently developed to justify their use in practice. Others might be poorly suited to a particular practice area. The guidelines we suggest in the following section can be used to make this decision. Once you decide to use the theory in practice, you can then design research methods to demonstrate how well the theory contributes to your practice goals through the validation of theory.

How to Determine Whether a Theory Should Be Validated in Practice

Theory ideally serves to improve nursing practice. Usually this goal is achieved by using theory or portions of theory to guide practice. Because theory can be used prematurely or inappropriately, it is important to consider how sound judgments are made regarding the validation of theory in practice.

Contrary to a common notion in nursing that theory is not relevant to nursing practice, nurses increasingly are expected to practice from a scientific foundation and from research and theory derived directly from nursing practice (Fulbrook, 2003; Whittemore & Grey, 2002). Early in nursing education programs, students are taught that empiric knowledge is the foundation for the nursing process. Nurses often are called on to provide a scientific rationale for nursing care, and the best practices in nursing are founded on scientific theories. In practice, judgments often are made without conscious effort or explicit explanation of the basis for the judgment, but most experienced nurses can cite valid empiric reasons for their judgments. Currently, the focus on evidence-based practice carries with it the expectation that nurses will integrate research evidence into clinical decision-making processes. This focus is creating a demand for research that clearly links with theory and practice in a way that is significant for meeting care goals.

Despite a focus on evidence-based practice, many common practices in nursing have emerged from sound principles or standards based in fundamental truths that have not yet come under sufficient challenge to be a focus for knowledge development. As Beckstrand (1980) has noted, "Principles of practice are shorthand ways of referring to fundamental truths to be considered and general customs to be followed" (p. 73). Standards of practice reflect valued actions that generally are accepted in a given situation. Principles and standards are judged by their consistent outcomes; for example, do they consistently yield desired results in practice? They are changed not by systematically challenging the standards or the principles themselves but rather by discovering another approach that better achieves the desired outcome (Beckstrand, 1980). Although facts, theories, or models that are cited as the basis of care may provide explanations that seem rational and well founded, it is important to consider how adequate the ideas are as a basis for making judgments and for directing nursing actions.

Theory cannot be assumed to predict a desired outcome and does not exist to give specific guidelines for what should be done in a given situation. Rather, theory explains possible relationships that can be questioned. The goal of a theory and goals of practice should be consistent, but this cannot be assumed to be the case. If the relationships predicted by a theory are inadequate or do not accurately represent what is typical of nursing practice, the theory may not be effective in achieving practice goals. Theory can be used effectively to describe, explain, predict and provide understanding of situations that occur in practice but may not adequately contribute to the goals of practice when it is used. Because any utilization of theory will affect practice, deliberative use of theory cannot be undertaken lightly.

The questions we suggest in the following section can be used to reach an informed decision about the use of the theory so that its practice value can be assessed.

Are the Theory Goals and Practice Goals Congruent? To answer this question, examine the goal of the theory and compare it with the outcomes or goals that you see as valuable for nursing practice. The existing standards of practice can be used as one basis for clarifying the values on which your practice is based and the overall goals that your practice should be reflecting. Another basis for identifying practice goals is your own view of nursing and that of nurses with whom you work. If a theoretic goal would lead to a situation that is not congruent with your idea of optimal health, you may not want to use the theory. Sometimes this judgment is not easy because of conflicting or difficult philosophic assumptions about nursing, health, the individual, the environment, and society. For example, validation of a theory may be undertaken to determine whether the theoretic goal is consistent with the goal of optimal health. If the theoretic goal is adaptation and you are uncertain whether this concept is consistent with your idea of optimal health, you could design a trial that uses the theory in practice, observe the outcomes, and then evaluate the consistency of the outcomes in light of your practice goals.

Is the Intended Context of the Theory Congruent with the Practice Situation? This question addresses how well suited the theory is for your situation, given the general ideas of context that are stated or implied theoretically. A theory of pain alleviation, for example, may explain the processes involved in alleviating pain in any instance in which it occurs. As you become familiar with the theory, you realize that it was developed with reference to mature adults, and you work with children. You and your colleagues would need to explore how well the ideas of the theory might transfer to your own situation before you make a decision to use the theory.

Is There, or Might There Be, Similarity Between Theory Variables and Practice Variables? This question compares the important theoretic variables, expressed as concepts in the theory, with the variables recognized to be directly influencing the practice situation. In some instances important practice variables may not be included in the theoretic relationship statements. For example, a learning theory may not consider the health status of the learner, and the learner is assumed to be a healthy individual. If practice variables are not accounted for in the theory or if there are substantial differences between the theoretic variables and the practice variables, the theory should be used with caution, if at all. If the theory appears to have value and satisfies the considerations of most people who will be involved in the deliberative validation process, it might be used with systematic observation of the effect on outcomes, considering the differing variables that occur in practice. Given your observations, you may have a basis to propose revision of the theory to include important practice variables.

Are the Explanations of the Theory Sufficient to Be Used as a Basis for Nursing Action? Responses to this question must be based on expert judgment about the particular nursing actions that are implied within the theory. As an expert nurse, you may find it difficult to describe the basis on which you would judge a theory to be sufficient or not sufficient. One specific approach in forming your ideas is to examine the correspondence between theoretic and practice variables. If variables in the nursing situation are similar to those that are suggested in the theory, you then can consider the nature of the relationships between the concepts of the theory. Examine the extent to which the explanation makes sense in light of your practice. You may feel guarded about the sense of the theory for practice, but you can see that the perspective of the theory is reasonable. In this case, the theory is probably sufficient as a basis for nursing action, but your tentativeness about it leads you to be cautious as you proceed to use it and to plan careful documentation of the relationships you observe in practice.

An example of a theoretic explanation sufficient for application in practice is the theory of parent-child interaction that has undergone extensive development and refinement through the work of Dr. Kathryn Barnard (Barnard, 1981, 1996; Barnard, Eyres, Lobo, & Snyder, 1983). The Barnard theory has been refined through a program of theory development and research spanning several years that still is active. In the Barnard model, the following three-way conceptual relationship is central to the theory. In Barnard's theory (1) the child, (2) the caregiver or parent, and (3) specific environmental factors interact. The interaction of these three elements determines how a parent/caregiver and child will relate interpersonally. For example, features of the *child* (fussy? docile?) and features of the *caregiver/parent* (oversolicitous? nonattentive?) as well as features of the *environment* (child care classes available? other family available for care relief?) create interpersonal interaction patterns. A fussy child being cared for by an oversolicitous parent in an environment where alternative sources of care support are not available will create a certain type of parent–child interaction. Conversely, other combinations of factors within these three broad concepts will create different qualities of parent–child interaction. The practice value of Barnard's model comes from research that has described which factors and combination of factors interfere with normal infant development. Normal infant development is a goal in which nurses have much interest. The theoretical relationships justify the importance of assessing caregiver/parent–child interaction and providing early intervention when interaction is problematic. Checklist scales have been developed that a nurse can use to observe and assess parent–child interaction during activities of feeding or when caregiver/parents teach the child a developmentally appropriate skill. The Barnard theory and accompanying assessment tools have been used extensively to benefit families and children. This theory can be used widely because research was employed to identify and validate which factors were significant in creating problematic parent/caregiver–child interaction. Furthermore, factors of significance were represented in a way that could be easily assessed in clinical practice. Research evidence that is generated with an insensitivity to whether variables and assessments are practical for nurses to use runs the risk of creating theory and models that require further development prior to practice utilization.

Is There Research Evidence Supporting the Theory? One very influential source of information for deciding whether a theory can be used in practice is research evidence, as noted in the example of Barnard's work just described. Sometimes a theorist, in presenting the theory, provides research evidence to support the initial theoretic formulation. If the evidence is convincing and attracts sufficient attention in the discipline, the professional literature will report research that either validates the initial theoretic relationships or does not support the theory. Research that reports findings in theory validation studies often suggests limits on the range of contexts in which theory can be utilized or flaws in the initial theoretic construction, which are based on the research evidence generated.

Because theories are not unequivocally supported by research evidence, practitioners have the responsibility to determine whether the evidence is sufficient to justify use of the theory in practice. This judgment is best made on the basis of several research studies. If there is little or no research evidence to justify utilization in practice but most of the other concerns have been satisfied, you can feel reasonably comfortable about utilizing the theory. In this case, give particular attention to observing and recording relevant information regarding corresponding theoretic and situational variables and the limits and outcomes of the theory's use in practice.

How Will the Use of This Theory Influence the Practical Function of the Nursing Unit? Before using a theory in practice, you need to consider the ways in which this approach will affect the functioning of the

---

Box 10-1

Questions to Be Addressed in Planning
for Theory Utilization

Do nursing personnel need to be oriented to the theory and its application?

Does the approach require adjustments in the function or processes of the nursing unit?

Does the approach require additional time or an adjustment in the allocation of time for nurses and other unit personnel?

Will the approach require new equipment or other material resources?

What practical arrangements and materials are needed to enhance the ease and accuracy of making and recording observations?

Are administrative personnel supportive of the approach being used?

How will trial application affect other activities in the setting?

Are special provisions needed for gathering and storing information?

How will patients be informed of the approaches that will be used?

How will the data that are obtained be assessed and analyzed?

If the theoretic goal is attained or not attained, how will the results be explained or accounted for?

Have alternative explanations been projected in order to provide sufficient information to make a judgment about outcomes?

How will the results of the experience be compiled to communicate them to others?

---

nursing unit and assess the potential for observing and recording factors that are relevant to the theory's application. Because practice utilization and validation will be disruptive, support of administrative personnel is important. Successful use of a theory in practice depends on planning for the changes that are required, including the changes that will be needed to gather the required research data. Questions to be addressed in planning for theory utilization are shown in Box 10-1. If each of these questions can be answered in such a way that makes the research seem feasible and desirable, then theory utilization and validation processes should proceed.

METHODOLOGIC APPROACHES TO VALIDATION OF RELATIONSHIPS AND OUTCOMES

Methods that are used in the validation of theory are drawn from evaluation research (Posavac & Carey, 1992; Schroeder & Maibusch, 1984; Smeltzer, Hinshaw, & Feltman, 1987). These methods depend on knowing what outcomes you wish to achieve and on having a well-planned approach for achieving your goal. Evaluation research methods depend on having some means for assessing pertinent circumstances that exist before deliberative utilization of a theory and then reassessing those same circumstances for change following utilization of the theory. Factors associated with the outcomes usually are identified and assessed before beginning theory validation and again after the approach has been in place for a specified period. The following sections describe quality-related outcomes that you might consider in planning for validation of theoretic relationships.

EXPECTED OUTCOMES THAT FLOW FROM THEORETIC REASONING

At the heart of validation of theory is the idea that the theory suggests goals or outcomes that the profession values and that the fundamental purpose for using the theory is to achieve these goals. The outcomes you identify as flowing from theoretic reasoning are likely to represent a key concept of the theory that requires sound empiric indicators and operational definitions. Your choice of empiric indicators and operational definitions may come from prior research, in which case you need to determine their adequacy for your purposes. If existing empiric indicators and operational definitions are not readily available, you will need to invest preliminary time and effort to develop your own. It is important to choose or create empiric indicators that can be, and are likely to be, assessed easily within the nursing context for theory validation.

Scientific Competence of Nurses

Although the primary aim in deliberatively utilizing theory in practice is improved quality of outcomes for those receiving care, it also is important to verify that the scientific competence of nurses is enhanced. This "outcome" serves to ensure that the positive benefits of utilizing theory in practice can be sustained over time.

Standards of nursing practice that are accepted by your nursing practice unit can contribute to your choice of ways to assess nurse scientific competence, but if your standards of care only reflect minimum acceptable practice, you may need to consider what extensions of the standards are implied within the theoretic reasoning. For example, a key element of your theory could be specific nursing care actions that signify the concept of *caring*. If your standards of care do not reflect or require these actions as part of minimum acceptable practice, you will need to integrate empiric indicators for these actions and plan a way to assess these nurse actions as an outcome.

Functional Outcomes

Nursing goals sometimes are defined in terms of how efficiently the work of nursing is done, how cost-effective it is, or how smoothly the work of each individual coordinates with others' work. If environmental factors impeding nurse efficiency have been identified as needing improvement for a particular unit, the environmental changes needed and the factors that are indicative of improvement need to be clearly specified and assessed before utilizing theory to improve nursing effectiveness. Once the baseline data are obtained and the approach based on the theory has been in place for a period, the measures of functional effectiveness are obtained and compared.

Nurse Satisfaction

Satisfaction with respect to nursing job responsibilities can be closely related to functional outcomes. Nurse job satisfaction can be assessed by factors such as working conditions, relationships with colleagues, personal fulfillment, various types of perceived benefits, and perceived dissatisfactions. A premise underlying the selection of this type of outcome is that if nurses are satisfied with their work situation, the quality of care they provide will improve.

Quality of Care Perceived by Those Who Receive Care

People who receive care can be interviewed or surveyed to ascertain their perception of the quality of their care. There are several aspects of perceived quality of care that can be assessed, including satisfaction with specific dimensions of care, perceived benefits from the care, and perceived dissatisfactions. If your nursing approach is guided by a particular theory, then consider asking specific questions based on the practices, ideas, goals, and processes that the theory directs you to use.

IMPLEMENTING A FORMAL METHOD OF STUDY

The approaches used to validate theory in practice can draw on traditional research methods but often shift to include the methods of evaluation and quality-assurance research (Posavac & Carey, 1992). In this type of research, the method is designed to provide evidence of the effect of theoretic knowledge on the overall well-being of people who receive care, on the scientific competence of those who practice nursing, and on the practice setting. Ideally, this type of investigation includes measurement of the key outcomes before application of the selected theory in practice to demonstrate what changes in practice occur after the theory has been applied.

If, for example, research evidence available suggests you need to validate a theory of pain alleviation in practice, you might design a study that first would estimate the quality of nursing care and patients' experiences of pain before the theory is used in practice. Your assessment could include the perspectives of nurses, people receiving nursing care, and others involved in caring for people who experience pain. After you have this information, you would begin to use the theory in practice and over time continue to observe the same outcome indicators of quality of care. On the basis of your findings, you could make recommendations for practice and for revisions in the conceptualizations of the theory.

When it is not possible to obtain data before utilizing the theory, alternative approaches include obtaining population or epidemiologic data related to selected outcomes or obtaining measures from a comparable population or group of people. You then compare your outcomes with the population statistics. This approach is necessary in many types of situations. One such circumstance is nursing care that is directed toward prevention of a negative health experience, such as child abuse. If you have selected a theory that you project will influence the parenting abilities of mothers who are at risk for abusing their children, you are not likely to be able to obtain reliable measures of the outcomes you are seeking to achieve. The mothers you are working with may not have had prior parenting experience, or you may not have been involved in their care before they were identified as high-risk parents. You can obtain population statistics concerning the incidence of child abuse, monitor the incidence of abusive behaviors among the mothers for whom you are providing care, and compare your outcomes with the population statistics. You also might identify a group of mothers who are receiving a different type of care to compare your outcomes with those of a different group.

THEORY- AND EVIDENCE-BASED PRACTICE

The major focus of this chapter is on the utilization and validation of theory in practice settings. We have maintained in Chapter 9 that linking theory with research is critical for practice utilization. The current professional trend to embrace evidence-based practice as a standard for professional nursing is an important trend that has potential to significantly change how theory is used in practice. Evidence-based practice is being taught to nursing students and is expected in a variety of health care settings. This emphasis raises the question: If practice is to be both evidence based and theory based, what sorts of research evidence will contribute to theory-based practice?

DiCenso, Guyatt, and Ciliska (2005) propose a definition of evidence-based practice that we favor. For these authors, evidence-based practice integrates best research evidence, health care resources, patient preferences and actions, clinical setting and circumstances, and the clinician's judgment in clinical decision making (pp. 4–5) Thus, evidence-based practice is not simply the utilization of research in practice as it is sometimes characterized. Although evidence-based practice requires consideration of best research evidence, it also must consider an array of circumstances where clinical decision making occurs including clinician expertise (DiCenso et al., 2005, p. 5). This characterization of evidence-based practice is highly compatible with the knowing patterns because it requires integrating empiric knowledge forms with knowledge and knowing located within all of the knowing patterns.

Although evidence-based practice requires integration of all knowing patterns, the definition privileges empirics when definitions identify best research evidence as a central feature to be integrated in evidence-based approaches to nursing practice. Further, research evidence is usually depicted in a hierarchy where "strong" or best evidence is identified as randomized clinical trials and meta-analyses of randomized clinical trials, whereas "weak," presumably the worst, forms of evidence include such things as case studies, qualitative studies, and reasoned opinions (Fulbrook, 2003; Melnyk, 2004; Melnyk & Fineout-Overholt, 2005; Rutledge & Grant, 2002; Sackett, Straus, & Richardson, 2000). Although hierarchies of best evidence abound, many resources acknowledge that best evidence in nursing may be found in research and other knowledge forms that are lower in the hierarchy, such as case studies or clinical observations. Because evidence hierarchies exist, we believe they suggest that nursing evidence should eventually move toward higher levels. Also, the acknowledgment that best research evidence for nursing may not be at those high levels suggests that much of nursing's knowledge is of an inferior nature.

As might be expected, qualitative researchers have challenged the privileging of knowledge located at the upper levels of strength-of-evidence hierarchies. These researchers maintain that carefully conducted qualitative, naturalistic studies are equally valuable. The hierarchical nature of evidence has also been criticized as supporting a particular methodological approach to creating research evidence in professional disciplines that all but ensures any evidence generated will not be useful in practice (Holmes, Perron, & O'byrne, 2006; Jensen, Weersing, Hoagwood, & Goldman, 2005). These criticisms offer the suggestion that a practice-based evidence approach be utilized. Practice-based evidence is an approach that acknowledges the environment of practice is important. Practice-based evidence values knowledge that generates from practice, versus knowledge that conforms to hierarchies of evidence and is created apart from the reality of practice. Practice-based evidence also connotes evidence that practitioners create as they move research into practice and make necessary modifications based on context variables. Practice-based evidence, then, is not decontextualized, universal knowledge—rather, it is quite the opposite (Fox, 2003; Krakau, 2000; Margison et al., 2000; Simons, Kushner, Jones, & James, 2003).

The focus on use of best research evidence in nursing and the existence of evidence hierarchies has positive aspects that will promote the linking of theory, research evidence, and practice. This is because evidence-based practice requires that practitioners frame the question to be answered, search out best research evidence, and use an approach to clinical decision making that integrates research evidence with other requisite features of context and client. Because evidence-based nursing practice is becoming widely advocated in nursing, it has potential to contribute to the development of evidence-based theory in several ways.

Evidence-based practice can be expected to strengthen the ability of nurses in practitioner and researcher roles to frame clinically important questions. Although asking a question for the purpose of gathering or creating evidence seems easy enough, this sort of activity requires a high degree of precision and sophistication. For practitioners the challenge is not just to find information about "obesity" but to ask a clinically important question that links "obesity" of a certain type to some significant nursing outcome, such as development of diabetes. Further, practitioners must focus in on whether the question has to do with obesity's link to risk for developing diabetes, prevention strategies, or actual morbidity statistics. Without a degree of precision, evidence uncovered will be too extensive to be practical and not focused on the problem or situation for which the evidence was sought. Practitioners will also need to have skill in evaluating the quality and limitations of research evidence that might be used as a basis for practice.

For researchers a significant challenge is to formulate questions that are clinically important to ask and to complete research in a way that will generate evidence that is usable in practice. This will require communication between researchers and practitioners in a way that has been largely absent in the past. Such communication has potential to erase role dichotomies and create expectations for integration of research and practice roles. When research evidence important to practice is addressed in ways that help ensure ease of movement between research and practice, the potential for creating more generalizable and usable theory for practice is enhanced. The valuing of meta-analyses and synthesizing reviews in the evidence hierarchy provide another way to create theory that has potential for use in practice.

As practitioners strive to locate best research evidence appropriate to managing care and attempt to use that knowledge, the extent to which research evidence is available and usable will become more obvious. The difficulties and benefits of various methodological approaches to generating empiric research evidence will be made visible. As practitioners discover well-conceived and well-carried-out research evidence that requires, for example, use of assessment tools that are impractical to use clinically, researchers will begin to understand the importance of considering how research is conducted. The importance of relating clinically important concepts and assessing conceptual relationships and outcomes in ways that allow clinicians to make use of the findings for practice will become clearer. This, in turn, will assist clinicians to identify, for formal knowledge developers, what are reasonable and useful variables for study and how to best assess and link variables for clinical utility.

Evidence-based practice also has potential to bring to light areas where even well-conceived and well-developed evidence for nursing practice cannot be easily utilized because of lack of resources, patient or client factors, and other contextual factors. The focus of research evidence may be appropriate for practice, and concepts in relationship may have been assessed and validated in a way that makes them well suited for use in practice. However, features of context, for example high nurse–patient ratios, insurance reimbursement patterns, or institutional policies around security, may make it difficult to use best evidence in practice. These situations bring to light the need for emancipatory knowledge to create a care context that will allow and encourage the use of best evidence, or the need for researchers to consider such features of context during the research process.

The move toward evidence-based practice, then, has potential to strengthen the linkages between roles in nursing that have heretofore been separate: the roles of practitioner and researcher. To summarize, the value of evidence-based practice is its potential for:

- Strengthening the practitioner's and researcher's ability to frame clinical questions to be answered
- Improving the skills of practitioners around determining the quality and limitations of research evidence and synthesizing research
- Supporting a decision-making infrastructure and database generation appropriate for the context of nursing practice
- Making visible the challenges inherent in utilizing knowledge not developed with practice in mind
- Providing researchers with information about the types of knowledge structures that are required to meet care goals
- Creating practical theory-building activity
- Bringing to light contextual factors related to resources and setting that affect evidence-based practice

- Energizing theory and research practices that are politically motivated
- Enhancing the potential for academic researchers and clinicians to work together and share roles—in fact, dissolving distinctions among research, practice, and theory

When best evidence as required in evidence-based practice is created using research processes that are sensitive to the context and goals of practice, in consideration of clinical nurses who use research evidence, and with critical consideration of context, there exists the possibility to transform practice. The features that link best research evidence and practice are the same features that will help encourage research and theory developed out of best evidence that will be useful in practice.

REFLECTION AND DISCUSSION

In this chapter we discussed the deliberative utilization and validation of empiric knowledge in practice, including refining conceptual meaning and validating theoretic relationships and outcomes in practice. We posed questions that you can consider before selecting a theory for validation in practice and considered how evidence-based practice has potential to contribute to theory for practice.

A centrally important message of this chapter is that theory must be developed in concert with practice and validated in practice. To deepen your appreciation of processes for utilizing and validating theory in practice consider the following related to the content of this chapter:

1. As you work in nursing, consider the various ways you might utilize and validate theory or how others might do this. What possibilities does the workaday world allow?
2. Consider what makes theories, formal empiric descriptions, and other types of empiric research useful. When these are not useful, why is that the case?
3. Search for best evidence in relation to some problem or situation you have encountered. Was the information useful to you? What, in particular, made it useful? How generalizable was the evidence?
4. Locate some research evidence that was useful to you. Consider how the research might have been refined, or done differently, to make it even more useful. What would you like to tell the researcher about the work?
5. Consider a theory-validating research project you would like to conduct in a clinical nursing environment. Would necessary resources be available? If not, why not?
6. Locate some credible evidence for a clinical situation that is real to you. Who or what is left out of the research? To whom might the evidence not apply? Consider its utility for marginalized groups.

Reference List

Barnard, K. E. (1981). An ecological approach to parent–child relations. In C. C. Brown (Ed.), *Infants at risk: Assessments and interventions*. Madison, CT: Johnson & Johnson Pediatric Round Table.

Barnard, K. E. (1996). *Influencing parent–child interactions for children at risk*, (7th ed.). New York: Brookes.

Barnard, K. E., Eyres, S., Lobo, M., & Snyder, C. (1983). An ecological paradigm for assessment and intervention. In T. B. Brazelton & B. M. Lester (Eds.), *New approaches to developmental screening of infants* (pp. 199–218). New York: Elsevier.

Beckstrand, J. A. (1980). A critique of several conceptions of practice theory in nursing. *Research in Nursing and Health, 3*(2), 69–79.

Carpenito-Moyet, L. J. (2006). *Handbook of nursing diagnosis*. Philadelphia: Lippincott Williams & Wilkins.

DiCenso, A., Guyatt, G., & Ciliska, D. (2005). *Evidence-based nursing: A guide to clinical practice*. St. Louis: Elsevier-Mosby.

Ellis, R. (1969). The practitioner as theorist. *American Journal of Nursing, 69*, 1434.

Fox, N. J. (2003). Toward collaborative and transgressive research. *Sociology, 17*(1), 81–102.

Fulbrook, P. (2003). Developing best practice in critical care nursing: Knowledge, evidence and practice. *Nursing in Critical Care, 8*(3), 96–102.

Holmes, D., Perron, A., & O'byrne, P. (2006). Evidence, virulence, and the disappearance of nursing knowledge: A critique of the evidence-based dogma. *Worldviews on Evidence-Based Nursing, 3*(3), 95–102.

Jensen, P. S., Weersing, R., Hoagwood, K. E., & Goldman, E. (2005). What is the evidence for evidence-based treatments? A hard look at our soft underbelly. *Mental Health Services Research, 7*(1), 53–74.

Krakau, I. (2000). The importance of practice-based evidence. *Scandinavian Journal of Primary Health Care, 18*(3), 130–131.

Margison, F. R., McGrath, G., Barkham, M., Clark, J., Audin, K., Connell, J., & Evans, C. (2000). Evidence based practice and practice-based evidence. *British Journal of Psychiatry, 177*, 123–130.

Melnyk, B. M. (2004). Evidence-based practice: Integrating levels of evidence into clinical decision-making. *Pediatric Nursing, 30*(4), 323–325.

Melnyk, B. M., & Fineout-Overholt, E. (2005). *Evidence-based practice in nursing health care: A guide to best practice*. Philadelphia: Lippincott Williams & Wilkins.

Posavac, E. J., & Carey, R. G. (1992). *Program evaluation: Methods and case studies*, (4th ed.). Englewood Cliffs, NJ: Prentice-Hall.

Rutledge, D. N., & Grant, M. (2002). Evidence-based practice in cancer nursing. *Seminars in Oncology Nursing, 18*(1), 1–2.

Sackett, D. L., Straus, S. E., & Richardson, W. S. (2000). *Evidence-based medicine: How to practice and teach evidence-based medicine*, (2nd ed.). London: Churchill-Livingstone.

Schroeder, P. C., & Maibusch, R. M. (1984). *Nursing quality assurance*. Rockville, MD: Aspen.

Simons, H., Kushner, S., Jones, K., & James, D. (2003). From evidence-based practice to practice-based evidence: The idea of situated generalization. *Research Papers in Education, 18*(4), 347–364.

Smeltzer, C., Hinshaw, A., & Feltman, B. (1987). The benefits of staff nurse involvement in monitoring the quality of patient care. *Journal of Nursing Quality Assurance, 1*(3), 1–7.

Whittemore, R., & Grey, M. (2002). The systematic development of nursing interventions. *Image—The Journal of Nursing Scholarship, 34*(2), 115–120.

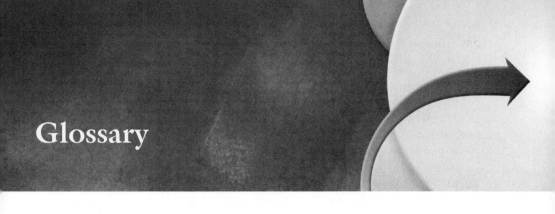

Glossary

The glossary contains definitions that we have created for the purposes of this book. Some are common definitions that are consistent with meanings generally found in the nursing literature. Other definitions are consistent with generally accepted meanings but adapted (we think appropriately) to suit our purposes and perspectives. We ask you to use the glossary with the understanding that we are not the final authority on meanings. Our definitions are reasonable and carefully formulated, but other nuances of meaning for many of these terms are possible.

abstract concept   Mental image derived largely from indirect evidence that is not easily presented by a specific empiric indicator.

academic analysis   Formal methods drawn from various academic disciplines that contribute to the process of praxis; these methods are used to critique oppressive social practices and imagine alternatives to end injustices. Examples of academic analysis methods include critical discourse analysis, critical feminist analysis, and critical social analysis.

accessibility   Trait of theory useful for questioning and clarifying the degree to which concepts have indicators in observable reality and, subsequently, how attainable are the outcomes, goals, and purposes of the theory.

aesthetics   Fundamental pattern of knowing in nursing related to the perception of deep meanings, calling forth inner creative resources that transform experience into what is not yet real, but possible. Expressed as knowledge through works of art and criticism and integrated in practice as transformative art/acts.

allies   Persons not directly affected by a particular disadvantage, injustice, or unfair practice, but who join those who are; allies honor the perspectives of the disadvantaged while they assist in their effort to rectify injustices and create a more equitable situation.

appreciation   Process of focusing and reflecting on aesthetic knowledge as it is understood and valued by members of the discipline. Interacts with the process of inspiration to challenge and authenticate aesthetic knowledge.

assumption   One of the structural components of theory that is taken for granted or thought to be true without systematically generated empiric evidence. Theoretic assumptions may be value statements or have potential for empiric testing but are assumed true within the theory because they are reasonable.

atomistic theory Theory that deals with a narrow scope of phenomena. The term often implies, in addition, an assumption that the whole may be understood from a study of the parts.

authentication Processes within each of the patterns of knowing for evaluating and assessing the soundness of knowledge that is formally expressed. Each pattern requires specific approaches for authentication that reflect the pattern's form of expression and knowing.

axiom Type of premise used in deductive logic, often one that is not tentative but relatively firm. Axioms as premises are used for deducing theorems, especially in mathematics.

centering Process that involves a deliberate focus on inner feelings, perception, and experience and involves contemplation and introspection to form deep inner personal meaning from life experiences. Interacts with the process of opening to create personal knowledge.

clarifying Process involving a deliberate focus on understanding the nature of ethical decisions and dilemmas and on bringing to full understanding those actions that are right and good. Interacts with the process of valuing to create ethical knowledge.

clarity Trait of theory useful for questioning and understanding the degree to which a theory is semantically and structurally lucid and consistent.

codes A form of knowledge expression within the ethics pattern. Codes are shorthand expressions of prescribed professional behaviors that generally are accepted as right and good. Codes primarily describe behaviors that represent the nurse's accountability as expressed in rights, duties, and obligations.

components of theory Features of theory that are useful for describing theory and that form a template for critically reflecting theory. Components include purpose, concepts, definitions, relationships, structure, and assumptions.

concept Complex mental formulation of experience. Concepts are a major component of theory and convey the abstract ideas within the theory.

conceptual framework A logical grouping of related concepts or theories, usually created to draw together several different aspects that are relevant to a complex situation such as a practice setting or an educational program. Term used synonymously with *theoretic framework*. A knowledge form within the empirics pattern.

conceptualizing General process within empiric pattern that focuses on identifying, defining, and creating meaning for concepts within theory. Conceptualizing includes, but is not limited to, the focused process of creating conceptual meaning.

conclusions Relationship statements that are derived from premises in a deductive logic system. Conclusions are a type of proposition and may take the form of a theorem or hypothesis.

confirmation In qualitative research, the processes of establishing the validity of empiric theory and research. In some qualitative methods, confirmation may be assumed a result of the methodology used; confirmation also may require the theory and research to be utilized in additional settings.

consistency Theory trait related to clarity. Consistency may be semantic or structural and refers to the general agreement, harmony, and compatibility of components within the theory.

construct Type of highly abstract and complex concept. Constructs are formed from multiple less-abstract or more-empiric concepts.

creating conceptual meaning Theory development process of identifying, examining, and clarifying the mental images that comprise the elements, variables, or concepts within theory. Conveys the thoughts, feelings, and ideas that reflect the human experience of the concept.

criteria for concepts Essential features of a concept formed by examining conceptual meaning. Criteria are designed with reference to the purposes for which the concept is being used and should be useful to both identify the concept and differentiate it from other concepts.

criteria for nursing diagnoses Essential features for a specific diagnosis to be used in a given instance or situation encountered in nursing practice.

critical analysis (noun) A form of formal expression of emancipatory knowledge. Critical analyses illuminate meanings that would otherwise remain hidden and can be informed by multiple perspectives including feminist, liberal, poststructural, or postcolonial.

critical multiplism An approach to inquiry that integrates multiple methodologic processes within the research inquiry process. Sometimes refers to the combining of qualitative and quantitative approaches to data collection to reduce bias.

critical reflection Process that questions the function, purposes, and value of empiric knowledge structures, especially theory, as reflected in the clarity, generality, simplicity, accessibility, and importance of the structure. The questioning process does not imply an expected response; for example, inquiring about clarity does not imply that clarity is desirable.

critical theory A broad term used to describe both the process and the product of analyses that take a historically situated and socio-political perspective. Critical theory seeks to undermine dominant power structures that create inequities and that maintain oppression and other forms of social injustice.

critical thinking The deliberate use of clear, concise, and thorough thought processes that consider diverse elements of a broad array of existing problems with the intent of solving the problem. Emancipatory knowing builds on critical thinking but focuses on problems related to social and political inequities. Emancipatory knowing, unlike critical thinking, requires examination and understanding of how sociopolitical networks sustain unfair institutionalized practices.

criticism A form of knowledge within the aesthetics pattern that is a discursive representation of meaning for expressions of aesthetic knowledge. Criticism is formed from aesthetic methods that are designed to deepen shared meanings for aesthetic knowing.

critiquing A creative inquiry process for emancipatory knowing that exposes the hidden dynamics and meanings that are structured and institutionalized by social, cultural, and political practices and ideologies.

deconstruction Taking apart assumptions, ideologies, and frames of reference in text; making explicit features of text that cannot be warranted as a basis for truths for the purpose of undermining language and social contexts that promote inequities and injustices.

deduction Form of reasoning that moves from the general to the specific. In deductive logic, two or more premises as relational statements are used to draw a conclusion; in deductive research processes, an abstract theoretic relationship is used to derive specific questions or hypotheses.

definition Component of theory that indicates the empiric basis for a concept. Definitions are statements of meaning that provide a link between theoretic abstrac-tions and empiric indicators. Definitions may be relatively general or specific.

deliberative utilization and validation of theory Theory development process that refines and develops empiric knowledge in relation to practice. Involves processes that refine conceptual meaning and validate theoretic relationships and outcomes within practice contexts.

demystification The process of making things visible, especially oppressive social practices; the open disclosure of that which was formerly hidden from understanding.

descriptive relationships Statements that provide an account of what something is. Descriptive relationships provide an image or impression of the nature or attributes of a phenomenon.

dialogue Process of exchanging various points of view concerning what is right, good, or responsible. Interacts with the process of justification to challenge and authenticate ethical knowledge.

discipline Group of individuals engaged in developing knowledge; the structured knowledge within an area of concern or domain of inquiry.

discourse Interconnected systems or patterns of language, symbols, and human communications that create meanings and behavior.

discourse analysis An inquiry approach that focuses on understanding patterns of language as well as other symbolic systems of communication (television, artwork, advertisements) as constitutive of meanings and behavior. In discourse analysis, interconnected symbolic systems (discourses) are assumed to create historically situated meanings and behavior. Critical discourse analysis focuses on de-centering dominant discourses that perpetuate power and justice inequities.

emancipatory knowing The pattern of knowing that makes social and structural change possible. It is the ability to recognize barriers that create unfair and unjust social conditions and to analyze complex elements of the social and political context, to change a situation to one that improves people's lives. Praxis, which is value-motivated, constant reflection and action to transform the world, is the fundamental process of emancipatory knowing.

empiric indicators   The sensory experience linked to a concept. More empirically grounded concepts have more direct empiric indicators; abstract concepts require the construction of indirect measures or tools that provide an approximate empiric measurement of some feature of the phenomenon.

empiric–abstract continuum   Means to visualize or represent the extent to which concepts have a basis in empiric reality. Empiric concepts have a direct reality basis and are more directly experienced, whereas abstract concepts have an indirect basis in empiric reality and are more mentally constructed.

empirics   Fundamental pattern of knowing in nursing focused on the use of sensory experience for creation of mediated knowledge expressions. Expressed as knowledge by theories and formal descriptions and integrated in practice as scientific competence.

empowerment   The growing capacity of individuals and groups to exercise their will, to have their voices heard, and to claim their full human potential; addressing and changing conditions to remove barriers that thwart an individual or group's ability to claim their full potential.

envisioning   Process of imagining forms, ways of being, actions, and outcomes into a possible future. Interacts with the process of rehearsing to create aesthetic knowledge.

epistemology   Pertaining to the "stem" or basis of knowledge; perspectives on how knowing becomes knowledge or how knowledge is created.

ethics   Fundamental pattern of knowing in nursing, focusing on matters of moral and ethical significance. Expressed as knowledge by principles and codes and integrated in practice as moral/ethical comportment.

evidence-based nursing practice   Nursing practice grounded in the integrated consideration of the following: (1) patient/client preferences, (2) sound clinical judgment of the nurse, (3) best research evidence, and (4) health care context.

explaining   Statements that provide an account of how something came to be. Explanatory relationships provide an image or impression of how the nature or attributes of a phenomenon interrelate.

explanatory relationships   Statements that provide ideas about how events happen, indicating how related factors affect or result in certain phenomena.

fact   Objectively verifiable event, object, or property; a phenomenon that is experienced and named similarly by others in a similar context.

feminism   Philosophic perspectives and methods that focus on the oppression of women as a class, a perspective that values women and women's experience; actions of feminist scholars and activists who are committed to a variety of social and political changes that improve women's lives and in turn the lives of all people.

formal descriptions   Expressions of knowledge within the empiric knowing pattern. A rigorous and confirmable accounting of perceptions, inferences and understanding expressed in a variety of written formats. Some formal descriptions may not be structured as theory but they reflect the components of theory.

formal expressions of knowledge   Written documents that convey in systematic ways what is known, the content of which can be examined and authenticated. Each pattern of knowing has specific forms of expression that are appropriately suited to the pattern.

general definition A statement of the meaning of a term or concept that sets forth characteristics of the phenomenon or indicates what the phenomenon is associated with. A specific definition, by contrast, states particular characteristics, or indicators, that name what the phenomenon is.

generality Trait of theory useful for questioning, clarifying, and understanding the range of phenomena to which the theory applies. Generality combined with simplicity yields parsimony.

generalizability Extent to which research findings can be applied to or used as a basis for making decisions in like situations. Generalizability is affected by the soundness of the conceptualization process, the research design, and the analysis of the data.

genuine self A form of nondiscursive knowledge expression within the personal knowing pattern. Refers to the self, whole, and entire, as understood by self and others.

grand theory Theory that deals with broad goals and concepts representing the total range of phenomena of concern within a discipline. This term may be used to imply macro theory and molar and wholistic theory.

grassroots activism An approach to the creative critiquing and imagining processes of emancipatory knowing; grassroots activism implies involvement of persons who are directly disadvantaged or who align themselves closely with those who are directly disadvantaged by unfair practices that need to be changed.

grounded theory Theory generated from inductive research processes; the source of data is empiric evidence.

hegemony An interconnected network of dominant views, values, assumptions, ideologies, and patterns of thought that benefit privileged groups. Hegemonic structures are taken to be "the way things are" without question while they unfairly separate and continue to disadvantage certain groups; hegemony is difficult to challenge because of its institutionalization in the social order.

hermeneutic inquiry Inquiry approach for interpreting text (language based) that considers the historical situation in which the text was produced. Approaches to hermeneutic inquiry vary but in general require movement between text and the historical context for the researcher to understand embedded meanings.

holism See *wholism*.

holistic theory See *wholistic theory*.

hypothesis Tentative statement of relationship between two or more variables that can be empirically tested. The term *hypothesis* generally is used to refer to a relationship statement that is tested by using specific research methods.

ideology Ideals and values that dominate the discourses of a culture or society, which are often unfair and unjust, and which typically go unquestioned.

imagining A creative development process for emancipatory knowing; focuses on envisioning and communicating how social and political structures must change to remove conditions of injustice and inequity, creating conditions that enable full human potential.

importance Trait of theory useful for questioning, clarifying, and understanding the extent to which a theory is clinically significant or has value for the profession.

induction Form of reasoning that moves from the specific to the general. In inductive logic a series of particulars are combined into a larger whole or set of things. In inductive research particular events are observed and analyzed as a basis for formulating general theoretic statements, often called grounded theory.

inspiration Process of responding to aesthetic knowledge to imagine new possibilities and directions. Interacts with appreciation to challenge and authenticate aesthetic knowledge.

interpretive research General inquiry approach that assumes "truth" is constructed from the frame of reference of the knower, including both research participants and researcher. Interpretive research approaches can be contrasted with objectivist research approaches, which assume an "out there" reality with truth value independent of the knower.

isolated research Research that is completed without recognized reference or linkage to theory.

justification Process of developing explicit descriptions of the values on which an ethical ideal rests and the line of reasoning toward which an ethical conclusion flows. Interacts with the process of dialogue to challenge and authenticate ethical knowledge.

knowing Individual human processes of perceiving and understanding self and the world in ways that can be brought to some level of conscious awareness. Not all that is comprehended in the processes of knowing can be shared or communicated. What is shared, communicated, and expressed in words or in actions becomes the knowledge of a discipline.

knowledge Awareness or perception acquired through insight, learning, or investigation expressed in a form that can be shared. Knowledge is a reasonably accurate accounting of the world as known and shared by members of a discipline. Knowledge is a representation of knowing that is collectively judged by shared standards and criteria.

law Relationship between variables that has been thoroughly tested and confirmed. Laws are said to be highly generalizable and are relatively certain.

logic System of reasoning that deals with the form of relationships among propositions without specific regard to their content.

macro theory Theory that deals with a broad scope of phenomena. This term may be used to imply grand, molar, and wholistic theory.

manifesto A form of formal expression of emancipatory knowledge; action-oriented and impassioned portrayals of that which is problematic, descriptions of the ideals envisioned, and actions required to effect change.

metatheory Theory about the nature of theory and the processes for its development.

metalanguage   In general, language that encompasses or transcends other language; in nursing the broad concepts of nursing, person, society and environment, and health that are commonly referred to as nursing's metaparadigm.

micro theory   Theory that is relatively narrow in scope or deals with a narrow range of phenomena. This term may be used to imply atomistic and molecular theory.

middle-range theory   A relative classification for theory that embodies concepts, relationships, and purposes that reflect limited aspects of broad phenomena. Concepts in middle-range theory can be more easily linked to perceptible events and situations.

model   Symbolic representation of empiric experience in words, pictorial or graphic diagrams, mathematic notations, or physical material (such as a model airplane). When represented in written language, models are form of knowledge within the empiric pattern.

modernism   In knowledge development, the period beginning in the early 1900s after the widespread abandonment of metaphysical and religious explanations of knowing. Modernism is characterized by the rise of traditional science with a focus on objectivism and a reliance on reason for the creation of knowledge.

molecular theory   Theory that is relatively narrow in scope or deals with a narrow range of phenomena. This term may be used to imply micro theory and atomistic theory.

moral distress   The distress that results when ethically significant moral behavior is blocked, for example by institutional or legal factors.

moral/ethical comportment   Expression of ethical knowledge and knowing in nursing practice, integrated with emancipatory, personal, aesthetic, and empiric knowledge and knowing.

morals, morality   The expression of ethical precepts in behavior and actions. Ontologic or behavioral expression of what is good and right.

multivocality   The use of many "voices" for methods, data sources, and interpretations in research and knowledge development. The gleaning of different interpretations from the same data set to form multiple understandings rather than a single "correct" interpretation.

narrative analysis   A research approach that typically uses a story, told chronologically, as data. Narrative analysis focuses on the meaning of interrelationships among elements in the story.

nursing practice   Experiences a nurse encounters in the process of caring for people. Experiences include those of the person receiving care, the nurse, others in the environment, and their interactions.

objectivity/objectivism   Assumption on which methods of science are based, in which truth is thought to exist apart from or outside the person who knows. Based on a dualistic view of the rational mind, the existence of a reality that is separate from the person who knows.

ontology   Pertaining to ways of being in the world; perspectives on the existence and experience of being.

opening   Process that involves the taking in of experience fully and with conscious awareness. Interacts with the process of centering to create personal knowledge.

operational definition   Statement of meaning that indicates how a term or concept can be assessed empirically. Operational definitions are inferred from theoretic definitions. They specify as exactly as possible the empiric indicators used to observe, assess, or measure the concept empirically. The standards or criteria to be used in making observations.

paradigm   A world view or overarching frame of reference. A paradigm implies standards or criteria for assigning value or worth to both the processes and the products of a discipline, as well as for the methods of knowledge development.

parsimony   Trait of theory that incorporates degrees of both simplicity and generality. A highly parsimonious theory is one that has a broad range or generality yet is stated in very simple terms.

patterns gone wild   The distortion of understanding that occurs when one pattern of knowing is not critically examined and integrated with the whole of knowing. Overemphasis on one pattern without integration leads to uncritical acceptance, narrow interpretations, and partial utilization of knowledge.

personal knowing   Fundamental pattern of knowing in nursing focused on the inner experience of becoming a whole, aware self. Expressed as knowledge through autobiographic stories and the genuine self and integrated in practice with other patterns as therapeutic use of self.

philosophy   Form of disciplined inquiry for the purpose of discerning general traits of reality and principles of value.

postcolonialism   An approach to understanding the relationship between culture and imperialistic colonization (the takeover and domination of the powerless by the powerful). Generally, postcolonial thought is concerned with reversing the effects of political and/or ideological colonization.

postmodernism   The period after modernism in which confidence in the achievement of objective knowledge through reason was eroded. Postmodernism generally rejects universal truths and the idea that truth is possible, but embraces multiple approaches to knowledge generation.

poststructuralism   In linguistics, the view that language is not reflective, but constitutive, of meaning. For poststructuralists there is no "reality" or truth and the humanist idea of an autonomous knower is rejected. We do not have language; rather, language "has us" in the sense that it constructs our experiences and understandings.

practice-based evidence   Evidence that comes from validation of clinically used approaches and techniques known to be effective in promoting health-related goals; emphasizes investigating and confirming what seems to be effective in practice as a way to generate research evidence.

praxis The critical action/reflection dimension of emancipatory knowing; value-grounded, thoughtful reflection and action that occurs in synchrony, integrating ontology and epistemology; a value-motivated process that changes nursing practice and the larger social and political environment to end injustices and inequities; praxis creates conditions where all people can reach maximum well-being and full potential, integrated with ethical, aesthetic, personal, and empiric knowledge and knowing in nursing practice.

predicting Process used for the creation of empiric knowledge. Prediction involves a focus on interrelating concepts and variables to create understanding of when and how phenomena and events will occur and recur. Used in conjunction with *explaining*.

predictive relationships Set of statements that interrelates variables so that a specified outcome can be expected when the theory is used.

premises Relationship statements used in deductive logic as a basis for forming a conclusion. In logic the form of the argument must be valid, regardless of how sound the premises are. Examples of types of premises are hypotheses and axioms.

principles A form of knowledge expression within the ethics pattern. Principles are general statements that reflect general and fundamental precepts of value or truths that are adhered to in providing nursing care, such as "do no harm."

problem solving The process of identifying a discrete difficulty or dilemma and finding situation-specific corrections or solutions.

processes for theory development In a practice discipline the processes for theory development are creating conceptual meaning, structuring and contextualizing theory, refining and validating concepts and theoretic relationships, and deliberatively utilizing and validating theory.

profession Vocation that requires specialized knowledge, provides a role in society that is valued, and uses some means of internal regulations of its members.

proposition Statement of relationship between two or more variables. The term *proposition* is a general category that includes postulates, premises, suppositions, axioms, conclusions, theorems, and hypotheses. When a distinction in meaning is made between these various terms, the distinction reflects the form or purpose of logic used or the context in which the proposition occurs. For example, *hypothesis* generally is used in the context of a research study. *Axiom* and *theorem* are used to refer to the relationship statements made in a particular type of deductive logic.

purpose A component of theory that establishes reasons underlying a theory's development; the outcome or outcomes expected to emerge if the relationships of the theory are valid. The purpose of the theory also suggests the range of situations in which the theory is expected to apply.

qualitative methods Methods of data collection and analysis that depend on talk; language expressions of talk; or observations expressed in language, with interpretations presented by non-numerical (usually language) means.

quantitative methods Methods of data collection and analysis that depend on measurement and are expressed in numerical terms.

reductionism Philosophic stance that the whole can be partitioned and understood through generalizations made from a study of the parts.

refining concepts and theoretic relationships A process for linking research and theory that focuses on the correspondence between the ideas of the theory and accessible experience that involves both qualitative and quantitative approaches. Includes validating empiric indicators for concepts, grounding emerging relationships empirically, and validating relationships through empiric methods.

reflection Process that requires integrating a wide range of perceptions to realize what is known within the self. Interacts with the process of response to challenge and authenticate personal knowledge.

reflective practice A necessary component of best practices that requires practitioners to thoughtfully consider and adopt ways to improve practice over time; part of the process of praxis, but praxis requires bringing oppressive social and political practices to the center of concern in transforming practice to end injustices and inequities.

rehearsing Process of creating and re-creating narrative, body movements, gestures, and actions in relation to an anticipated situation. Interacts with the process of envisioning to create aesthetic knowledge.

relationship statement Any statement that sets forth a connection or association between two or more phenomena. This general term is used to denote both tentative and confirmed types of statements, such as propositions, laws, axioms, and hypotheses. As a more general term, it does not imply a particular form of logic or a particular context in which the statement is used.

relationships Component of theory that refers to the interconnections between concepts.

replication Process that draws on methods of science to determine the extent to which an observation remains consistent from one situation or time to another. Interacts with the processes of validation and confirmation to challenge and authenticate empiric knowledge.

research Application of formalized methods of obtaining confirmable and valid knowledge about empiric experience.

response Process of interacting with one's own self and others to provide insight concerning the meanings conveyed in experience. Interacts with the process of reflection to challenge and authenticate personal knowledge.

science As a product, the knowledge forms generated by the use of rigorous and precise empirically based methods (e.g., facts, formal descriptions, models, and theories). As a process, the utilization of empirically based methods to generate theories, models, and descriptions of reality.

scientific competence Expression of empiric knowledge and knowing in nursing practice, integrated with emancipatory, ethics, aesthetics, and personal knowing and knowledge.

simplicity Trait of theory used in critical reflection for questioning, clarifying, and understanding the degree to which a theory reduces complexity by using a minimum number of descriptive components, especially concepts, to accomplish its purpose. Simplicity combined with generality yields parsimony.

situation-specific theory Theory that is developed with sensitive consideration of context. Assumes that theory, even mid-range formulations, generally cannot be used without taking into account important differences across populations. Draws attention to the variables that significantly affect successful utilization of theory.

social equity A criterion for authentication of emancipatory knowledge; the demonstrable elimination or reduction of conditions that create disadvantage for some, and advantage for others.

specific definition Statement of the meaning of a term or concept that names the associated object, property, or event and assigns it particular characteristics, as opposed to saying what the concept is like or associated with in reality.

stories Tangible expressions of personal knowledge that are discursive in form and can be shared within the discipline.

structuralism In linguistics, the view that the meanings of word and language are not universally understood but derived from the language structure within which the word(s) is found. More broadly, language practices are structured by the context of use and reflect the broader social and political environments.

structure A component of theory that refers to the overall morphologic arrangement of specific elements, especially concepts, within the theory.

structuring Process that involves forming empiric concepts into formal expressions such as theories, models, or frameworks. Interacts with the process of explaining to create empiric knowledge.

structuring and contextualizing theory Theory development process of forming relationships between and among concepts in a unique, creative, rigorous, and systematic way, consistent with the purposes of the theory. This process also includes identifying and defining the concepts, identifying assumptions, clarifying the context of the theory, and designing relationship statements.

substantive middle-range theory In nursing, theory that tends to cluster around a concept (usually clinical) of interest to nursing; theories of pain alleviation, fatigue, or uncertainty represent theory in the middle range.

sustainability A criterion for authentication of emancipatory knowledge; establishes how well the envisioned and implemented social change survives and thrives.

theoretic definition Statement of meaning that conveys essential features of a concept in a manner that fits meaningfully within the theory. A theoretic definition specifies conceptual meaning and implies empiric indicators for concepts. This term may be used synonymously with *conceptual definition*.

theoretic framework A logical grouping of related concepts, usually created to draw several different aspects together that are relevant to a complex situation such as a practice setting or an educational program. Term used synonymously with *conceptual framework*. A knowledge form within the empirics pattern.

theory An expression of knowledge within the empirics pattern. Creative and rigorous structuring of ideas that project a tentative, purposeful, and systematic view of phenomena.

theory-linked research Research that is designed with reference or linkage to theory. Theory-linked research may be theory testing or theory generating. Theory-testing research ascertains how accurately existing theoretic relationships depict reality-based events. Theory-generating research is designed to discover and describe relationships by observing empiric reality and then constructing theory based on empiric data observed.

therapeutic use of self Expression of personal knowledge and knowing in nursing practice, integrated with emancipatory, ethics and empiric and aesthetic knowledge and knowing.

transformative art/act Expression of aesthetic knowledge and knowing in nursing practice, integrated with emancipatory, empiric, aesthetic, and personal knowing and knowledge.

translational research Research designed to move evidence into the clinical arena by evaluating outcomes in the practice setting; research to connect basic discoveries to patient/client care.

validation Process that draws on the traditional methods of science to substantiate the accuracy of conceptual meanings in terms of empiric evidence. Interacts with replication to challenge and authenticate empiric knowledge. Validation also may refer to newer methods for establishing credibility or truth value of knowledge structures within the empiric pattern.

values analysis A technique for objectively examining and seeking to understand the values operative in a situation as a basis for questioning the responsibleness of moral/ethical decisions.

values clarification A technique for subjectively examining, understanding, challenging, and embracing one's personal values. Values clarification provides a basis for questioning the responsibleness of moral/ethical decisions.

valuing Process of examining motives, actions, outcomes, and other dimensions of experience to embrace and reflect chosen values as a basis for understanding moral/ethical behavior. Interacts with the process of clarifying to create ethical knowledge.

wholism Perspective that is based on the assumption that a whole is emergent and cannot be reduced to discrete elements or be analyzed without residue into the sum of its parts. *Wholism* also may refer to an emphasis on the value of the whole but with consideration of discrete parts that are interrelated.

wholistic theory Theory that deals with a broad scope of phenomena. Use of the term *wholistic theory* often implies, in addition, an assumption that the whole is greater than the sum of its parts. This term may be used to imply macro and grand theory.

work of art Tangible expression of knowledge within the aesthetic patterns that is not discursive in form and that can be communicated and shared within the discipline. The term includes aesthetic expressions such as poetry, drawings, music, dance, and other forms of art as generally understood.

Index

Page numbers followed by *f, t,* or *b* indicate
figures, tables, or boxed material, respectively.